New Insights into Oral and Maxillofacial Surgery

New Insights into Oral and Maxillofacial Surgery

Edited by Gideon Schmidt

hayle
medical

New York

Hayle Medical,
750 Third Avenue, 9th Floor,
New York, NY 10017, USA

Visit us on the World Wide Web at:
www.haylemedical.com

ISBN: 978-1-63241-775-6

Cataloging-in-Publication Data

New insights into oral and maxillofacial surgery / edited by Gideon Schmidt.
    p. cm.
Includes bibliographical references and index.
ISBN 978-1-63241-775-6
1. Face--Surgery. 2. Mouth--Surgery. 3. Maxilla--Surgery. I. Schmidt, Gideon.
RD523 .N49 2019
617.520 59--dc23

Table of Contents

Preface

Oral and maxillofacial surgery is a surgical specialty which deals with the treatment of the defects, diseases and injuries related to the face, jaws, head, neck, and the hard and soft tissues of the oral and maxillofacial region. Rhytidectomy, orthognathic surgery, blepharoplasty, genioplasty, otoplasty, chin augmentation, septoplasty, rhinoplasty, reconstructive surgery, and dentoalveolar surgery are some common oral and maxillofacial surgeries. It may be performed for the treatment of cutaneous malignancy, chronic facial pain disorders, temporomandibular joint disorder, etc. This book is a valuable compilation of topics, ranging from the basic to the most complex advancements in the field of oral and maxillofacial surgery. The ever growing need of advanced technology is the reason that has fueled the research in the field of oral and maxillofacial surgery in recent times. This book aims to equip students and experts with the advanced topics and upcoming concepts in this area.

This book unites the global concepts and researches in an organized manner for a comprehensive understanding of the subject. It is a ripe text for all researchers, students, scientists or anyone else who is interested in acquiring a better knowledge of this dynamic field.

I extend my sincere thanks to the contributors for such eloquent research chapters. Finally, I thank my family for being a source of support and help.

Editor

Novel Techniques in Dentoalveolar and Implant Surgery

Mohammad Hosein Kalantar Motamedi and
Ali Hassani

Abstract

The topics of this chapter can help manage or prevent several common intraoperative problems facing clinicians during dentoalveolar and implant surgery. Three novel techniques are presented: (1) a technique for the stabilization of mucoperiosteal flaps following exposure of an impacted tooth requiring the apical repositioning of the gingival flap to allow for bonding of an orthodontic bracket, (2) a technique for the management of bone loss after tooth extraction and immediate dental implant placement, and (3) a technique to repair maxillary sinus membrane perforations during sinus lifting for implant placement.

Keywords: apical reposition flap, sinus membrane repair, bone grafting, implants, dentoalveolar surgery

1. Introduction

Dentoalveolar surgery may be associated with intraoperative complications; these complications may impede treatment, hinder healing, preclude immediate implant placement, or complicate delayed implantation [1–3]. Several new concepts and techniques presented in this chapter can help manage or prevent some of the common intraoperative sequels facing clinicians during dentoalveolar surgery. Three novel techniques in dentoalveolar surgery are presented herein, including "bone anchorage" (the stabilization of mucoperiosteal flaps following exposure of an impacted tooth requiring the apical repositioning of the gingival flap to allow for bonding of an orthodontic bracket), "crescent graft" (a technique to manage bone loss after tooth extraction and immediate dental implant placement), and "sinus membrane repair" [a simple technique to repair maxillary sinus membrane perforations (SMPs) during sinus lifting].

2. Bone anchorage: a fail-proof technique for the apical repositioning of the gingival flap following exposure of impacted teeth

Exposure of impacted teeth is a prerequisite for bracket bonding and orthodontic therapy. Sometimes, exposure of an impacted tooth requires the apical repositioning of the gingival flap to allow for bonding of an orthodontic bracket. In some cases, this procedure can be very difficult; this is particularly true in the posterior regions of the mandible where anatomical hindrances such as the external oblique ridge and muscle insertions are obstacles preventing the apical fixation of the flap [1]. In the anterior regions, we may also face difficulties if the impacted tooth requiring exposure is in the depth of the oral vestibule. In these cases, the mobility of the oral mucosa and muscle pull in the vestibule precludes the fixation and stabilization of the gingival flap impeding orthodontic bracket bonding. We present an effective approach by which these obstacles can be overcome. Our technique can effectively reposition the attached gingival flap apically after exposing the crown of the impaction and secure it until orthodontic bracket bonding.

2.1. Technique

To apically reposition the gingival flaps of attached gingiva after exposure of an impacted tooth and allow for orthodontic bracket bonding, surgery is indicated. After injection of local anesthesia, a full-thickness trapezoid-shaped mucoperiosteal flap is reflected using periosteal elevators to expose the bone. Buccal bone removal is then started laterally over the impacted tooth using an electric-driven hand piece and a rose bur. After tooth exposure, the buccal cortical bone is removed towards the cervix to sufficiently expose the crown. Care is taken not to remove the bone over or below the cervix of the tooth, as this may endanger the bifurcation or trifurcation in molar teeth. Using a 704 fissure or rose bur, a hole is drilled through the buccal cortex; this is often possible when there is a gap created via the dental follicle separating the tooth from the buccal bone or when a tooth adjacent to it has been removed (i.e. third molar). This gap provides room for passing the suture. Next, a 3-0 silk or polyglactin suture is passed through the superior part of the flap and then through the buccal cortex and tied securely to

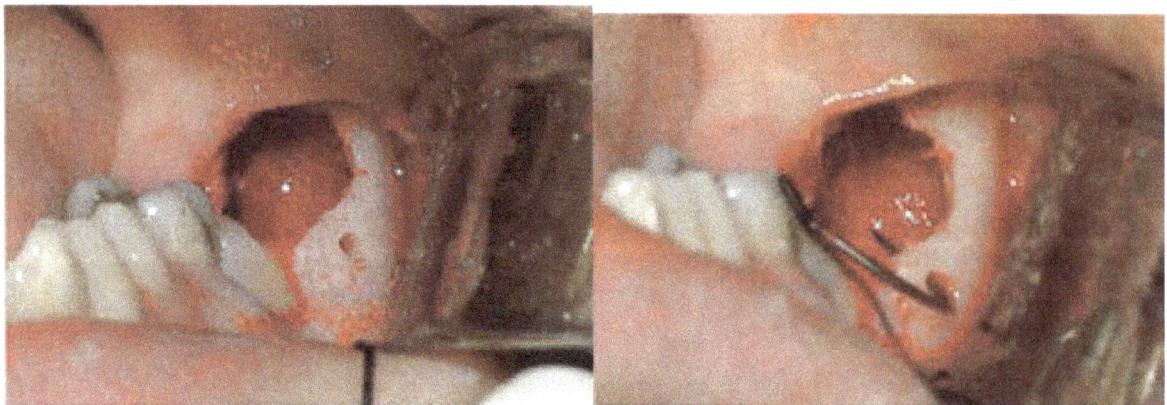

Figure 1. Bur hole drilled through the buccal cortex after the removal of an impacted third molar. A polyglactin or silk suture is passed through the mucosa and then through the hole drilled in the buccal cortex.

the bone to anchor down the flap apically below the crown of the tooth. The crown should be exposed sufficiently for bracket bonding (**Figures 1** and **2**).

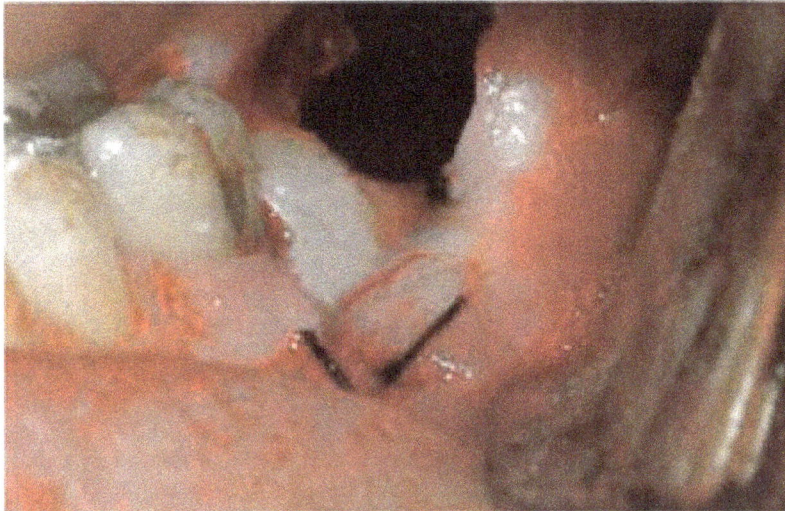

Figure 2. The suture is tied down to anchor the flap securing the exposure of the horizontally impacted second molar tooth for orthodontic bracketing.

2.2. Discussion

The apical repositioning of the gingiva for orthodontic bracketing is problematic in the posterior part of the mandible because of the external oblique ridge and shallow vestibule. The disruption of the gingival attachments and flap reflection of the attached gingiva will cause an immediate loss in vestibular depth due to the upward pull of facial muscles, such as the buccinator. In the anterior regions, we may also face difficulties if the impacted tooth requiring exposure is in the depth of the oral vestibule, because, in these cases, the mobility of the oral mucosa and muscle pull in the vestibule precludes the fixation and stabilization of the gingival flap impeding orthodontic bracket bonding. Securing the flap to the overlying bone is an optimal way to manage such cases [1].

3. Managing alveolar bone loss after tooth extraction for immediate implant placement: the "crescent graft"

3.1. Introduction

Although immediate implantation after tooth extraction has its merits, it may not always be feasible. The most common dilemma in such cases is the confrontation of postextraction bone loss due to difficult extraction of the tooth or preexisting periodontal disease. Many techniques exist with which to manage such complications, namely, autogenous bone grafts (the gold standard), which possess osteoinductive properties and other graft materials with osteocon-ductive properties. There are numerous sites from which to harvest autogenous bone, each having inherent advantages and disadvantages. Chronic periodontitis is one of the major causes of excessive bone loss. After initial evaluations, the pocket depth must be assessed upon tooth extraction; periodontal bone defects may be encountered (vertical defects, crater defects, bone dehiscence, etc.) in the tooth socket of the extracted tooth. Defects may also be caused by traumatic extraction of a tooth without a defect preoperatively. Such defects may preclude immediate insertion of dental implants and require reconstruction either before or simultaneously upon insertion of the implant. It is generally believed that autogenous bone grafts are better than alloplasts; this is because of their osteoconductive and, more importantly, osteoinductive properties [4, 5]. Many sites exist from which to harvest bone and many techniques exist from which to do so. Herein, we present a new site and a novel technique for graft harvesting and restoring bone loss in implantology.

3.2. "Crescent graft" technique to manage bone loss after tooth extraction and immediate implant placement

When the clinical and radiographic examination of a tooth shows evidence of cortical bone loss, the patient may be a candidate for corrective bone grafting of the defect site after tooth extraction and immediate implant placement (**Figure 3**).

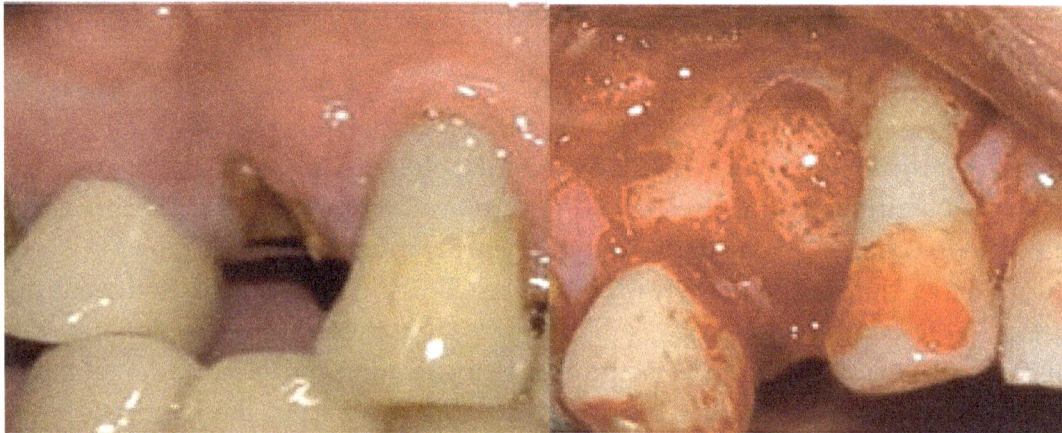

Figure 3. Patient requiring extraction of a hopeless "first" maxillary premolar. After the reflection of a mucoperiosteal trapezoid flap, a large cortical bone defect was seen.

After tooth extraction, the recipient site must be assessed and the amount of autogenous bone needed should be determined. Cross-sectional tomography or cone beam computerized tomography can be used to estimate the amount and thickness of available bone and the safest graft harvesting site.

3.3. Surgical technique

After local anesthesia and tooth extraction, a buccal mucoperiosteal flap is reflected. The defect is exposed and measured with a periodontal probe. The implant is inserted into the extraction socket. Then, the exposed implant surface area needing coverage is assessed; the volume of bone needed is reestimated (**Figure 4**).

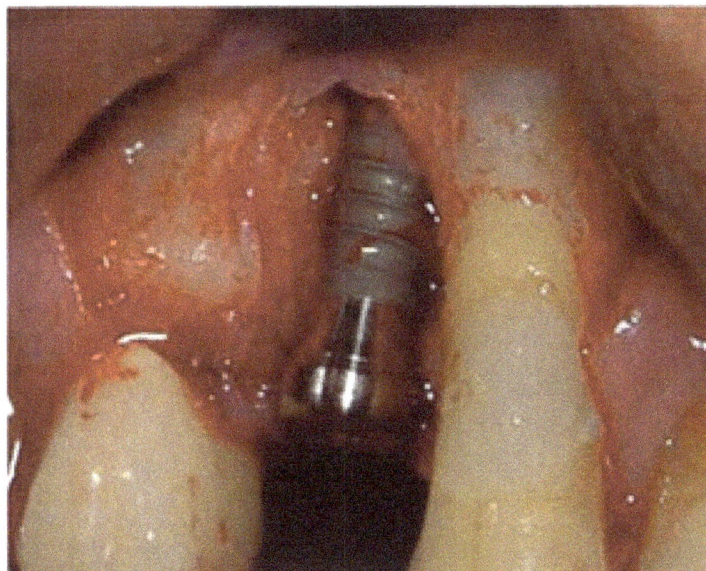

Figure 4. Implant inserted into fresh tooth socket.

The donor site and the size of the trephine bur are determined and a mucoperiosteal envelope flap in the palate is reflected. In our case, we used a trephine bur (5 mm in diameter); two overlapping insertions of the trephine are made parallel to the roots of the incisors and 2 to 4 mm away from them (**Figure 5**).

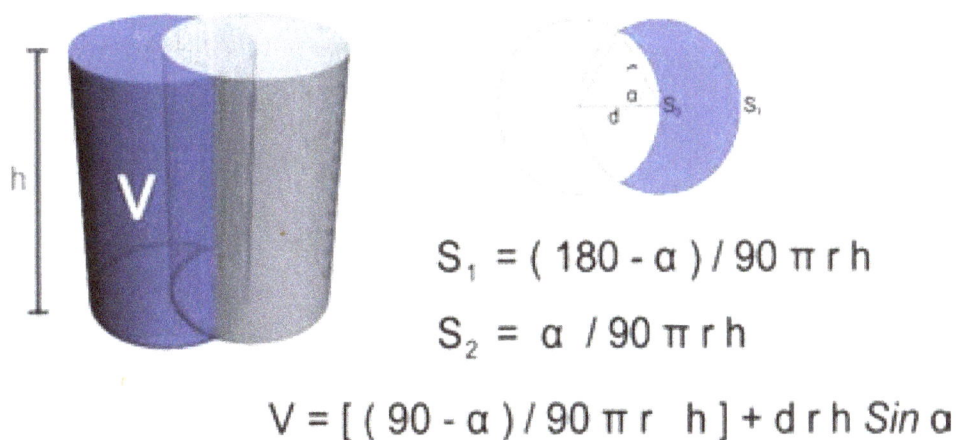

$$S_1 = (180 - a)/90 \, \pi \, r \, h$$

$$S_2 = a/90 \, \pi \, r \, h$$

$$V = [(90 - a)/90 \, \pi \, r \quad h] + d \, r \, h \, Sin \, a$$

Figure 5. Two circles overlapping each other shape two crescents. S_1, area of outer surface of graft; S_2, area of implant facing surface of graft; V, volume of graft; h, depth of bur penetration; r, radius of trephine bur; d, intercentral distance; a, arcos $(d/2r)$.

The trephine penetration depth is predetermined according to the sagittal tomogram. Extreme care should be taken not to penetrate the nasal floor by perforating the anterior palate. However, should this occur, it is not a problem because the palatal mucosa is intact and this precludes the formation of an oronasal fistula. It is essential to have a proper three-dimensional concept of the incisor roots to prevent iatrogenic damage [4]. A periodontal probe is used to determine the bur penetration depth during bone removal. Bone harvesting from the palate produces two crescents, one of which is used in the procedure as a free graft with the concave inner side of the graft placed to cover the convex outer surface of the implant (**Figure 6**).

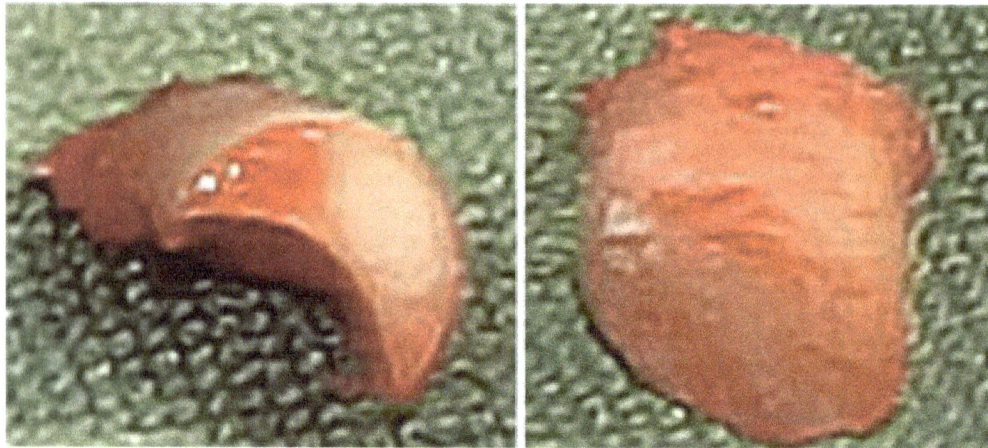

Figure 6. Two insertions of the trephine bur are done to harvest bone; two crescents are produced, one of which is used in the procedure as a free graft. The remaining harvested bone is blended and placed over the recipient site.

The crescent graft is placed into the recipient site (**Figure 7**). The remaining harvested bone is blended and placed over the recipient site.

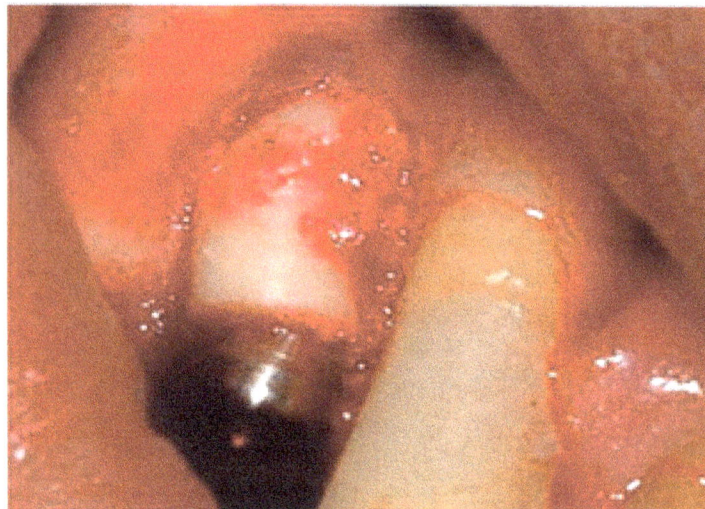

Figure 7. Crescent graft placed into the recipient site.

The small size of the graft precludes fixation with mini-screws. Therefore, a slot is made in the defect via a fissure bur, and the crescent graft is wedged into it. Then, the flap is repositioned and sutured. Postoperatively, the patient is prescribed antibiotics and instructed to use normal saline rinses the next day. The sutures are removed after 7 to 10 days. After 3 months, the cover screw is removed, and the abutment is placed and restored by the use of a cement-retained metal-ceramic crown. The patient is examined at 6 and 12 months after surgery. Vitality tests of the maxillary canines and incisors are performed to ensure vitality.

3.4. Discussion

Dental implants can improve the quality of life, especially in edentulous patients [6]; however, implants are not without complications [4, 7, 8]. A common problem is bone loss or defects. Many studies have assessed the use of different grafts in such defects [9]. Several have shown advantages in using guided bone regeneration on autogenous grafts to avoid soft-tissue ingress [10–12]. Behneke et al. [13] advocated the use of autogenous bone grafts. Common sites in the jaws used as donor sites in autogenous harvesting procedures include the anterior border of the external oblique ridge, lingual exostosis, maxillary tuberosity, and the chin (**Figure 8**) [5, 14–16].

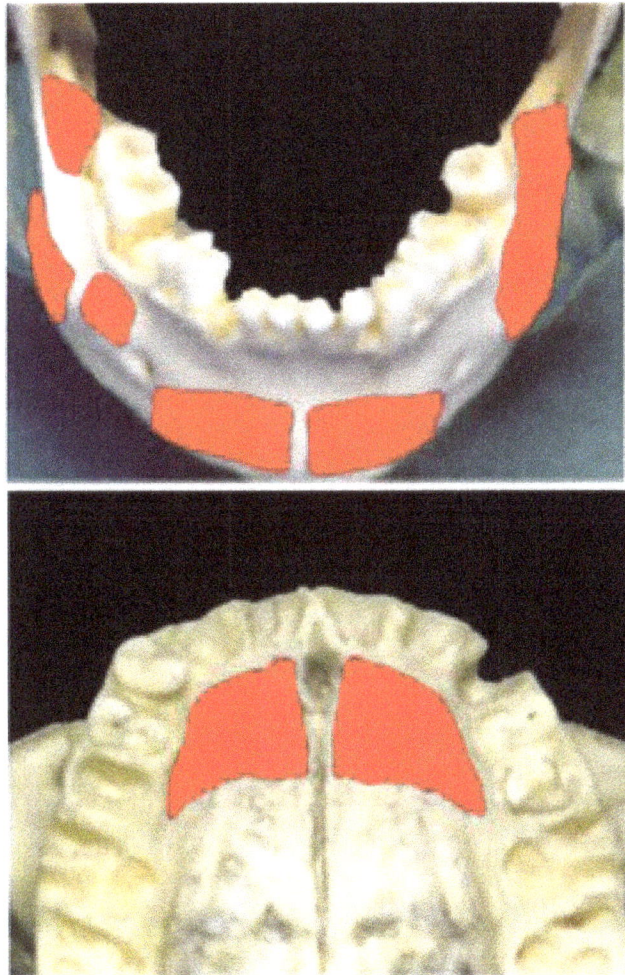

Figure 8. Intraoral donor sites.

The anatomic form of the donor site is as important as the bone quantity and quality [16]. Hassani et al. [17] first introduced the anterior palate of the maxilla as a quantitative donor site in cadavers. The bone is corticocancellous in nature despite its small volume. However, the curvature of the hard palate conforms conveniently to the implant. When two circles with equal radii cross each other in such a way that the perimeter of one circle crosses the center of the other, two crescents result. The use of a trephine bur to achieve this produces a favorably shaped bone graft for implants. This design (the "crescent" graft) has a concave surface (cortex) that conforms nicely to the dental implant surface for coverage. Harvesting chin grafts should be done primarily in those presenting with an edentulous anterior mandible or a large chin protuberance with short roots of the anterior mandibular teeth [18]. Using a local donor site has the advantage of convenient surgical access, which means shorter duration of surgery and anesthesia [19, 20]. Bone harvesting can be performed in the office setting or at the hospital. The procedure is more cost-effective and is estimated to have less donor site morbidity than procedures involving extraoral approaches. Cross-sectional tomograms and lateral skull images can help prevent injury to the anterior maxillary teeth. The intramembranous origin of the harvested bone causes rapid vascularization and improves bone formation [17]. The bone harvested from the anterior palate has a corticocancellous nature. Revascularization occurs more rapidly with cancellous autografts than with cortical grafts. Cancellous autografts tend to be completely integrated with time, whereas cortical grafts tend to remain as admixtures of necrotic and viable bone [21, 22].

4. Sinus membrane repair: a novel technique to repair maxillary sinus membrane perforations during sinus lifting

4.1. Introduction

Boyne and James [23] first reported maxillary sinus lifting in an atrophic maxilla. Sinus lifting for implant placement has now become an established procedure in implantology. It is a predictable method used to augment bone in the posterior maxilla. Increased sinus lifting procedures and bone grafting for the implant placement in the posterior maxilla has in turn increased the complication rate. The most common complication in sinus lifting is the inadvertent perforation of the sinus membrane; if left untreated, it may result in the loss of graft material into the sinus cavity, infection, oroantral fistula, or impairment of the physiologic function of the antrum [24–27]. Fugazzotto and Vlassis [28] classified sinus membrane perforations or SMPs into three groups (class I, class II, and class III) based on their location [29, 30]. The most common location of perforation is the apical wall of the cavity (class I) followed by the mesial surface of the lateral wall (class II) and within the window extension (class III). SMPs are usually classified based on two factors, namely, perforation size and site. SMP has been reported to be as high as 58%, and it is more common in cases where the membrane is too thin or when septae are present [31, 32]. Thus, a method to manage this complication is warranted. We introduce a new, simple, feasible, and effective method to manage SMPs during sinus lifting.

4.2. Technique

Should inadvertent SMP occur after access to the maxillary antrum, the initial step is to evaluate the perforation size and determine whether biomaterials are necessary or not. After severe perforation (class I or II) of the sinus membrane (class II, mesial wall) during sinus lifting, if the quality of the sinus membrane is acceptable, first the membrane margins are gently released. For class II perforations or class I perforations in the apical wall, two holes are made 3 to 4 mm from one another using a fissure bur in the lateral wall near the access window. Next, a 4-0 absorbable suture with a round needle is passed through one of the cortical holes from the outer surface then into the antrum and then passed through 2 sites in the membrane (to reduce tension and prevent membrane tearing). The suture is then passed through the other hole, exiting from inside of the sinus outward; the knot is tied outside the antrum via a horizontal mattress technique; the sinus membrane abuts the bone as a result of the tension applied (**Figures 9** and **10**).

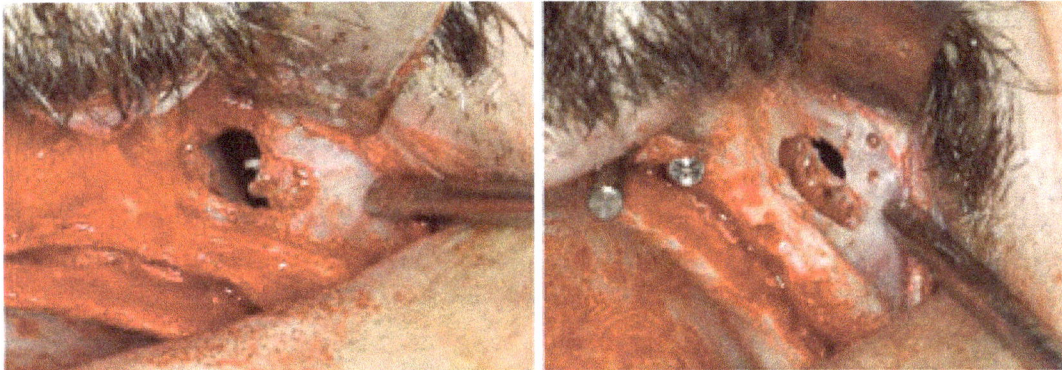

Figure 9. The sinus membrane is carefully released. Two holes are gently made 3–4 mm from one another using a fissure bur.

The perforation is closed in this manner; the integrity of the maxillary sinus floor is preserved, and the sinus lift procedure is resumed; bone grafting and the insertion of biomaterial under the sinus membrane can be done and implants may also be placed. For large perforations, it is prudent to place a membrane to ensure the closure and prevention of graft material from migrating into the sinus cavity. Alternatively, buccal fat can be used for perforation closure or as a barrier between the sinus membrane and the graft material. This fixation method can be used along with a variety of biomaterials.

4.3. Discussion

The growing popularity of implant treatment runs hand in hand with procedural complications. One example is SMP during sinus lifting in the atrophic posterior maxilla, complicating implant placement. In 1980, Boyne and James [23] performed the first sinus lift procedure. Since then, sinus lifting has been the treatment of choice for implant placement in an atrophic maxillary ridge. Like every other conventional treatment, sinus lifting has its inherent risks and complications. The most common potential complication of open sinus lift surgery is SMP intraoperatively, which if left untreated, may result in the leakage of graft material into the sinus, infection, oroantral fistula, and impairment of physiologic sinus function [24–27]. The risk of SMP has been reported to be as high as 58%, especially when the membrane is thin or when bone septae are present [31, 32]. The most common factor that can cause SMP is the use of excessive force upon elevation of the sinus membrane [33] or the inadequate reflection or release of the periphery [29]. Anatomic variations can also increase the risk of SMP [30]. These anatomic variations associated with the risk of SMP are as follows: thin sinus membrane (28%), presence of septae (22%), membrane adhesion (17%), previous surgery (17%), presence of scar tissue(11%), and presence of cysts (5%) [11].

4.4. Repair

In SMPs smaller than 5 mm, the perforation can usually be closed by applying a direct suture, covering it with a collagen membrane or fibrin tissue sealant [34–36]. Larger perforations require application of other techniques. Various methods have been used [35–40]. Some recommend to abort the procedure and postpone it for 6 to 9 months to let the membrane heal [41]. In contrast, others believe that the perforation can be managed efficiently using biomaterials and grafts placed at the same time of repair [42]. Shin and Sohn [43] repaired SMPs using fibrin adhesive and implant placement. These were only for small perforations and not medium or large perforations. Pikos [27] offered a method for the repair of sinus perforations. He created four notches in four corners of the membrane, adapted it to the cavity, and used a tack to stabilize it. Testori et al. [32] introduced a method for repair of large SMPs. They used a few stitches on the sinus wall and created a strut for placement. However, a membrane was not attached to these sutures, and the stitches only worked as a strut. In general, suturing the two edges of the perforated membrane inside the sinus or keeping them close to each other for use of fibrin adhesive is not an easy task. In contrast, fixing the perforated membrane to the bone is simple.

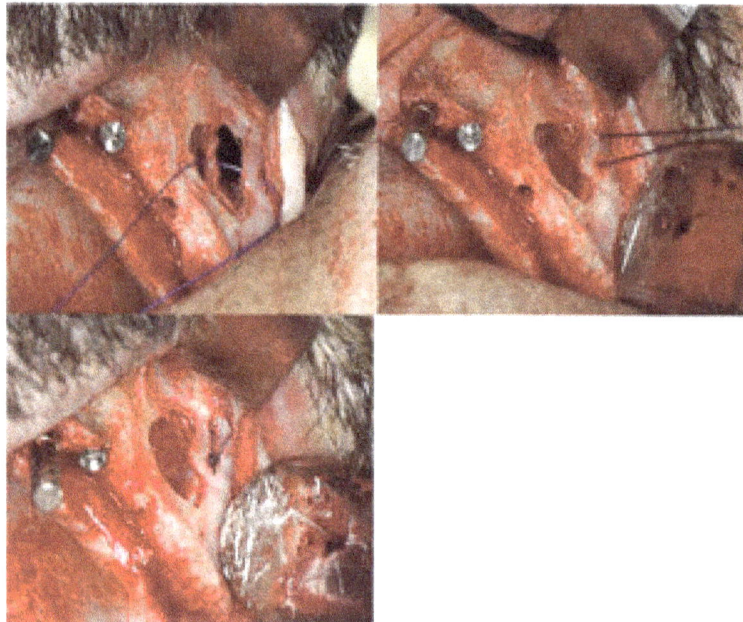

Figure 10. The suture enters through the first hole from the outside, towards the inside of the cavity and traverses the sinus membrane. The suture exits through the second hole. After tension is applied, the membrane is pulled adjacent to the bone.

The suture is tied and the knot is tightened on the external sinus wall. The perforation is completely closed. The perforated membrane will be fixed to the bony sinus wall. In our study,

14 patients in whom perforations of maxillary sinus membrane developed and who were treated using our technique were assessed; perforations developed after sinus lifting in 10 patients, after the removal of impactions in 3 patients, and after cyst removal in 1 patient. There were six perforation sites on the apical part of the window (class I), six on the lateral part (class II), and two within the window extension (class III). Patients were followed for an average of 13.7 months (range, 12–18 months). All were treated and complications were minor.

5. Conclusion

Our technique is an easy, feasible, and predictable technique that helps the surgeon easily manage SMP during sinus lifting. Other operations not related to implant placement might also be associated with this complication. In such situations, it is necessary to use a simple applicable method for management. Using the double-hole bone fixation technique allows for safe repair.

Author details

Mohammad Hosein Kalantar Motamedi[1*] and Ali Hassani[2]

*Address all correspondence to: motamedical@lycos.com

1 Trauma Research Center, Baqiyatallah University of Medical Sciences, Department of Oral and Maxillofacial Surgery, Azad University, Dental Branch, Tehran, Iran

2 Azad University, Dental Branch, and Buali Hospital, Tehran, Iran

References

[1] Motamedi MH. Concepts to consider during surgery to remove impacted third molars. Dent Today. 2007 Oct;26(10):136, 138–41; quiz 141, 129.

[2] Motamedi MH. Preventing periodontal pocket formation after removal of an impacted mandibular third molar. J Am Dent Assoc. 1999 Oct;130(10):1482–4.

[3] Motamedi MH, Shafeie HA. Technique to manage simultaneously impacted mandibular second and third molars in adolescent patients. Oral Surg Oral Med Oral Pathol Oral Radiol Endod. 2007 Apr;103(4):464–6. Epub 2006 Oct 16.

[4] Hassani A, Kalantar Motamedi MH, Tabeshfar S, Vahdati SA. The "crescent" graft: A new design for bone reconstruction in implant dentistry. J Oral Maxillofac Surg. 2009;67:1735–8.

[5] Laskin DM, Edwards JL. Immediate reconstruction of an orbital complex fracture with autogenously mandibular bone. J Oral Surg. 1977;35:749.

[6] Strassburger C, Heydecke G, Kerschbaum T. Influence of prosthetic and implant therapy on satisfaction and quality of life: A systematic literature review. Part 1— Characteristics of the studies. Int J Prosthodont. 2004;17:83.

[7] Tomson PLM, Butteworth CJ, Walmsley AD. Management of peri-implant bone loss using guided bone regeneration: A clinical report. J Prosthet Dent. 2004;92:12.

[8] Fugazzotto PA, Baker R, Lightfoot S. Immediate implant therapy in clinical practice: Single tooth replacement. J Mass Dent Soc. 2007;56:28.

[9] Nemcovsky CE, Artzi Z, Moses O, et al. Healing of marginal defects at implant placed in fresh extraction sockets or after 4–6 weeks of healing: A comparative study. Clin Oral Implants Res. 2002;13:410.

[10] Lorenzoni M, Pertl C, Keil C, et al. Treatment of peri-implant defects with guided bone regeneration: A comparative clinical study with various membranes and bone grafts. Int J Oral Maxillofac Implants. 1998;13:639.

[11] Khoury F, Buchmann R. Surgical therapy of peri-implant disease: A 3 year follow-up study of cases treated with 3 different techniques of bone regeneration. J Periodontol. 2001;72:1498.

[12] Wikesjö UM, Qahash M, Thomson RC, et al. rhBMP-2 significantly enhances guided bone regeneration. Clin Oral Implants Res. 2004;15:194.

[13] Behneke A, Behneke N, d'Hoedt B. Treatment of peri-implantitis defects with autogenous bone grafts: 6 Month to 3 year results of a prospective study in 17 patients. Int J Oral Maxillofac Implants. 2000;15:125.

[14] Lozada JL, James RA, Boskovic M, et al. Surgical repair of peri-implant defects. J Oral Implantol. 1990;16:42.

[15] Mish CM. The harvest of ramus bone in conjunction with third molar removal for onlay grafting before placement of dental implant. J Oral Maxillofac Surg. 1999;57:1376.

[16] Khoury F, Khoury C. Mandibular bone block grafts: Diagnosis, instrumentation, harvesting techniques and surgical procedures, in Khoury F, Antoun H, Missika P, Bone Augmentation in Oral Implantology. Hanover Park, IL: Quintessence, 2007, pp. 115–212.

[17] Hassani A, Khojasteh A, Shamsabad AN. The anterior palate as a donor site in oral and maxillofacial bone grafting procedure. A quantitative anatomic study. J Oral Maxillofac Surg. 2005;63:1196.

[18] Khoury F. The late transposition of wisdom teeth. Dtsch Zahnärztl Z. 1986;41:1061 (in German).

[19] Gapski R, Wang HL, Misch CE. Management of incision design in symphysis graft procedures: A review of the literature. J Oral Implantol. 2001;27:134.

[20] Girdler NM, Hosseini M. Orbital floor reconstruction with autogenous bone harvested from mandibular bone. Br J Oral Maxillofac Surg. 1992;30:36.

[21] Brian C, Harsha A, Timothy A, et al. Use of autogenous cranial bone graft in maxillofacial surgery. J Oral Maxillofac Surg. 1980;44:11.

[22] Burchardt H, Ennerking WF. Transplantation of bone. Surg Clin North Am. 1978;58:2.

[23] Boyne PJ, James RA. Grafting of the maxillary sinus floor with autogenous marrow and bone. J Oral Surg. 1980;38:613.

[24] Mazor Z, Peleg M, Gross M. Sinus augmentation for single-tooth replacement in the posterior maxilla: A 3-year follow-up clinical report. Int J Oral Maxillofac Implants. 1999;14:55.

[25] Misch CE. The maxillary sinus lift and sinus graft surgery, Carl Misch *in* Contemporary Implant Dentistry. St Louis: Mosby, 1999, pp. 469–495.

[26] Jensen J, Sindet-Pedersen S, Oliver AJ. Varying treatment strategies for reconstruction of maxillary atrophy with implants: Results in 98 patients. J Oral Maxillofac Surg. 1994;52:210.

[27] Pikos MA. Maxillary sinus membrane repair: Report of a technique for large perforations. Implant Dent. 1999;8:29.

[28] Fugazzotto PA, Vlassis J. A simplified classification and repair system for sinus membrane perforations. J Periodontol. 2003;74:1534.

[29] Vlassis JM, Fugazzotto PA. A classification system for sinus membrane perforations during augmentation procedures with options for repair. J Periodontol. 1999;70:692.

[30] Proussaefs P, Lozada J. The "Loma Linda pouch": A technique for repairing the perforated sinus membrane. Int J Periodont Restor Dent. 2003;23:593.

[31] Krennmair G, Ulm C, Lugmayr H. Maxillary sinus septa: Incidence, morphology and clinical implications. J Craniomaxillofac Surg. 1997;25:261.

[32] Testori T, Wallace SS, Del Fabbro M, et al. Repair of large sinus membrane perforations using stabilized collagen barrier membranes: Surgical techniques with histologic and radiographic evidence of success. Int J Periodont Restor Dent. 2008;28:9.

[33] Becker ST, Terheyden H, Steinriede A, et al. Prospective observation of 41 perforations of the Schneiderian membrane during sinus floor elevation. Clin Oral Implants Res. 2008;19:1285.

[34] Hernández-Alfaro F, Torradeflot MM, Marti C. Prevalence and management of Schneiderian membrane perforations during sinus-lift procedures. Clin Oral Implants Res. 2008;19:91.

[35] Van den Bergh JPA, ten Bruggenkate CM, Disch FJM, et al. Anatomical aspects of sinus floor elevations. Clin Oral Implants Res. 2000;11:256.

[36] Chanavaz M. Maxillary sinus: Anatomy, physiology, surgery, and bone grafting related to implantology—Eleven years of surgical experience (1979–1990). J Oral Implantol. 1990;16:199.

[37] Fugazzotto PA, Vlassis J. Long-term success of sinus augmentation using various surgical approaches and grafting materials. Int J Oral Maxillofac Implants 1998;13:52.

[38] Ardekian L, Oved-Peleg E, Mactei EE, et al. The clinical significance of sinus membrane perforation during augmentation of the maxillary sinus. J Oral Maxillofac Surg. 2006;64:277.

[39] Simunek A, Kopecka D, Cierny M. The use of oxidized regenerated cellulose (Surgicel) in closing Schneiderian membrane tears during the sinus lift procedure. West Indian Med J. 2005;54:398.

[40] Avera SP, Stampley WA, McAllister BS. Histologic and clinical observation of resorbable and nonresorbable barrier membrane used in maxillary sinus graft containment. Int J Oral Maxillofac Implants 1997;12:88.

[41] Karabuda C, Arisan V, Özyuvaci H. Effects of sinus membrane perforations on the success of dental implants placed in the augmented sinus. J Periodontol. 2006;77:1991.

[42] Wallace SS, Froum SJ, Tarnow DP. Histologic evaluation of sinus elevation procedure: A clinical report. Int J Periodont Restor Dent. 1996;16:47.

[43] Shin HI, Sohn DS. A method of sealing perforated sinus membrane and histologic finding of bone substitutes: A case report. Implant Dent. 2005;14:328.

2

Ridge Augmentation Techniques in Preprosthetic Implant Surgery

Bahattin Alper Gultekin, Erol Cansiz and
Serdar Yalcin

Abstract

Rehabilitation of missing teeth with dental implant-supported restorations has become a predictable treatment option in dentistry. The stability of hard and soft tissues around the implant is fundamental for long-term success. However, due to factors such as trauma, oncologic diseases, and missing teeth, vertical and horizontal bone loss is expected, and the available bone may not be suitable for optimum implant placement. Ridge augmentation procedures are applied to increase in the volume of the deficient sites for implant treatment. Autogenous block bone augmentation and guided bone regeneration (GBR) are two surgical approaches for implant placement. Autogenous bone is widely used for augmentations because of its osteogenic potential. A myriad of biomaterials, including xenografts, allografts, alloplasts, and composite grafts, are available for GBR. The aim of this chapter is to provide a brief summary of these methods and to discuss the advantages and pitfalls of ridge augmentation techniques.

Keywords: Alveolar ridge deficiency, guided bone regeneration, iliac block bone augmentation, biomaterials, autogenous bone

1. Introduction

Rehabilitation of edentulous sites with implant-supported restorations is a reliable technique with a predictable outcome. Alveolar ridge resorption after tooth loss is very common and may compromise the placement of implants. Trauma, oncologic diseases, oral infections, and congenitally missing teeth may also cause severe bone deficiency. A wide range of surgical procedures, such as guided bone regeneration (GBR) through the use of resorbable and non-resorbable membranes, intra- and extra-oral block grafting, and distraction osteogenesis, can be applied for reconstruction of alveolar ridge deficiencies [1–3].

Defect morphology plays an important role in the success of alveolar ridge augmentation techniques. Defects can basically be classified as intrabony or extrabony defects [4]. It is easier to maintain space, stabilize the augmented site, achieve primary soft tissue closure, and protect the grafting site in intrabony defects than in extrabony defects. Therefore, intrabony defects are much easier to augment through techniques such as socket augmentation and sinus floor elevation. Extrabony defects can be more challenging in cases such as lateral and vertical augmentations (**Figure 1**) [5].

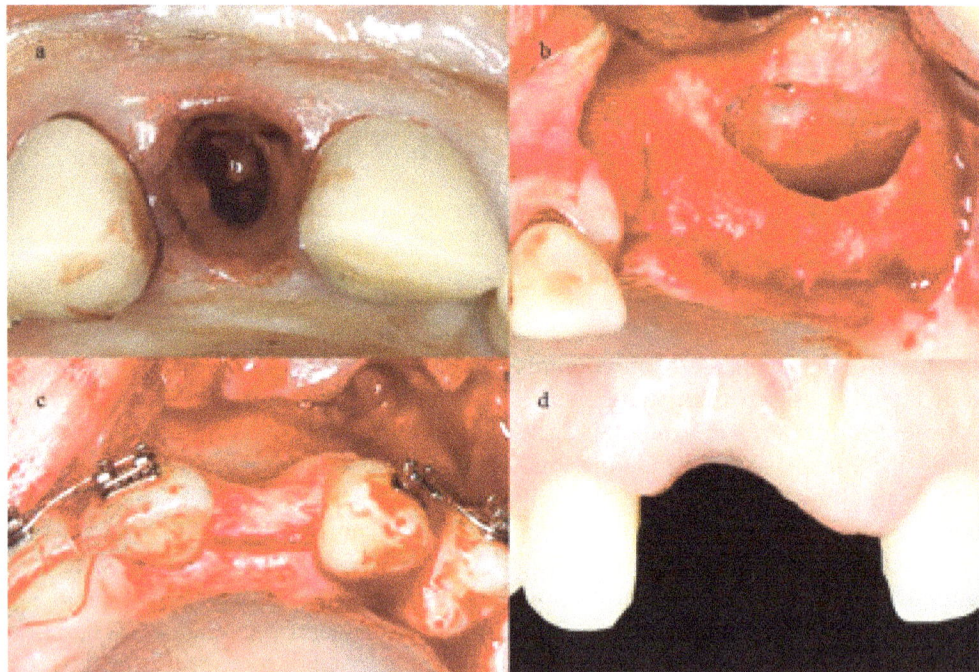

Figure 1. Intrabony (a, b) and extrabony (c, d) alveolar ridge defects.

The amount of augmentation may also influence the risk assessment of the operation. Particularly for vertical augmentation, complications are more likely if a large amount of height is needed outside the natural bone after bone regeneration.

This chapter is focused on GBR and extra-oral bone block techniques that are widely used for ridge augmentation.

2. Alveolar ridge augmentation techniques

2.1. Guided bone regeneration (GBR)

GBR is a surgical technique that increases the amount of alveolar ridge for implant placement using barrier membranes with or without bone substitutes [4]. Regeneration at the deficient site depends on the exclusion of soft tissue (epithelial cells and fibroblasts) from osteogenic tissue (osteoblasts) during organization of the bone [6]. Osteoblasts are mainly responsible for increasing the amount of regenerated alveolar ridge. However, osteoblasts do not regenerate the alveolar ridge as quickly as epithelial and connective tissue cells grow. The success of the GBR approach mainly depends on the exclusion of soft tissue cells during bone remodeling by slowly working osteoblasts [6]. Aghaloo et al. evaluated the success of ridge augmentation techniques (GBR, onlay block grafting, distraction osteogenesis, ridge splitting, and mandibular interpositional grafting) based on implant survival in a systematic review [7]. They found that GBR may be the best way to augment the ridge according to implant survival.

The GBR technique can be applied in two stages (delayed approach) or in one stage (simultaneous approach with implant placement). If the bone deficiency is low and implant stability can be achieved, the one-stage approach can be applied (**Figure 2**).

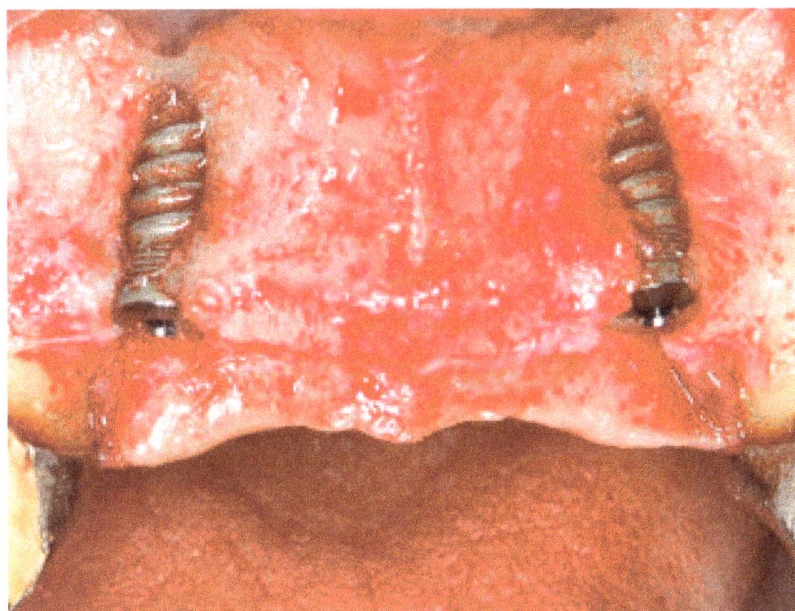

Figure 2. Labial bone deficiency.

However, if a greater amount of bone must be regenerated, then the two-stage approach is preferable and the complication risk will be reduced.

The predictability of GBR is based on several principles, such as space maintenance, stability, nutrition, and primary closure [5]. In this section, these principles are introduced in detail according the morphology of the bone defects, the grafting material, and the chosen technique.

2.2. Space maintenance

Maintenance of space at the augmented site is one of the fundamental principles of the GBR technique. A protected space is needed for hard-tissue cells to regenerate bone that excludes soft-tissue cells during healing and maturation.

Bone substitutes, membranes, tenting screws, titanium, and bone plates are suggested for the maintenance of space. Jovanovic et al. evaluated the treatment groups in a pre-clinical study on GBR. They found that significant bone gain could be achieved when membrane and graft material were used than when no membrane was used [8]. Space maintenance can be challenging depending on the properties of the defect site. When significant bone augmentation is required in a severely resorbed alveolar ridge, creating space is more critical for the success of GBR.

2.3. Grafting biomaterials

Currently, the use of a bone substitute material in GBR applications is the standard of care. The primary types of bone substitutes are autogenous bone, xenografts, allografts, and alloplasts [4]. An ideal biomaterial for bone regeneration should have the ability to form new bone, and bone formation must be balanced with the speed of resorption [4, 6]. Autogenous bone is the gold standard for augmentation because of its osteogenic potential. It has the ability to regenerate bone through the mechanisms of osteogenesis, osteoinduction, and osteoconduction [4, 6]. Osteogenesis is the production and evolution of bone at every site, even in the absence of local undifferentiated mesenchymal stem cells. Osteoinduction is the transformation of undifferentiated mesenchymal cells into pre-osteoblasts and osteoblasts. Therefore, the graft material should be in contact with living bone. Osteoconduction provides a non-living scaffold for the regeneration of bone [9]. By using local bone harvesting techniques, morbidity can be lowered during autogenous bone collection. Scraping autogenous bone from a location near the recipient site may simplify bone harvesting, decrease morbidity, and reduce the treatment time (**Figure 3**).

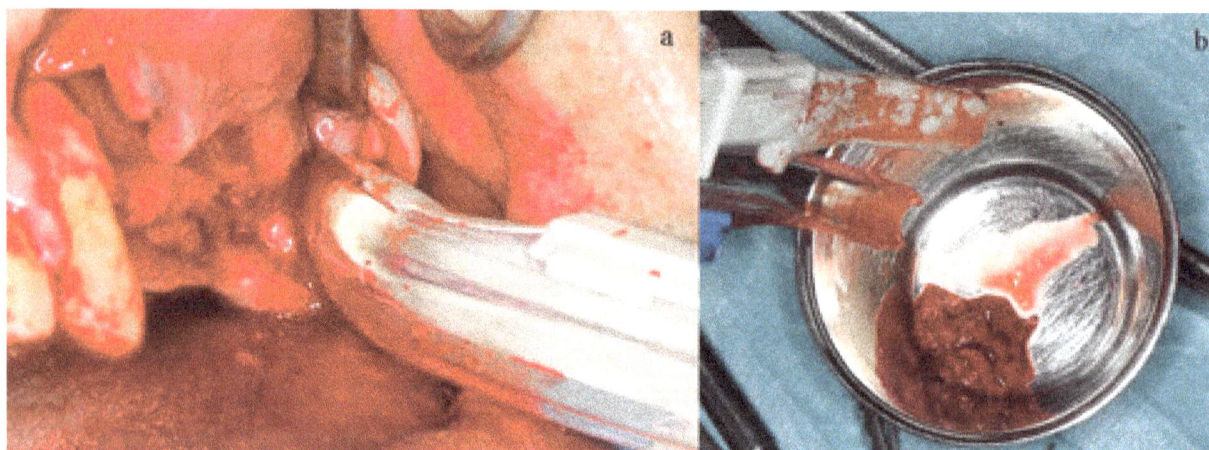

Figure 3. Bone harvesting from tuber site.

Peleg et al. found that the use of a bone scraper to harvest autogenous bone at the ramus resulted in no neurosensory injuries to the anatomical tissues and minimal morbidity in the patients [10]. There are also novel rotary tools to harvest bone easily from local sites (**Figure 4**).

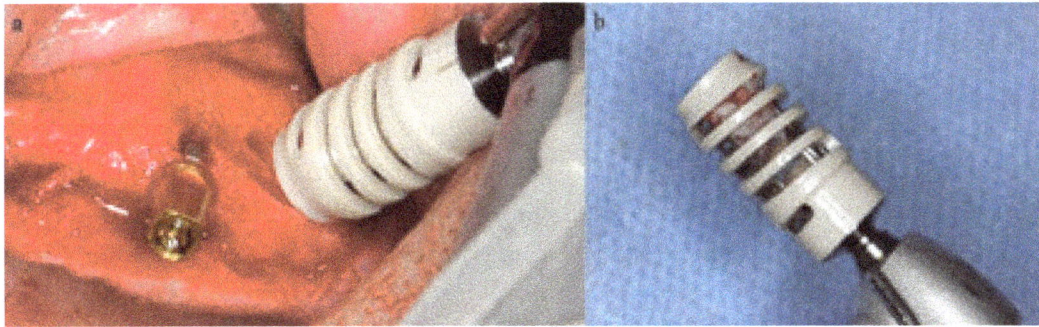

Figure 4. Bone harvesting rotary instrument.

These autogenous particulate grafts can be used alone or with biomaterials as a composite. Composite grafts greatly reduce the amount of autogenous bone required and therefore reduce morbidity.

Bone graft substitutes have osteoconductive properties. However, the use of bone grafting material is very popular among clinicians because of benefits such as the unlimited availability, lack of a need to harvest bone (hence, reduced donor-site morbidity), reduced operation time, and reduced risk of postoperative complications [4, 6].

Xenografts are bone grafts obtained from animals such as cows, horses, or species other than human [4, 6]. Deproteinized bovine bone (DBB) is a xenograft material that is frequently used in GBR applications. DBB is osteoconductive and has an interconnecting pore system that serves as a scaffold for the migration of osteogenic cells; the inorganic bone substance has a microscopic structure similar to that of natural cancellous bone [11, 12]. DBB particles are incorporated over time within the living bone, and DBB resorbs very slowly and has low-substitution rates. Therefore, it can provide space maintenance over a very long term [4, 6]. It was shown that DBB graft particles remain present even after 10 years postoperatively [13]. Chackartchi et al. reported that the mean percentage of new bone was $28 \pm 6\%$ using DBB alone 6–9 months after sinus augmentation [14]. Materials with low-substitution rates are good scaffolds for host bone growth during healing, and they inhibit resorption of the augmented site [4, 6]. However, increased amounts of residual graft particles may negatively impact the healing of the augmented site and decrease the rate at which the implant surface area is integrated with the newly formed bone [15]. In challenging cases that require a greater amount of bone augmentation, such as vertical, horizontal, or both, DBB can be mixed with autogenous particulate bone and applied as a composite [2]. The authors recommend allowing 6–9 months for healing of lateral/vertical augmentations before implant placement. During long-term healing, DBB particles prevent the shrinkage of the augmented site, and autogenous particles facilitate the incorporation of this scaffold with the living natural bone. The authors do not recommend implant placement during the early stages of bone healing (less than 4–5 months) for two-stage augmentations because implant stability may be compromised or severe marginal bone loss may occur before loading [4, 6].

Allografts are bone grafts obtained from the same species but are genetically dissimilar from the recipient [4, 6]. Allograft donors are meticulously screened, and specimens are carefully processed to reduce the possibility of disease transmission. Freeze drying is a commonly used process. Mineralized allografts (MAs) provide stability and space by maintaining their physical properties during the bone remodeling phase [4, 6]. Osteoconductive scaffolds provide volume enhancement and effective site management for successful dental implant placement after augmentation [16]. MAs can be composed of cortical and cancellous particles. Mineralized cortical particles with slow resorption rates offer a scaffold, whereas cancellous particles that have faster resorption rates and are prone to resorption may provide a space for the ingrowth of bone cells and angiogenesis. Therefore, if the amount of cortical graft particles is increased in the composite, less resorption can be expected [17]. Demineralized allograft (DA) contains bone morphogenic proteins and stimulates osteoinduction. However, DA is highly biodegradable and has less compressive strength than DBB and MA. Therefore, it is often mixed with other slowly resorbed graft materials to maintain space [18]. The authors recommend using MAs in challenging cases, and demineralized grafts are recommended in well-protected defects such as socket augmentation. Implants can be placed safely after 4 months of healing in well-protected defects [17, 18]. The authors do not recommend using DA in challenging cases, such as vertical and lateral augmentation, because a great amount of bone loss can be expected after long-term healing [17, 18].

The possibility of disease transmission from xenografts and allografts to humans has drawn attention to synthetic bone graft substitutes [19]. Alloplasts are synthetic and also have osteoconductive properties that provide a scaffold for bone regeneration [20]. Various synthetic graft materials have been developed for crestal ridge augmentations, such as synthetic hydroxyapatite (HA), beta-tricalcium phosphate (β-TCP), and calcium sulfate (CS) [4]. HA has a low or very limited resorption rate [4]. β-TCP and CS are highly biodegradable and have less compressive strength than synthetic HA and DBB [21, 22]. CS can be completely resorbed within 1 month [23]. Therefore, according to the defect properties, these materials can be mixed with slow resorbable materials in different ratios to maintain space during healing [21, 22]. By increasing the amount of resorbable material in the composite, the rate of new bone formation can also be increased. However, the space maintenance capacity will be reduced, even in sinus augmentation applications [24].

The particle size in the graft may also affect the resorption time and the success of the procedure. There are conflicting articles in the literature regarding graft particle usage [14, 25]. Particles that are too small may be resorbed too rapidly, and advanced shrinkage of the augmented site can be observed. Particles that are too large may prevent angiogenesis and delay and/or reduce new bone formation [25]. Chackartchi et al. compared the use of small and large particles in grafts during two-stage sinus floor augmentation with regard to new bone formation and vertical bone height stability. The authors could not detect any statistically significant differences between the small and large graft particles [14].

Several factors, such as the graft properties, membrane choice, surgical technique, use of compression during packing of the graft material, availability of natural bone, composition of the graft, and activity of the host bone, may influence the resorption rate at the augmented site and may therefore affect space maintenance [26].

2.4. Barrier membranes

Barrier membranes are routinely used to maintain space. There are two kinds of barrier membranes: resorbable and non-resorbable [4, 6].

2.5. Resorbable membranes

The most important advantages of resorbable membranes are the elimination of membrane removal after healing, resulting in decreased morbidity, easy manipulation, and lower rate of complications. However, resorbable membranes are not very successful in comparison with non-resorbable membranes with regard to space maintenance. These membranes must be used with bone graft substitutes and additional tools, such as tenting screws or plates for space maintenance.

Resorbable membranes that are made of native collagen (non-cross-linking) show high biocompatibility resulting in good tissue integration and rapid vascularization (**Figure 5**) [27].

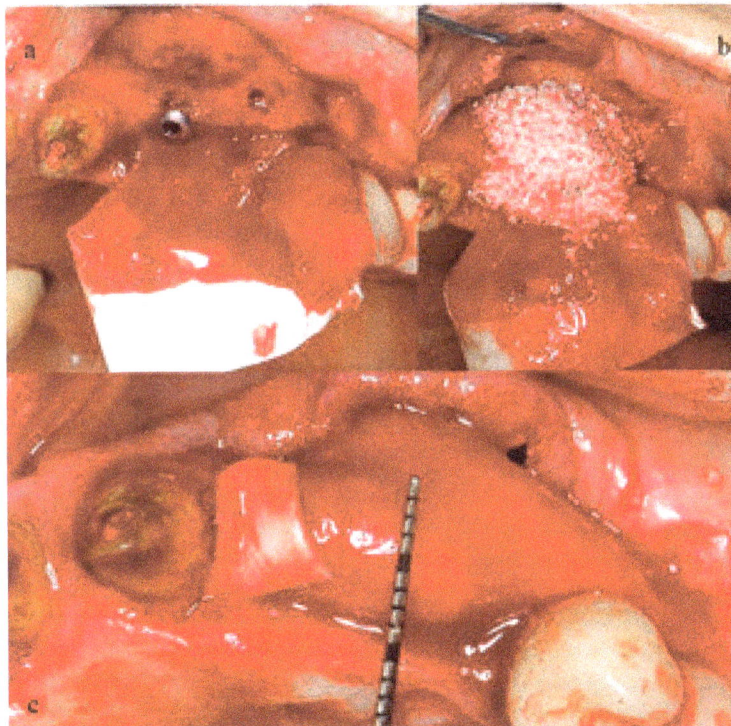

Figure 5. Native collagen resorbable membrane.

However, these membranes may lose their barrier function early due to rapid biodegradation [28]. The resorption time depends on the membrane's properties, the cellular activity of the native bone, and exposure [29]. One of the most important benefits of non-cross-linked collagen membranes is the spontaneous closure of membrane exposure during the healing period [30]. Epithelization of the exposed membrane occurs within weeks after mucosal dehiscence. Although spontaneous healing of the exposure occurs, the grafting volume may be negatively affected during healing, and some bone loss may be expected

[4, 6]. Simion et al. compared the effects of exposed and non-exposed membranes on bone regeneration at the site of implant insertion [31]. Bone regeneration was 99.6% with non-exposed membranes and 48.6% with exposed membranes [31]. There are also studies showing predictable results with late membrane exposures up to 6 months [5]. Therefore, every effort should be made to ensure primary closure of the grafted site during healing. Some clinicians recommend using double non-cross-linked membrane over the grafted site to extend the resorption time for better barrier function [6].

Cross-linking resorbable collagen membranes were produced to extend the degradation time in GBR applications. In a preclinical study, different collagen membranes were compared to evaluate the resorption time [32]. It was found that if the amount of cross-linking collagen fibrils was increased, the resorption time was also extended. However, tissue biocompatibility was decreased. There are also studies showing good results regarding tissue integration and bone regeneration using these membranes [33, 34]. Various types of cross-linked membranes may affect biocompatibility and tissue integration differently [6].

Membranes made of polylactic acid/polyglycolic acid copolymer (PGLA) are also available. These synthetic membranes simplify the clinical manipulation and reduce the application time [6]. Although studies have shown that this material is highly biocompatible and degrades without acidic products, concerns about the healing mechanism remain (**Figure 6**) [35, 36].

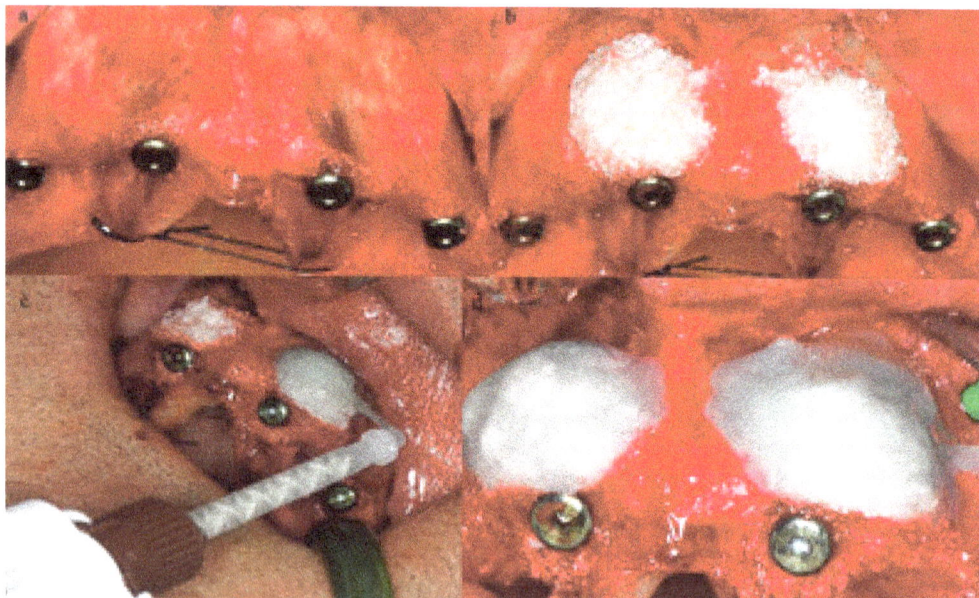

Figure 6. PGLA resorbable membrane.

2.5.1. Non-resorbable membranes

When a higher amount of bone augmentation is required, reinforced non-resorbable membranes are used. Reinforced membranes withstand the pressure from the surrounding tissues, resulting in the prevention of membrane collapse and allowing the bone to be regenerated during healing. Titanium mesh, titanium-reinforced expanded polytetrafluoroethylene (e-PTFE), and dense polytetrafluoroethylene (d-PTFE) membranes are most commonly used, and their benefits have been demonstrated in published studies [2, 4, 6]. Urban et al. augmented alveolar ridges vertically using e-PTFE membranes [37]. The mean vertical augmentation was 5.5 mm after 6–9 months of healing. They concluded that vertical augmentation with e-PTFE membranes and particulate autografts are a reliable method for the reconstruction of deficient alveolar ridges.

Currently, e-PTFE membranes are not used in oral surgery due to high rates of complications related to membrane exposure. d-PTFE membranes are novel titanium-reinforced non-resorbable membranes that have replaced e-PTFE membranes and are used for the reconstruction of critical-sized defects, such as sites requiring vertical augmentation. The highly porous structure of e-PTFE membranes allows ingrowth of the oral microflora when the membrane is exposed. Exposure results in high rates of infection, regardless of whether it occurs early or late during healing. Due to the high porosity of the membrane, it is almost impossible to mechanically or chemically clean the exposed site of the membrane; therefore, early removal of the membrane is required. After removal, it is generally discovered that GBR has failed due to infection, and re-augmentation is needed. e-PTFE membranes must be completely healed in primary closure, and they have no tolerance for exposure [4, 6].

Novel d-PTFE membranes are manufactured in a dense micro-porous form that prevents oral bacteria from entering the grafted site when exposed. These membranes are also easy to mechanically and chemically clean. The removal of a d-PTFE membrane after healing is also easy to perform and takes less time than the removal of titanium-mesh membranes (**Figure 7**).

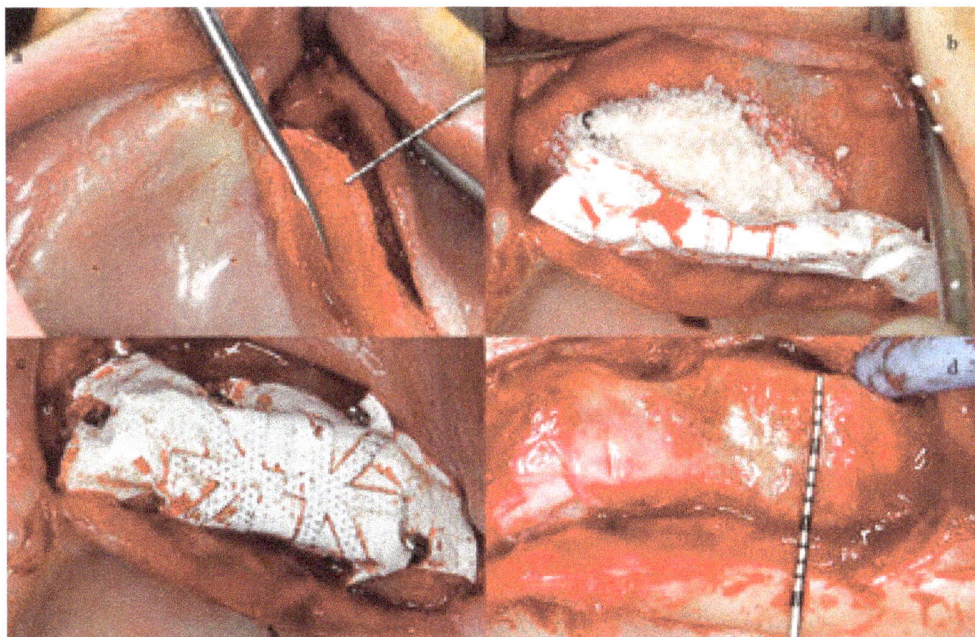

Figure 7. Titanium reinforced non-resorbable membrane.

Ronda et al. reported a mean defect fill of 5.49 mm after 6 months of healing at vertically augmented sites using d-PTFE membranes [38]. Urban et al. observed an average bone gain of 5.45 mm using d-PTFE membrane with a mixture of bovine bone and autogenous particulate bone [2]. They also found a high rate of new bone formation (36.6%) on core biopsies that were taken at the time of implant placement. They concluded that treatment of vertically deficient alveolar ridges with GBR using a mixture of particulate autogenous bone and bovine grafts with d-PTFE membrane is a reliable method.

Although a high level of success with non-resorbable titanium-reinforced d-PTFE membranes has been reported in the literature, these membranes must be applied cautiously in selected patients. Non-resorbable membranes have higher complication rates than resorbable membranes [39]. If a d-PTFE membrane begins to be exposed, the amount of exposure can increase incrementally during healing [5]. Therefore, if early exposure of this membrane occurs, the prognosis may not be predictable. However, late exposures may be better tolerated with meticulous mechanical cleaning. If an infection does not occur 3–4 months after grafting, removal of the membrane may preserve the regenerated bone [5]. Complications regarding membrane exposure are less likely with resorbable membranes. The cost of GBR with titanium-reinforced membranes may also be higher than with resorbable membranes. Jensen et al. reported comparable amounts of bone gain between resorbable and non-resorbable membranes used for horizontal augmentation [40]. If minor augmentation is planned at a deficient site, resorbable collagen membranes should be considered first due to their low risk of complications. If the natural bone is not too thin, lateral augmentation can be successfully performed using collagen membranes with mixed autogenous particulate grafts and low-substitute graft materials such as DBB.

Titanium mesh is another alternative to non-resorbable membranes, and this type of mesh has a good space maintenance advantage [41]. It can be easily trimmed and bent according to the defect site. Another advantage, and also a disadvantage, of mesh over a PTFE membrane is that the holes within the membrane allow vascularization and nutrition from the periosteum to the grafting site [4–6]. However, bone can also grow from inside these holes over the mesh. After healing, the mesh can integrate with newly formed bone and complicate removal during surgery at the second stage [42, 43].

2.6. Stability

The stability of the augmented site in GBR applications during healing is an important factor for achieving success. The initial blood clot formation and stabilization of graft particles will result in predictable bone formation [5]. Although barrier membranes will cover the augmented site and exclude epithelial and connective tissue cells from the regenerating bone, additional tools are needed to provide stability and also to increase the resistance of the augmented site from the flap, lip, and mastication force pressure [5].

Membrane fixation systems can be used to secure resorbable membranes effectively. By using manual or automatic handles, tacks stabilize the membrane to the natural bone and prevent migration of the graft and soft tissue invasion (**Figure 8**).

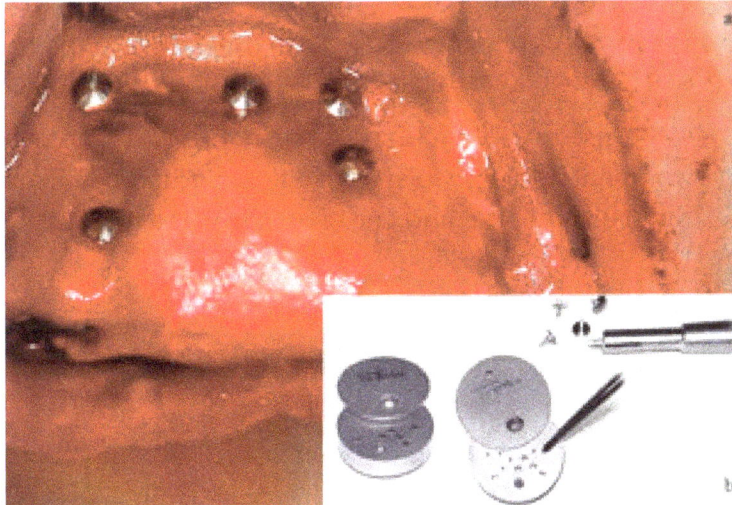

Figure 8. Bone tacks.

Another advantage is that tacking membranes simplify suturing because the membrane does not move during suturing. If lingual or palatal tacking is needed, the angled neck of the handle can be used to simplify the application. Generally, the tacks are made of titanium, and they do not need to be removed at the second-stage surgery. The authors recommend removing tacks that are placed coronally and leaving apically positioned ones to reduce morbidity from excessive flap elevation at the time of implant placement. If tacks are left, they may disturb the patient in the future, and they can be easily removed using a small circular incision around the tack.

Tacks may not be strong enough to secure non-resorbable membranes. Generally, membrane fixation screws are used for stabilization. The aggressive tip and thread design engage the membrane and bone and allow for precise placement in soft and dense bone (**Figure 9**).

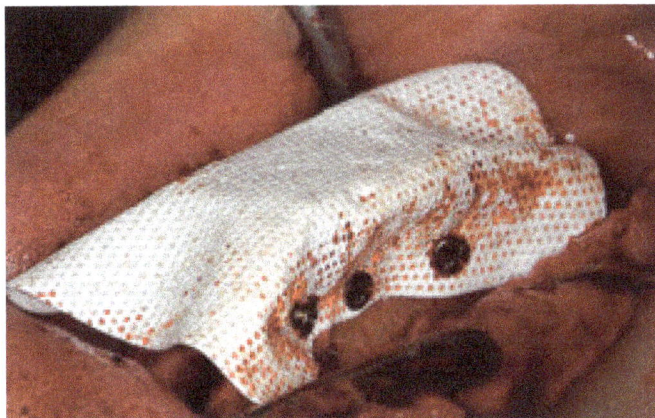

Figure 9. Bone screws.

The authors recommend using short screws in the mandible and longer screws in the maxilla due to its low density; it is easier to engage longer screws in soft bone. If lingual or palatal screwing is needed, surgical hand pieces can be used to simplify the application. At the second surgery, the non-resorbable membrane and all screws must be removed. If any screw is left, the membrane may not be removed easily.

Tenting screws can also be used under resorbable or non-resorbable membrane to prevent pressure from the environment and also to stabilize the augmented site. The treaded part of these screws engages the natural bone, and the smooth part remains at the augmented site (**Figure 10**).

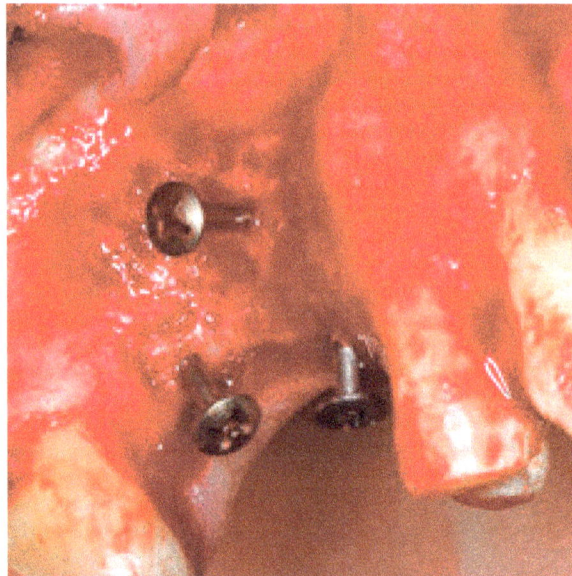

Figure 10. Tenting screws.

Another advantage of using tenting screw is that the clinician may estimate the amount of future bone gain at the time of the operation based on the length of the smooth part. For example, if 5 mm of bone gain is needed, an 8-mm tenting screw can be used and 3 mm of bone will stabilize the screw.

Metal plates that are generally used for orthognathic or trauma surgery can be used for space maintenance [4, 6]. The plate is fixed to the natural bone with screws, and the space between the bone and plate is filled with graft material. A resorbable membrane covers the augmented site. The authors recommend avoiding the use of overly thick plates to prevent soft tissue exposure during healing. Thin cortical strut allografts can also be used for space maintenance in a method known as the Shell technique. Space is created between the cortical strut and the host bone as with metal plates, but there is no need to remove the cortical struts during the second-stage surgery. However, these bone struts are very vulnerable during screwing, and they can be easily broken into pieces [4, 6].

2.6.1. Nutrition

The osteogenic potential of the defect site is also very important for the success of GBR. At the augmented site, the formation of a blood clot begins and granulation tissue invades over the following days and weeks [44]. Blood vessels that are in the granulation tissue serve in osteoid formation and subsequently bone formation. Therefore, the remaining bone walls are an important source of vessels and native cell transformation. When there are fewer walls around the defect, the regenerative capacity is reduced and the total treatment time is increased [5]. Hammerle et al. observed that grafted sites were regenerated with new bone at least 6–9 months after surgery [45].

Buser at al. recommend perforating the cortical bone before bone grafting for better migration of vessels to the augmented site [46]. There are also conflicting studies suggesting that decortication is not needed for better augmentation [47, 48]. Decortication of both the buccal and lingual aspects of the recipient site has been shown to increase the bone healing capacity by 2–10 times when compared to non-decorticated sites [49]. Several benefits of decortication of recipient site have been demonstrated [50]. First, revascularization is increased after decortication, particularly in the mandible. Second, the release of growth factors can improve healing. Finally, the roughed surface of the recipient site may integrate with the graft materials and increase the stability [50]. If the osseous defect is in the mandible, the authors recommend decortication of the recipient site with a drill under copious cold sterile irrigation (**Figure 11**).

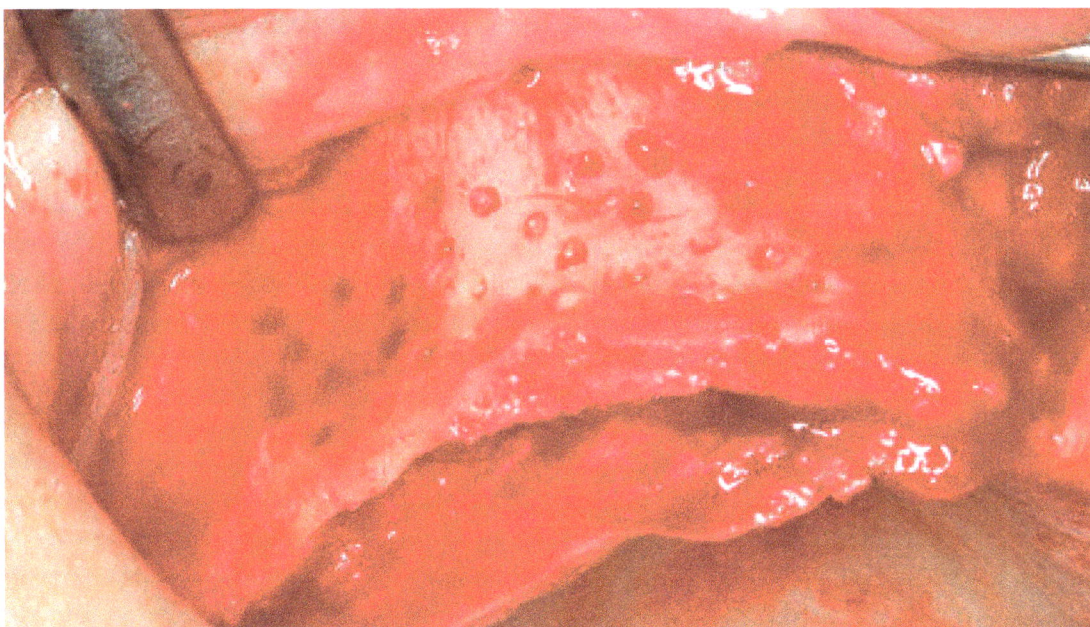

Figure 11. Decorticated bone.

Generally, decortication does not take a considerable amount of time or prolong the operation.

2.6.2. Primary closure

Protection of the grafted site during is an important factor. Wound healing in soft tissue can be achieved by primary or secondary intention. In primary intention, the edges of the flap are brought close and are in the same position as before the incision (**Figure 12**).

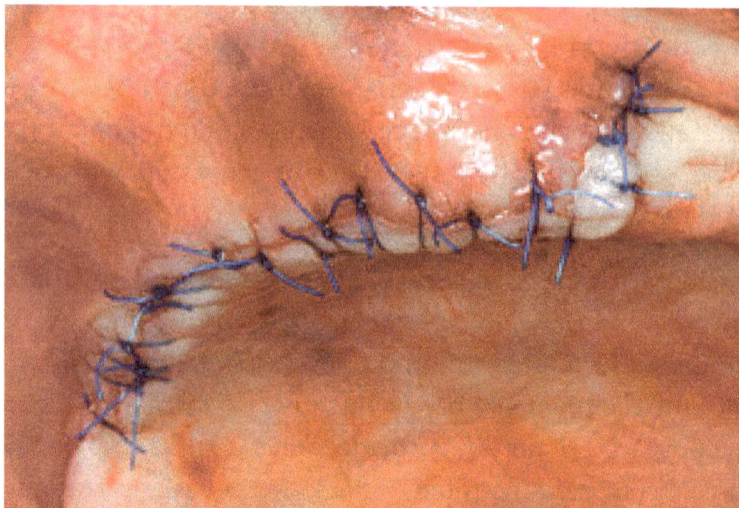

Figure 12. Primary closure.

In secondary intention, the edges of the flap are not closely approximated, and the membrane or grafting material can be seen visually [5]. Secondary intention prolongs the healing and increases the risk of infection at the grafted site [4–6]. Protection of the augmented site begins from a primary tension-free flap closure. If secondary intention healing occurs inadvertently, a series of complications may be encountered, and re-augmentation may be required [5].

Many factors may affect the predictability of GBR outcomes upon primary closure, including the grafting volume of the deficient site. The rate of soft tissue complications may increase in direct proportion with the grafting volume [4, 6]. Therefore, in challenging cases such as vertical augmentation, failures due to soft tissue dehiscence are more frequently seen [6]. Another factor that may affect the clinical outcome is the usage of the appropriate materials and technique. Multifilament sutures, such as silk sutures, are not recommended to use in augmented sites due to the high incidence of infection. Monofilament sutures may help to reduce the infection rate [4–6]. Most importantly, the clinician should be familiar with different suturing techniques to reduce the pressure on the edges of the flap. The authors recommend removing sutures 2–3 weeks after the operation. For vertical augmentations, sutures are generally removed after 3 weeks.

Incision design is also a key factor for tension-free flap closure. In particular, if large deficient sites are planned to be grafted, a greater number of releasing incisions will be needed for tension-free flap closure. Therefore, soft tissue surgical interventions may be needed before or after the operation to increase the vestibular depth and keratinized mucosa [6]. Clinicians should not only focus on hard tissue grafting. For the achievement and maintenance of success, soft tissue conditions such as the gingival biotype, the amount of keratinized mucosa, the vestibular depth, and previous surgical interventions due to failures should be evaluated meticulously during treatment planning [6].

Postoperative care during the initial weeks of healing may affect the outcome of GBR [51]. Chlorhexidine and hyaluronic acid mouthwash after the operation are recommended to reduce infection and improve soft tissue healing [5].

Postsurgical medications should also be prescribed, including antibiotics starting on the day of surgery and lasting for 7 days (1000 mg amoxicillin and clavulanic acid, twice daily), analgesics (to be taken as needed every 6 h), and corticosteroid (e.g., dexamethasone 4 mg daily) for 2–3 days to minimize edema [4, 6, 52]. Patients should be informed in detail with written postoperative instructions after the operation. Solely verbal instructions are not recommended because patients are generally tired after the operation and may forget these instructions.

2.6.3. Iliac crest block bone grafting

Iliac crest block bone grafting is widely used in oral and maxillofacial surgery for the reconstruction of major deficient alveolar ridges. Although both the anterior and posterior ilium can be a source of extra-oral bone grafts, clinicians generally choose the anterior ilium as a donor site because it allows convenient access to the recipient site. Patients remain in a supine position during the operation, and this approach reduces the operation time. Generally, the patient remains in a prone jackknife position during harvesting of the posterior iliac bone, and the patient must be switched to a supine position during the procedure. This may increase the operation time by at least 1–2 h. The anterior ilium can provide both cortical and cancellous bone blocks. Uni-, bi-, or tri-corticocancellous blocks can be harvested under general anesthesia. A bone volume of 50 cc or less can be harvested from a single anterior ilium [53]. If large corticocancellous blocks are needed, harvesting from the posterior iliac bone is appropriate.

The block is harvested according to the dimensions of the bone graft required for the reconstruction of the alveolar ridge. Under general or neuroaxial blockade anesthesia, a skin incision is made approximately 2 cm above the anterosuperior iliac spine, along the anterosuperior margin of the anterior iliac crest. The medial and lateral cortical surfaces of the iliac crest are exposed directly after the subperiosteal dissection. A micro-saw and chisel are used to harvest an autogenous bone block from the anterior iliac crest (**Figure 13**).

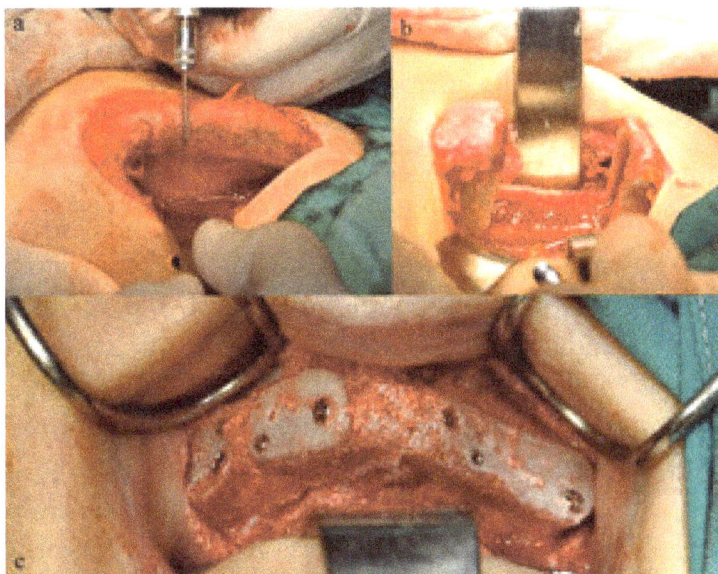

Figure 13. Iliac bone block application.

The block bone grafts are recontoured with diamond burs for optimum adaptation to the recipient site as an onlay technique, and they are fixed to the residual ridge with multiple screws to inhibit micro-movement during the healing process. The corners of the graft are smoothed out to avoid any undesirable exposure during the healing process. Suction drains can be used after harvesting before closure. The periosteum, fascia, and subcutaneous tissues are closed with sutures.

Numerous studies report low-to-moderate morbidity at the time of grafting. Major and minor complications, such as seroma, hematoma, fracture, paresthesia, pain, and gait disturbances, may occur after the operation [54]. Patients should remain in the hospital for at least 1 day; therefore, the total treatment cost is higher than the cost for intra-oral harvesting applications. Iliac bone block grafting morbidity is higher than that of local bone harvesting techniques, such as ramus or chin intra-oral autogenous block harvesting [54]. The experience of the surgeon and technique used plays important roles in reducing morbidity.

Sbordone et al. evaluated the resorption rate in alveolar ridge augmentation after iliac bone block grafting using computerized tomographic scans [53]. The authors reported an average resorption rate of 87% for maxillary grafts after 6 years follow-up [53]. Vermeeren et al. observed a resorption rate ranging from 44% to 50% after 5 years using two-dimensional images [55]. Other studies found a resorption rate ranging from 42% to 87% for onlay grafted bone [56, 57]. The use of a bone block for the reconstruction of a deficient alveolar ridge may be easier than GBR with regard to space maintenance. However, the use of a collagen membrane is still recommended, even in block grafting, to reduce bone resorption [4, 6]. The use of a collagen membrane with block grafting may reduce resorption by almost 25% [4, 6].

Jensen at al. compared GBR and block grafting techniques and found that in 11.1% of cases using GBR and in 2.8% of cases using block grafting, re-augmentation was needed [40]. Contour augmentation can be applied during the second-stage surgery, particularly during implant placement at an esthetically appropriate site. This second augmentation may not only limit bone resorption around implants in the future, but it may also support soft tissue and improve the esthetic appearance [4, 6]. The authors recommend using only slowly resorbable grafting materials such as DBB at the buccal site for re-augmentation with a collagen membrane. Tacked collagen membrane with grafting material will increase the bone thickness horizontally and facilitate anterior esthetic success.

More bone can be regenerated using iliac blocks than GBR [40]. However, iliac bone blocks may be more prone to resorption during healing [53]. Therefore, clinicians should estimate the rate of resorption and increase the amount of harvested bone block. Caution should be taken during treatment planning, and it is preferable to increase the number of implants used in iliac block-augmented patients to decrease the detrimental effects of loading forces [58]. Implant designs that include platform switching may also help to reduce marginal bone loss [52]. One important advantage of block grafting over GBR is the healing time. Four to five months are sufficient for a bone block integrates with the host bone and allow for implant placement [53, 54, 56]. However, particularly for vertical augmentations, 7–9 months are needed for the GBR technique to achieve implant stability [2, 37]. Therefore, it is easier for patients to accept a two-stage GBR treatment if temporary prostheses are provided during long-term healing. A temporary prosthesis can be manufactured using a provisional implant with a fixed or removable prosthesis. If the available bone is appropriate for the stabilization of four provisional implants, fixed temporary restorations can be provided during long-term healing. Soft tissue-supported removable prostheses are not recommended because they may adversely influence the stability of the augmented site.

According to the literature, the survival rates of dental implants inserted at augmented sites are similar to the survival rates of implants placed in natural bone [59, 60]. Marginal bone loss was also similar between implants placed in augmented and pristine bone [61, 62].

2.6.4. The future of tissue engineering

The field of biomaterials and tissue engineering is rapidly growing, and growth factors have great potential for promoting bone regeneration at the resorbed alveolar ridge. Among the various growth factors, recombinant human bone morphogenic protein-2 (rhBMP-2) and recombinant human platelet-derived growth factor (rhPDGF) have received a great deal of attention [63]. Although there are numerous graft materials available, such as xenograft, allograft, and alloplast, most have only osteoconductive properties and provide only a scaffold for bone regeneration during healing. Researchers are attempting to completely eliminate the use of autogenous bone at severe augmentation sites to decrease patient morbidity. Therefore, studies regarding growth factor use with graft materials are increasing [63, 64].

The bone morphogenetic proteins (BMPs) are members of the transforming growth factor-β superfamily. BMPs regulate differentiation, chemotaxis, growth, and apoptosis of osteogenic cells and induce significant bone regeneration [65, 66].

Platelet-derived growth factor (PDGF) is released from aggregated platelets during the early healing phase at the wound site and exerts chemotactic and mitogenic effects on inflammatory cells and undifferentiated mesenchymal cells [67]. PDGF-BB shows potential effects on cells that influence bone regeneration, and it stimulates type I collagen synthesis in osteoblasts, directs cell migration or chemotaxis of progenitor cells, and participates in the initiation angiogenesis [68, 69]. Of the five PDGF isoforms, PDGF-BB is the most biologically potent and has the greatest binding affinity for osteoblasts [69].

In a preclinical study, Simion et al. found that a significant amount of new bone formation was achieved using DBB blocks and rhPDGF-BB in the rehabilitation of severe mandibular ridge defects [70]. Wallace et al. applied rhBMP-2-wetted absorbable collagen sponges in extraction sockets [71], and they found 49.6% vital bone in core biopsies taken after 4 months of healing. These authors suggested that rhBMP-2 and collagen sponges may replace the use of barrier membranes and graft materials to rehabilitate extraction sockets for future implant placement. In another study, Misch et al. used rhBMP-2/collagen sponges and a titanium mesh for augmentation of the atrophic mandible prior to implant placement [72]. All dental implants were placed after 6 months of healing, and healing of the augmented sites was uneventful.

The Food and Drug Administration has approved the usage of rhBMP-2/collagen sponges (INFUSE Bone Graft kits; Medtronic, Minneapolis, MN, USA) in extraction socket and sinus floor augmentation (well-protected defects). The number of published pre-clinical and clinical articles regarding the use of growth factors in reconstruction of hard tissue defects is growing. The use of growth factor instead of autogenous bone offers several advantages, such as decreased patient morbidity, reduced operation time, increased amounts of vital bone at the augmented site in comparison with scaffold biomaterials, and simplification of the surgical technique [70–72]. Clinicians need to be familiar with properties, limitations, and techniques associated with these materials before application. In the future, there can be no doubt that growth factors will play an important role in hard and soft tissue engineering.

3. Conclusion

Many novel techniques, biomaterials, and tools have been described in the literature that clinicians may use to reconstruct bone deficiencies. However, most importantly, the success of alveolar ridge augmentation procedures mainly depends on clinician experience and skill. The surgical risks may be increased for challenging reconstructions. Therefore, the clinician and patient should carefully evaluate the benefits and risks of the operation and decide on the most ideal treatment option. Prosthetic-driven augmentation is recommended for a better outcome. If the clinician focuses only on ridge augmentation techniques to solve bone deficiency problems, he or she may overlook other treatment options that may have lower risks and less morbidity, such as using short, narrow, or tilted implants. After all, ridge augmentation is being performed for the ideal placement of dental implants.

Author details

Bahattin Alper Gultekin[1*], Erol Cansiz[2] and Serdar Yalcin[1]

*Address all correspondence to: alpergultekin@hotmail.com

1 Istanbul University, Faculty of Dentistry, Department of Oral Implantology, Istanbul, Turkey

2 Istanbul University, Faculty of Dentistry, Department of Oral and Maxillofacial Surgery, Istanbul, Turkey

References

[1] Chiapasco M, Consolo U, Bianchi A, Ronchi P. Alveolar distraction osteogenesis for the correction of vertically deficient edentulous ridges: a multicenter prospective study on humans. Int J Oral Maxillofac Implants. 2004;19:399–407.

[2] Urban IA, Lozada JL, Jovanovic SA, Nagursky H, Nagy K. Vertical ridge augmentation with titanium-reinforced, dense-PTFE membranes and a combination of particulate autogenous bone and anorganic bovine bone-derived mineral: a prospective case series in 19 patients. Int J Oral Maxillofac Implants. 2014;29:185–193. doi: 10.11607/jomi.3346.

[3] Urban IA, Nagursky H, Lozada JL, Nagy K. Horizontal ridge augmentation with a collagen membrane and a combination of particulate autogenous bone and anorganic bovine bone-derived mineral: a prospective case series in 25 patients. Int J Periodontics Restorative Dent. 2013;33:299–307. doi: 10.11607/prd.1407.

[4] Liu J, Kerns DG. Mechanisms of guided bone regeneration: a review. Open Dent J. 2014;16:56–65. doi: 10.2174/1874210601408010056.

[5] Wang HL, Boyapati L. "PASS" principles for predictable bone regeneration. Implant Dent. 2006;15:8–17.

[6] Benic GI, Hämmerle CH. Horizontal bone augmentation by means of guided bone regeneration. Periodontol 2000. 2014;66:13–40. doi: 10.1111/prd.12039.

[7] Aghaloo TL, Moy PK. Which hard tissue augmentation techniques are the most successful in furnishing bony support for implant placement? Int J Oral Maxillofac Implants. 2007;22:49–70.

[8] Jovanovic SA, Schenk RK, Orsini M, Kenney EB. Supracrestal bone formation around dental implants: an experimental dog study. Int J Oral Maxillofac Implants. 1995;10:23–31.

[9] Schenk RK, Buser D, Hardwick WR, Dahlin C. Healing pattern of bone regeneration in membrane-protected defects: a histologic study in the canine mandible. Int J Oral Maxillofac Implants. 1994;9:13–29.

[10] Peleg M, Garg AK, Misch CM, Mazor Z. Maxillary sinus and ridge augmentations using a surface-derived autogenous bone graft. J Oral Maxillofac Surg. 2004;62:1535–1544.

[11] Wallace SS, Froum SJ. Effect of maxillary sinus augmentation on the survival of endosseous dental implants. A systematic review. Ann Periodontol. 2003;8:328–343.

[12] Chiapasco M, Casentini P, Zaniboni M. Bone augmentation procedures in implant dentistry. Int J Oral Maxillofac Implants. 2009;24:237–259.

[13] Piattelli M, Favero GA, Scarano A, Orsini G, Piattelli A. Bone reactions to anorganic bovine bone (Bio-Oss) used in sinus augmentation procedures: a histologic long-term report of 20 cases in humans. Int J Oral Maxillofac Implants. 1999;14:835–840.

[14] Chackartchi T, Iezzi G, Goldstein M, Klinger A, Soskolne A, Piattelli A, Shapira L. Sinus floor augmentation using large (1–2 mm) or small (0.25-1 mm) bovine bone mineral particles: a prospective, intra-individual controlled clinical, micro-computerized tomography and histomorphometric study. Clin Oral Implants Res. 2011;22:473–480. doi: 10.1111/j.1600-0501.2010.02032.

[15] Jensen T, Schou S, Gundersen HJ, Forman JL, Terheyden H, Holmstrup P. Bone-to-implant contact after maxillary sinus floor augmentation with Bio-Oss and autogenous bone in different ratios in mini pigs. Clin Oral Implants Res. 2013;24:635–644. doi: 10.1111/j.1600-0501.2012.02438.

[16] Blomqvist JE, Alberius P, Isaksson S, Linde A, Obrant K. Importance of bone graft quality for implant integration after maxillary sinus reconstruction. Oral Surg Oral Med Oral Pathol Oral Radiol Endod. 1998;86:268–274.

[17] Avila G, Neiva R, Misch CE, Galindo-Moreno P, Benavides E, Rudek I, Wang HL. Clinical and histologic outcomes after the use of a novel allograft for maxillary sinus augmentation: a case series. Implant Dent. 2010;19:330–341. doi: 10.1097/ID.0b013e3181e59b32.

[18] Won YH, Kim SG, Oh JS, Lim SC. Clinical evaluation of demineralized bone allograft for sinus lifts in humans: a clinical and histologic study. Implant Dent. 2011;20:460–464. doi: 10.1097/ID.0b013e31823541e7.

[19] Sogal A, Tofe AJ. Risk assessment of bovine spongiform encephalopathy transmission through bone graft material derived from bovine bone used for dental applications. J Periodontol. 1999;70:1053–1063.

[20] Barrack RL. Bone graft extenders, substitutes and osteogenic proteins. J Arthroplasty. 2005;20:94–97.

[21] Degidi M, Daprile G, Piattelli A. Primary stability determination of implants inserted in sinus augmented sites: 1-step versus 2-step procedure. Implant Dent. 2013;22:530–533.

[22] Giannoudis PV, Dinopoulos H, Tsiridis E. Bone substitutes: an update. Injury 2005;36:20–27.

[23] Guarnieri R, Grassi R, Ripari M, Pecora G. Maxillary sinus augmentation using granular calcium sulfate (surgiplaster sinus): radiographic and histologic study at 2 years. Int J Periodontics Restorative Dent. 2006;26:79–85.

[24] Mazzocco F, Lops D, Gobbato L, Lolato A, Romeo E, del Fabbro M. Three-dimensional volume change of grafted bone in the maxillary sinus. Int J Oral Maxillofac Implants. 2014;29:178–184. doi: 10.11607/jomi.3236.

[25] Committee on Research, Science and Therapy of the American Academy of Peridontology. Tissue banking of bone allografts used in periodontal regeneration. J Periodontol. 2001;72:834–838.

[26] Kirmeier R, Payer M, Wehrschuetz M, Jakse N, Platzer S, Lorenzoni M. Evaluation of three-dimensional changes after sinus floor augmentation with different grafting materials. Clin Oral Implants Res. 2008;19:366–372. doi: 10.1111/j.1600-0501.2007.01487.

[27] Owens KW, Yukna RA. Collagen membrane resorption in dogs: a comparative study. Implant Dent. 2001;10:49–58.

[28] Miller N, Penaud J, Foliguet B, Membre H, Ambrosini P, Plombas M. Resorption rates of 2 commercially available bioresorbable membranes. A histomorphometric study in a rabbit model. J Clin Periodontol. 1996;23:1051–1059.

[29] Rothamel D, Schwarz F, Fienitz T, Smeets R, Dreiseidler T, Ritter L, Happe A, Zöller J. Biocompatibility and biodegradation of a native porcine pericardium membrane: results of in vitro and in vivo examinations. Int J Oral Maxillofac Implants. 2012;27:146–154.

[30] Riedmann A, Strietzel FP, Maretzki B, Pitaru S, Bernimou-lin JP. Observations on a new collagen barrier membrane in 16 consecutively treated patients. Clinical and histological findings. J Periodontol. 2001;72:1616–1623.

[31] Simion M, Baldoni M, Rossi P, Zaffe D. A comparative study of the effectiveness of e-PTFE membranes with and without early exposure during the healing period. Int J Periodontics Restorative Dent. 1994;14:166–180.

[32] Rothamel D, Schwarz F, Sager M, Herten M, Sculean A, Becker J. Biodegradation of differently cross-linked collagen membranes: an experimental study in the rat. Clin Oral Implants Res. 2005;16:369–378.

[33] Friedmann A, Gissel K, Soudan M, Kleber BM, Pitaru S, Dietrich T. Randomized controlled trial on lateral augmentation using two collagen membranes: morphometric results on mineralized tissue compound. J Clin Periodontol. 2011;38:677–685.

[34] Moses O, Pitaru S, Artzi Z, Nemcovsky CE. Healing of dehiscence-type defects in implants placed together with different barrier membranes: a comparative clinical study. Clin Oral Implants Res. 2005;16:210–219.

[35] Herten M, Jung RE, Ferrari D, Rothamel D, Golubovic V, Molenberg A, Hammerle CH, Becker J, Schwarz F. Biodegradation of different synthetic hydrogels made of polyethylene glycol hydrogel/RGD-peptide modifications: an immunohistochemical study in rats. Clin Oral Implants Res. 2009;20:116–125.

[36] Wechsler S, Fehr D, Molenberg A, Raeber G, Schense JC, Weber FE. A novel, tissue occlusive poly(ethylene glycol) hydrogel material. J Biomed Mater Res A 2008;85:285–292.

[37] Urban IA, Jovanovic SA, Lozada JL. Vertical ridge augmentation using guided bone regeneration (GBR) in three clinical scenarios prior to implant placement: a retrospective study of 35 patients 12 to 72 months after loading. Int J Oral Maxillofac Implants. 2009;24:502–510.

[38] Ronda M, Rebaudi A, Torelli L, Stacchi C. Expanded vs. dense polytetrafluoroethylene membranes in vertical ridge augmentation around dental implants: a prospective

randomized controlled clinical trial. Clin Oral Implants Res. 2014;25:859–866. doi: 10.1111/clr.12157.

[39] Zitzmann NU, Naef R, Schärer P. Resorbable versus nonresorbable membranes in combination with Bio-Oss for guided bone regeneration. Int J Oral Maxillofac Implants. 1997;12:844–852.

[40] Jensen SS, Terheyden H. Bone augmentation procedures in localized defects in the alveolar ridge: clinical results with different bone grafts and bone-substitute materials. Int J Oral Maxillofac Implants. 2009;24:218–236.

[41] Sumi Y, Miyaishi O, Tohnai I, Ueda M. Alveolar ridge augmentation with titanium mesh and autogenous bone. Oral Surg Oral Med Oral Pathol Oral Radiol Endod. 2000;89:268–270.

[42] Jovanovic SA, Nevins M. Bone formation utilizing titanium-reinforced barrier membranes. Int J Periodont Restorat Dent. 1995;15:56–69.

[43] Malchiodi L, Scarano A, Quaranta M, Piattelli A. Rigid fixation by means of titanium mesh in edentulous ridge expansion for horizontal ridge augmentation in the maxilla. Int J Oral Maxillofac Implants. 1998;13:701–705.

[44] Schmid J, Wallkamm B, Hämmerle CH, Gogolewski S, Lang NP. The significance of angiogenesis in guided bone regeneration. A case report of a rabbit experiment. Clin Oral Implants Res. 1997;8:244–248.

[45] Hämmerle CH, Schmid J, Olah AJ, Lang NP. A novel model system for the study of experimental guided bone formation in humans. Clin Oral Implants Res. 1996;7:38–47.

[46] Buser D, Dula K, Belser UC, Hirt HP, Berthold H. Localized ridge augmentation using guided bone regeneration. II. Surgical procedure in the mandible. Int J Periodontics Restorative Dent. 1995;15:10–29.

[47] Kostopoulos L, Karring T, Uraguchi R. Formation of jawbone tuberosities by guided tissue regeneration. An experimental study in the rat. Clin Oral Implants Res. 1994;5:245–253.

[48] Kostopoulos L, Karring T. Augmentation of the rat mandible using guided tissue regeneration. Clin Oral Implants Res. 1994;5:75–82.

[49] Nishimura I, Shimizu Y, Ooya K. Effects of cortical bone perforation on experimental guided bone regeneration. Clin Oral Implants Res. 2004;15:293–300.

[50] Lundgren AK, Lundgren D, Hämmerle CH, Nyman S, Sennerby L. Influence of decortication of the donor bone on guided bone augmentation. An experimental study in the rabbit skull bone. Clin Oral Implants Res. 2000;11:99–106.

[51] Bunyaratavej P, Wang HL. Collagen membranes: a review. J Periodontol. 2001;72:215–229.

[52] Gultekin BA, Gultekin P, Leblebicioglu B, Basegmez C, Yalcin S. Clinical evaluation of marginal bone loss and stability in two types of submerged dental implants. Int J Oral Maxillofac Implants. 2013;28:815–823. doi: 10.11607/jomi.3087.

[53] Sbordone C, Toti P, Guidetti F, Califano L, Santoro A, Sbordone L. Volume changes of iliac crest autogenous bone grafts after vertical and horizontal alveolar ridge augmentation of atrophic maxillas and mandibles: a 6-year computerized tomographic follow-up. J Oral Maxillofac Surg. 2012;70:2559–2565. doi: 10.1016/j.joms.2012.07.040.

[54] Barone A, Ricci M, Mangano F, Covani U. Morbidity associated with iliac crest harvesting in the treatment of maxillary and mandibular atrophies: a 10-year analysis. J Oral Maxillofac Surg. 2011;69:2298–2304. doi: 10.1016/j.joms.2011.01.014.

[55] Vermeeren JI, Wismeijer D, van Waas MA. One-step reconstruction of the severely resorbed mandible with onlay bone grafts and endosteal implants. A 5-year follow-up. Int J Oral Maxillofac Surg. 1996;25:112–115.

[56] Johansson B, Grepe A, Wannfors K, Hirsch JM. A clinical study of changes in the volume of bone grafts in the atrophic maxilla. Dentomaxillofac Radiol. 2001;30:157–161.

[57] Sbordone L, Toti P, Menchini-Fabris GB, Sbordone C, Piombino P, Guidetti F. Volume changes of autogenous bone grafts after alveolar ridge augmentation of atrophic maxillae and mandibles. Int J Oral Maxillofac Surg. 2009;38:1059–1065. doi: 10.1016/j.ijom.2009.06.024.

[58] Bayraktar M, Gultekin BA, Yalcin S, Mijiritsky E. Effect of crown to implant ratio and implant dimensions on periimplant stress of splinted implant-supported crowns: a finite element analysis. Implant Dent. 2013;22:406–413. doi: 10.1097/ID. 0b013e31829c224d.

[59] Donos N, Mardas N, Chadha V. Clinical outcomes of implants following lateral bone augmentation: systematic assessment of available options (barrier membranes, bone grafts, split osteotomy). J Clin Periodontol. 2008;35:173–202.

[60] Hammerle CH, Jung RE, Feloutzis A. A systematic review of the survival of implants in bone sites augmented with barrier membranes (guided bone regeneration) in partially edentulous patients. J Clin Periodontol. 2002;29:226–231.

[61] Gbureck U, Holzel T, Biermann I, Barralet JE, Grover LM. Preparation of tricalcium phosphate/calcium pyrophos-phate structures via rapid prototyping. J Mater Sci Mater Med. 2008;19:1559–1563.

[62] Jung RE, Fenner N, Zitzmann NU, Hammerle C. Long- term outcome of implants placed with guided bone regeneration (GBR) using resorbable and non-resorbable membranes after 12 to 14 years. Clin Oral Implants Res. 2013;24:1065–1073.

[63] Park SY, Kim KH, Shin SY, Koo KT, Lee YM, Seol YJ. Dual delivery of rh PDGF-BB and bone marrow mesenchymal stromal cells expressing the BMP2 gene enhance bone formation in a critical-sized defect model. Tissue Eng Part A 2013;19:2495–2505.

[64] Rocchietta I, Dellavia C, Nevins M, Simion M. Bone regenerated via rhPDGF-bB and a deproteinized bovine bone matrix: backscattered electron microscopic element analysis. Int J Periodontics Restorative Dent. 2007;27:539–545.

[65] Reddi AH. Bone morphogenetic proteins: from basic science to clinical applications. J Bone Joint Surg Am. 2001;83:1–6.

[66] Groeneveld EH, Burger EH. Bone morphogenetic proteins in human bone regeneration. Eur J Endocrinol. 2000;142:9–21.

[67] Canalis E, Varghese S, Mc Carthy TL, Centrella M. Role of platelet derived growth factor in bone cell function. Growth Regul. 1992;2:151–155.

[68] Andrew JG, Hoyland JA, Freemont AJ, Marsh DR. Platelet-derived growth factor expression in normally healing human fractures. Bone 1995;16:455–460.

[69] Centrella M, Mc Carthy TL, Kusmik WF, Canalis E. Relative binding and biochemical effects of heterodimeric and homodimeric isoforms of platelet-derived growth factor in osteoblast-enriched cultures from fetal rat bone. J Cell Physiol. 1991;147:420–426.

[70] Simion M, Rocchietta I, Kim D, Nevins M, Fiorellini J. Vertical ridge augmentation by means of deproteinized bovine bone block and recombinant human platelet-derived growth factor-BB: a histologic study in a dog model. Int J Periodontics Restorative Dent. 2006;26:415–423.

[71] Wallace SC, Pikos MA, Prasad H. De novo bone regeneration in human extraction sites using recombinant human bone morphogenetic protein-2/ACS: a clinical, histomorphometric, densitometric, and 3-dimensional cone-beam computerized tomographic scan evaluation. Implant Dent. 2014;23:132–137. doi: 10.1097/ID.0000000000000035.

[72] Misch CM, Jensen OT, Pikos MA, Malmquist JP. Vertical bone augmentation using recombinant bone morphogenetic protein, mineralized bone allograft, and titanium mesh: a retrospective cone beam computed tomography study. Int J Oral Maxillofac Implants. 2015;30:202–207. doi: 10.11607/jomi.3977.

3

Facelift: Current Concepts, Techniques, and Principles

Fereydoun Pourdanesh,
Mohammad Esmaeelinejad,
Seyed Mehrshad Jafari and Zahra Nematollahi

Abstract

The effects of aging on skin, including thinning and loss of muscle tone, result in a flabby or drooping appearance of the face. The demands of an attractive appearance and smooth skin are wanted all around the world. There are a lot of factors which influence the choice of rejuvenation techniques, including anatomy of the facial skeleton, the severity of aging changes, social and economic status of the patient, and structure of the skin. Facelifting is a facial rejuvenation procedure in which by dissection of subcutaneous layers and different suturing techniques we are able to stretch the skin and make the patient look younger. This chapter presents the technique, current concepts, complications, and indications of facelift surgery.

Keywords: aging, lifting, rhytidectomy, rhytidoplasty

1. Introduction

Facelifting, also known as a **rhytidectomy,** technically means removal of wrinkles by surgery to give a more youthful appearance to the face. Although the history of this surgery goes back to more than one hundred years ago, in recent decades it has become more popular because demands of being youthful in middle and senile ages have increased among people. Due to contemporary improvements in medical care and increased common knowledge about the importance of healthcare, the life-span of people all around the world, especially in the first world countries, has been significantly increased. As a result, the common problems associated with senility have gained more attention.

One of the main concerns is facial rejuvenation of wrinkles.

A wrinkle or **rhytide** is a crease in the skin. Skin wrinkles typically appear as a result of aging processes such as glycation [1]. There are other factors such as age spots, sun ray effects, tissue sagging, and volume loss, which may also lead to an aged face. The major role of each factor depends on the skin type of the patient. Sagging or drooping is more prominent in patients with thick skin whereas patients with thin skin usually manifest aging with wrinkles and volume loss.

Asian people have thicker skins than Caucasians; therefore, their chief problem is tissue drooping and have less wrinkles in their face. Due to their relatively thick skin, the weight of their tissue is considerably more than other groups and performing facelift surgery is more difficult. Wrinkles begin to form in the early 30s. They usually start in anatomic regions with the thinnest skin such as the periorbital area. As the body gets older, skin and subcutaneous fat loses its volume and the collagen and elastic fibers lose their elasticity, which results in superficial wrinkles.

This chapter briefly explains different approaches of facelifting as well as indications, advantages, and disadvantages of various modifications of facelift surgery, complications, and post-operative care.

2. History of facelift surgery

In early 1900, Hollander introduced the basic facelift surgery which only involved removal of excessive tissue along the hairline. In 1920, surgeons undermined the subcutaneous layer, which became the preferred technique. This method improved skin laxity, but it was unable to address the underlying soft tissues ptosis. Surgeons found that increased skin redundancy is not the only factor involved in aging processes and there are other factors such as ptosis of the deep soft tissues, skeletal deformities, and changes in skin texture which play a significant role.

In 1974, Skoog developed a technique which elevated a subdermal flap in continuity with the subplatysmal plane in the neck in order to address the deeper tissues. The skin and platysma muscle were elevated together as a unit to develop a more youthful jawline for the patient. Although Skoog's technique did not gain acceptance, it was a turning point in facelift surgery.

In 1976, Mitz and Peyronie defined the superficial musculoaponeurotic system (SMAS) [1]. In the late 1980s and early 1990s, based on Skoog's technique, Hamra introduced the deep plane rhytidectomy followed by composite facelift in order to improve the periorbital and nasolabial regions [2]. Owsley made this technique even better by describing the malar fat pad dissection and suspension to improve the nasolabial crease [3]. Ramirez introduced the subperiosteal rhytidectomy technique to improve the cheek, forehead, jowls, lateral canthus, and eyebrows [4].

---

[1] Non-enzymatic glycosylation is the result of typically covalent bonding of a protein or lipid molecule with a sugar molecule, such as glucose, without the controlling action of an enzyme.

There have been a lot of comparisons between the risks and benefits of these methods. Less invasive methods which only included the superficial plane dissection showed decreased risk, reduced complications, lower morbidity, decreased convalescence, and more patient satisfaction.

More invasive methods, which included deeper plane dissections, showed more stable long-term results, better control of the midface and similar risks and complication rates as less invasive techniques. During the past decade, surgeons tend to reduce the complexity of facelift procedure and patients demanded less invasive and less complicated surgeries. Nowadays, due to younger age of facelift procedure, less invasive methods such as endoscopic technique, minimal incision facelift surgery and suspension sutures have gained popularity.

3. Facelift anatomy

Any surgeon who wants to perform a facelift procedure must know the anatomy of the face. The first layer in facelift anatomy is the skin. The dermal plexus of blood vessels is responsible for the skin and facelift flap blood supply. Usually, fat is left adherent to the dermal under surface of the flap to enhance its viability.

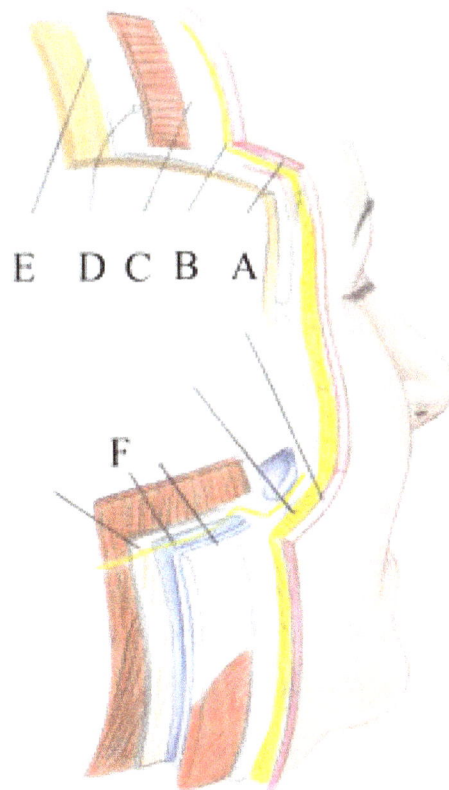

Figure 1. Anatomy of layers of the face. (A) Skin; (B) subcutaneous; (C) SMAS; (D) retaining ligaments; (E) deep fascia; (F) nerve.

The next layer is the subcutaneous layer. The fat in this layer is in close contact with deeper SMAS and superficial dermis. This layer can be safely undermined without damaging the anatomic structures. The subcutaneous layer has different thicknesses based on the location and patient. It becomes thickened over the malar region and is attached to it by ligaments running from the underlying periosteum through the malar pad and insert into the dermis. This area, also referred to as McGregor's patch, provides resistance when dissecting because of its fibrous nature.

The third layer is the SMAS layer. This layer separates the subcutaneous fat from the parotid-masseteric fascia and facial nerve branches. The SMAS layer is continuous with the galea in the scalp, the temporoparietal fascia in the temples, and the superior cervical fascia in the neck. SMAS is continuous with the platysma and separates two layers of fat in the face into superficial and deep layers. All of the facial muscle motor nerves are deep to this plane (**Figure 1**). When this layer is stretched or pulled, it moves the entire lateral face in the desired vector. In theory, this would allow the face to move more as a unit, thus making expression more efficient.

The fourth surgical plane is the sub-SMAS plane. It contains the facial nerve motor branches and the parotid duct. The parotidomasseteric fascia is the layer over the parotid gland and masseter muscle. By operating superior to this layer, the facial nerve branches are protected. Just as the SMAS is an extension of the superficial cervical fascia, parotidomasseteric fascia is also an extension of the superficial layer of the deep cervical fascia into the face and the deep temporal fascia above the zygomatic arch. By deeper and more anterior dissection beneath this layer, the chance of injury to the facial nerve branches increases.

There is a sub-SMAS loose areolar tissue plane extending from the anterior border of the parotid to the anterior border of the masseter. Blunt dissection in this plane gives the deep plane facelift (DPFL) dissection the ability to proceed safely even though it is almost intimate with the underlying facial nerve branches.

As the facial nerve branches move further anteriorly, they pass over the buccal fat pad and innervate the mimetic muscles. Facial nerve branches, parotid duct, buccal fat pad, and facial artery and vein are all part of the plane under the parotidomasseteric fascia. Dissection over the parotid gland must be done with great caution because although it is a safe plane, it may damage the facial nerve branches as they course out of the parotid gland and cross the masseter muscle.

Several other structures may be damaged in a routine facelift procedure. The greater auricular nerve and external jugular vein are in close contact with sternocleidomastoid muscle. The greater auricular nerve innervates the earlobe and cheek. These two are always superficial to the SMAS layer; hence, dissecting in the subcutaneous layer may preserve these structures.

4. Patient selection and evaluation

As any other cosmetic procedure, patient evaluation and selection are very important in the whole treatment plan. The surgeon should keep in mind that failing to plan is planning to fail.

During the asking of chief complaint and taking case history, evaluation of psychological aspect of the patient must be done carefully. Never treat a SIMON[2] patient.

At first, the surgeon and the patient must have complete understanding of the procedure and the risk and benefits. Second of all, the surgeon must know the chief complaint of the patient. Next, a thorough medical and habitual history must be taken from the patient. Some drugs such as isotretinoin and vitamin E have adverse effects on healing and must be noted in the patient's history. Vitamin E supplements and NSAIDs or aspirin should be avoided at least 2 weeks before the surgery. Smoking and alcohol consumption can further delay the healing period and increase the skin flap necrosis. The patient must be persuaded to quit smoking 2 months before surgery.

Areas such as the jowls, prominent bands in the platysma, and a collection of submental fat are the most improved areas in facelift procedure. Thorough examination of these regions gives valuable clues about the treatment plan.

The face is divided into thirds. The upper third consists of the forehead and upper and lower eyelids, which are not typically addressed in superficial plane rhytidectomy. The middle third includes ears and cheeks. The surgeon must assess the amount of skin laxity in this region. The initial position of the earlobe must be noted because there may be a displacement after closure. The lower third includes chin, jawline, and neck [5].

Dedo classified neck profiles into the following subtypes [6]:

- Class 1: No submental fat, good muscle tone, and a well-defined cervicomental angle.
- Class 2: Cervical skin laxity and an obtuse cervicomental angle.
- Class 3: Submental fat accumulation; may require submental lipectomy.
- Class 4: Platysmal muscle banding.
- Class 5: Retrognathia and/or microgenia.
- Class 6: Demonstrating a low hyoid.

Based on this classification, the surgeon chooses the best treatment modality possible. In some cases, facelift surgery alone is not enough for attaining proper results, so other resurfacing procedures must be discussed with the patient that might be needed in future. Good marking of the patient's face and neck in upright position before scheduling for anesthesia has an important role in facelift surgery.

4.1. Indications for facelift surgery

The appearance of wrinkles, folds, and creases on an individual's face is the primary basis for a surgeon to agree to the operation. Skin drooping of the cheeks and jowls are among the factors indicating a person as a prime candidate for the facelift procedure. Other factors include

[2] Single, immature, male, overly expectant, narcissistic is a patient with excessive concern of their surgery and usually exaggerates a minor physical defect.

predominant eye bags, folds in the eye area (crow's feet and laugh lines), and a permanent crease above the bridge of the nasal region and folds in the forehead. Ideally, the patient should be around the age of fifty or below. Above this age may not be ideal anymore, because the work may be more extensive than for younger individuals. This means that more surgeries may be needed.

Another indication for rhytidectomy is the state of skin in the surgical site. Sun exposure is one of the main reasons of wrinkles. The sun basically makes the skin look older and constant exposure of skin to sun exacerbates this matter. Facelift can rejuvenate patients. It is important to remember that normal looking appearance is one of the primary goals after this kind of surgery.

4.2. Contraindications of facelift surgery

Relative contraindications are poor medical health, patients who continuously consume blood-thinning medications, patients with unrealistic expectations, and heavy smokers. Fine wrinkles which can be managed by nonsurgical or conservative treatment very well are contraindications of facelift surgery. Secondary facelifts should also be done with caution because the scar from the primary procedure may disrupt the original tissue planes and increase the risk of facial nerve damage.

5. Facelift techniques

5.1. Subcutaneous facelift

5.1.1. Procedure

Subcutaneous facelift or skin-only facelift was initially the major concept of the facelift procedure. Lexer presented skin-only facelift as a procedure in which the dissection is in a subcutaneous plane [7]. Subcutaneous dissection is needed in this technique so that muscular structure and SMAS remain intact. Facelift in this technique is consisted mainly of skin excision with primary closure. This method was the most popular modification of facelift for a long time. Although the role of subcutaneous facelift has diminished after deep layer (i.e., SMAS layer) was presented, the skin-only facelift is still suggested in selected patients.

This procedure is indicated in thin women with good facial skeleton as well as appropriate skin tone. Actually, this technique is suitable when the surgeon needs to only reduce the facial skin excess. Previous facelift surgery with SMAS plication is an indication for subcutaneous facelift procedure. The results of skin-only facelift are limited because of not addressing other senile facial structures. This technique is contraindicated in obese patients, especially with a non-ideal facial skeleton. Besides, this procedure is not appropriate in elderlies with severe aging changes and sagging of deep facial structures [8]. It is also important to consider that excessive subcutaneous dissection medially especially in smokers make the skin flap at the risk of ischemia [9].

5.1.2. Advantages

This procedure is very simple and suitable for beginners. The dissection plane is above the SMAS layer which contains the facial nerve, so it decreases the risk of nerve injury in this technique. This procedure is associated with good recovery and is an appropriate technique in secondary facelift and after that [10]. The complications of this method are not significantly higher than other DPFL [10, 11].

5.1.3. Disadvantages

The long-term results of skin-only facelifts are not very good. This is a major concern for surgeons. This issue results from two reasons. First, skin viscoelasticity property causes loosening of tightened skin after a while [12]. Second, intact subcutaneous tissues are susceptible to ptosis after a period of time because they are not manipulated in this technique.

5.2. SMAS plication facelift

5.2.1. Procedure

Introducing and describing SMAS by Mitz changed the concepts of facelift [1]. This technique was suggested as a new method to manipulate the subcutaneous tissues to solve the senile changes of the face including skin wrinkles and deep soft tissue sagging simultaneously. The fibro-fatty composition of SMAS layer gives it greater strength against gravity than skin. The concept of SMAS plication technique was manipulating a stronger layer which can bear more loads than skin.

The dissection plane in this technique is supra-SMAS. After dissecting in the subcutaneous plane, SMAS layer is exposed. The mobile segment of SMAS layer is fixed to the posterior relatively immobile layer (i.e., parotidomasseteric fascia) by mainly three sutures in a vertical direction. The excess of SMAS layer could be trimmed after suturing to prevent bulging. This technique is indicated in middle-aged patients with thin skins and moderate to severe laxity. Obese patients with thick skin types are not candidates for this technique.

5.2.2. Advantages

SMAS plication seems to be an easy procedure with little risk for facial nerve damage. Despite manipulation of SMAS layer, the dissection plane is above this layer and the facial nerve plane which let this method to be a relatively safe procedure. The surgery time is short and the recovery would be good in this technique. This technique may have a better esthetic result in midface area than DPFL [13]. On the other hand, the surgeon may be able to manipulate skin movements by SMAS plication procedure comparing to MACS lift and less invasive than sub-SMAS procedures [14, 15].

5.2.3. Disadvantages

Resolving neck aging is more difficult by this technique than DPFL. This issue is related to the inadequate release of platysma facial attachments [16]. SMAS plication is more invasive than some other lifting methods such as MACS lift [14]. The surgeon is not able to manipulate deeply positioned soft tissues under SMAS layer, which results in relatively short-term outcomes comparing to DPFLs.

5.3. Minimal access cranial suspension (MACS) lift

5.3.1. Procedure

The main concept of MACS lift was the difference in vector of traction. The skin is re-draped in an oblique direction in traditional face lifting. In MACS procedure, the horizontal vector of traction is avoided and skins simultaneously with under soft tissues are moved vertically [17] (**Figure 2**). MACS procedure is mainly divided into two types: simple and extended. The simple variation of MACS technique is used to correct the lower third of the face and aging appearance of the neck including jowling and the cervicomental angle by using two purse-string sutures. Extended MACS lift was presented to correct nasolabial groove and midface and lower eyelid senile changes [18]. The incision in the latter form of MACS technique is

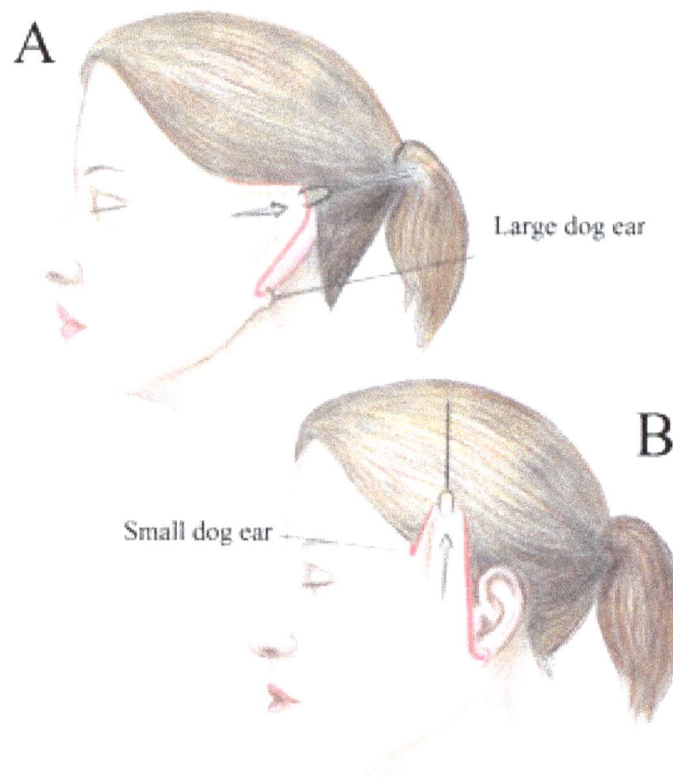

Figure 2. (A) The wrong direction of facelifting forms a large dog ear under the ear lobe. (B) The correct direction of lifting in MACS technique omits the dog ear.

extended along the temporal hairline and a third purse-string suture is used to suspend the malar fat pad (**Figure 3**).

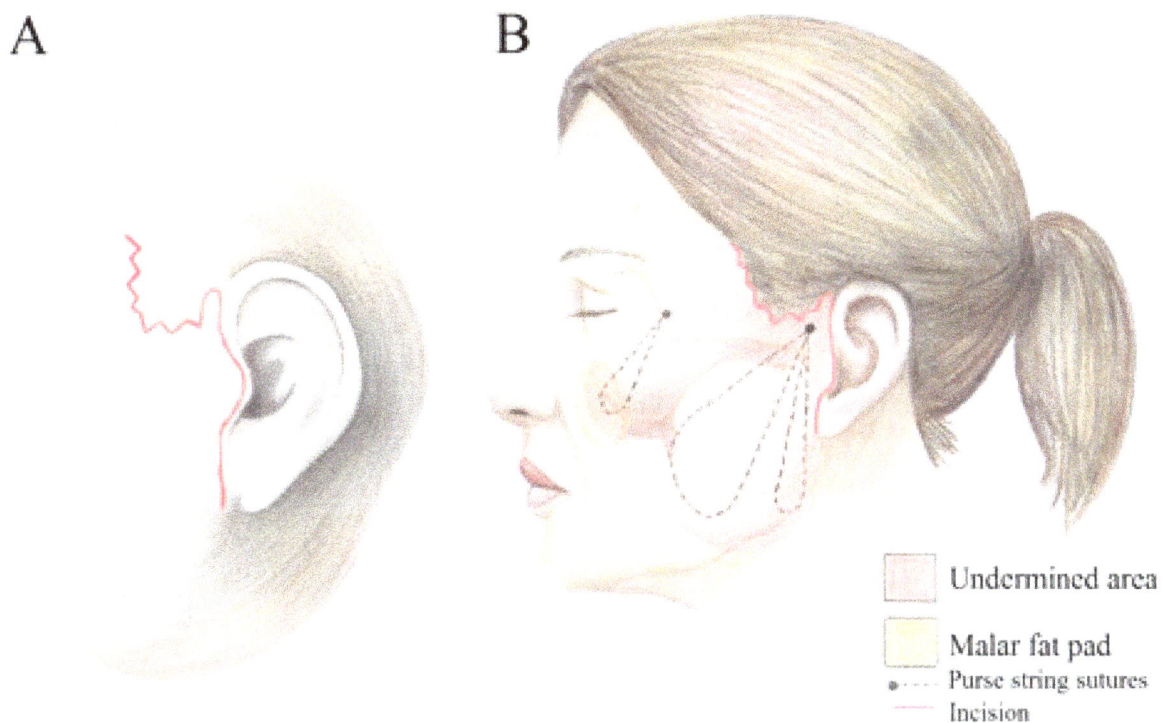

Figure 3. (A) Incision line in MACS technique. (B) Undermining area in MACS technique.

Submental liposuction is performed before starting MACS lift. The incision is made from lower limit of the lobule going through the pre-auricular crease upwards. The upper limits of the incisions in simple and extended variations are at the level of the lateral canthus and the level of the tail of the eyebrow, respectively. This procedure is performed in the pre-SMAS plane above the plane of facial nerve path. Dissection is performed two fingers below the angle of mandible. The purse-string sutures are used to fix the deep temporal fascia in the simple variation. In the extended variation, the third u-shaped purse-string suture is placed between the anterior part of the deep temporal fascia and the malar fat pad. The skin is excised after re-draping in a vertical direction.

5.3.2. Advantages

There are several advantages of MACS procedure suggested in the literature. Small skin incisions and limited subcutaneous dissection are the major advantages of this technique. The risk of facial nerve damage is low due to supra-SMAS dissection. The results are good and the recovery is rapid in this technique. The surgeon is able to re-drape the skin of the lower third of the face, correct the senile changes of the neck, and correct the cervicomental angle [19].

The MACS lift is a shorter procedure than SMAS imbrication with high patient satisfaction and low morbidity. The short incision in MACS lift is a major advantage in this technique, especially in young patients. Avoiding the postauricualr incision in this method makes this procedure acceptable in young patients who usually pull their hair up. The risk of hematoma is low in this technique. Besides, hematoma is easily evacuated and usually does not track into the neck. The dog ear formation under the ear lobe is prevented in this technique, owing to the vector of traction [20].

5.3.3. Disadvantages

The limitations of MACS lift procedure are mainly associated with the anatomy of the patient. The results of this technique are not very good in patients with a bulky neck and significant skin laxity [21]. The final neck contour is unsatisfactory in bulky neck patients due to limited skin excision and pure vertical vector of skin re-draping. The improvement would be less optimal in the latter group. There is a chance of skin flap irregularity regarding to the excessive bunching of the purse-string sutures. Avoiding the ligamentous lysis in this technique prevents the long-term results of MACS lift, especially if the sutures pull through. The cheese wiring effect is also more probable in this facelift modification.

5.4. Deep plane facelift (DPFL)

5.4.1. Procedure

Deep plane rhytidectomy was suggested in place of traditional face lifting to correct aging changes of midface (i.e., malar fat pad) and nasolabial grooves. The deep plane modification was presented by Hamra for the first time [2]. The main concept of this technique was based on reversing gravity's effect by manipulating deep soft tissues to make more satisfying changes in older patients.

In the beginning of the procedure, subcutaneous dissection is performed 2 to 3 mm anterior to the tragus. SMAS layer is then incised after a few millimeters exposure. The dissection plane is the sub-SMAS plane. There are three main reference points during dissection of DPFL (**Figure 4**). Orbicularis oris is the first reference point which should not considered as a part of the flap in deep plane dissection. Good esthetic results would be achieved by incorporating most of the soft tissue into the flap. The zygomatic major muscle is the second important reference point. Deep plane dissection is continued superiorly to the border of this muscle. The last reference point is the zygomatic minor muscle. Zygomatic cutaneous ligament as a major facial retaining ligament is lysed directly. It is necessary to release this ligament to mobilize the midface completely. The final flap consists of skin, subcutaneous tissue, and malar fat pad [22].

Patients with significant aging changes of midface and mentolabial fold are good candidates for this procedure. This method is not suggested for patients with irrational expectations and with poor medical health. This procedure is not suitable in secondary facelift unless the first one was not a sub-SMAS procedure. Although DPFL is indicated for smokers in some investigations [23], the surgeon should be aware of increased risk of wound-healing complications.

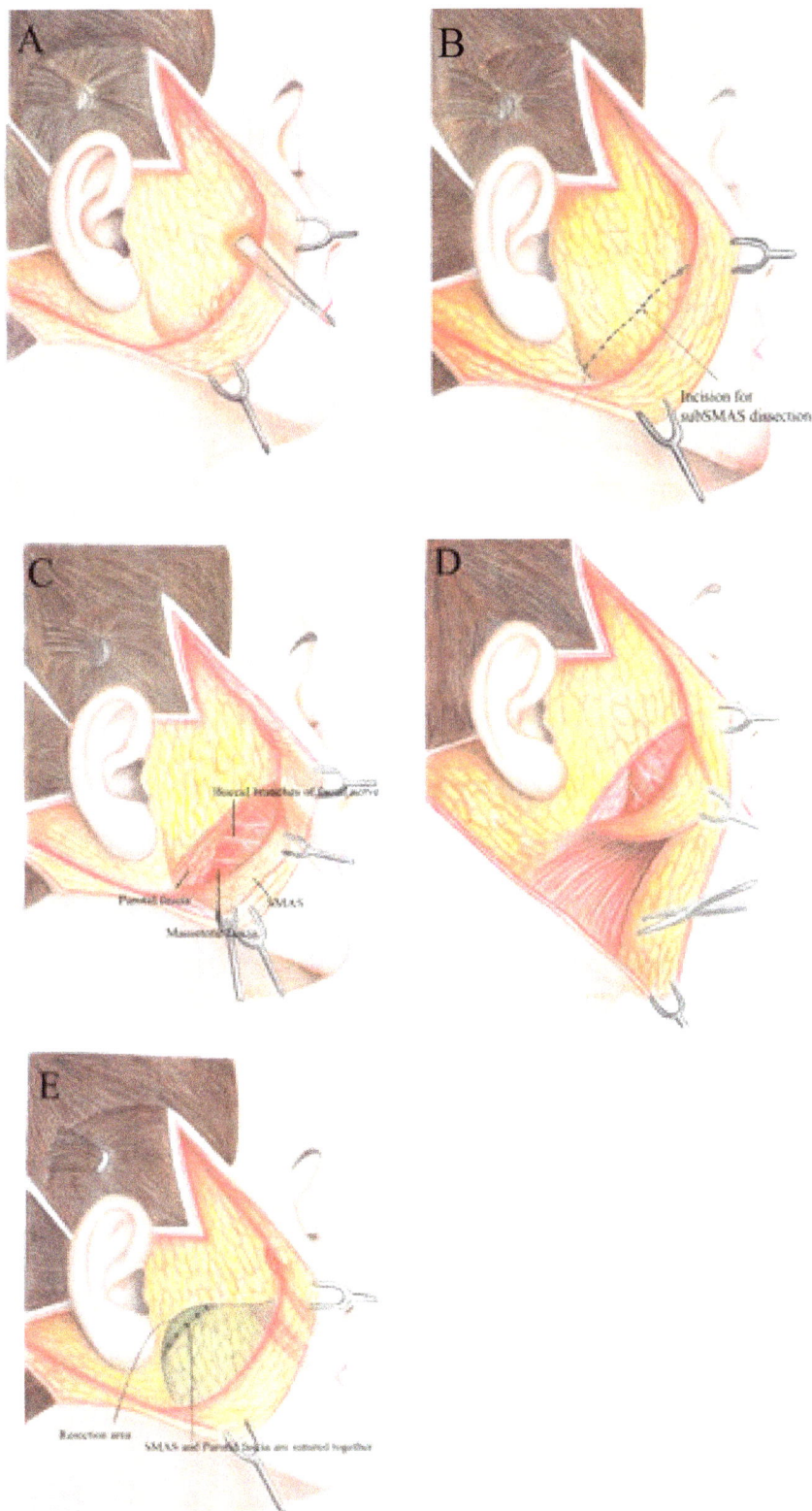

Figure 4. Deep plane rhytidectomy. (A) Subcutaneous dissection is performed 2–3 mm anterior to the tragus. (B) SMAS layer is then incised after a few millimeters exposure. (C) The dissection plane is the sub-SMAS plane. (D) Dissected SMAS layer is obvious. (E) The SMAS layer is sutured to the parotid fascia at the end.

5.4.2. Advantages

This procedure is performed to gain good results in improvement of nasolabial folds. The results of this technique are relatively longer than other supra-SMAS techniques [24]. The surgeon is able to lyse the major facial retaining ligament (i.e., zygomatic cutaneous ligament) and assess the herniation of buccal fat pad directly. Dissecting in sub-SMAS layer and manipulating deep soft tissues of the face give rise to major changes and improvements of senile faces.

5.4.3. Disadvantages

This facelift modification is associated with higher risk of facial nerve damage. Mono-plane dissection in this procedure does not give the surgeon the ability to move different layers including skin, subcutaneous, and SMAS layers in various directions.

5.5. Extended SMAS lift

5.5.1. Procedure

Presenting sub-SMAS dissection by Lemmon was rapidly accepted by cosmetic surgeons [25]. Supporting the overlying skin by manipulating deeper soft tissues (i.e., SMAS layer) is the key concept of sub-SMAS modifications. Although SMAS plication seems to provide better results where the SMAS layer is thin, dissection of thick SMAS layer obtains more satisfactory outcomes.

This technique was presented by Stuzin et al. in 1995 [26]. The main procedure protocol in this method is dissecting and drawing skin and SMAS flaps separately. At first, the skin flap is dissected in the subcutaneous plane. The SMAS layer is incised, after which dissection is continued in sub-SMAS plane.

There are five critical landmarks during performing extended SMAS facelifting [27]:

The first point is 1 cm inferior to the zygomatic arch, which is the origin of the frontal branch of the facial nerve. The incision to start sub-SMAS dissection is from this point.

The second important landmark is the beginning point of releasing and dissecting the platysmal auricular ligament. This second landmark is 3 cm below the earlobe.

The third point is 5 cm below the mandibular angle, which is the inferior extent of sub-platysmal dissection.

Fourth landmark is the anterior border of the sub-platysmal dissection, which is identified by the facial vein where it crosses the inferior border of the mandible.

The last landmark is the zygomaticus major muscle, which is the anterior limit of sub-SMAS dissection in the cheek.

The vector of stretching the SMAS layer is different from the skin's [28]. The vector of retracting the SMAS layer is more vertical than the skin flap. The SMAS and platysma flaps can be rotated in the postauricular area to improve the jowl and cervical contour. The SMAS flap is advanced superolaterally, perpendicular to the nasolabial fold in the malar fat pad area.

5.5.2. Advantages

The surgeon is more able to reverse the effects of the aging process by manipulating skin and SMAS flaps separately. The outcomes of this technique are long lasting due to releasing the facial ligaments and repositioning of the malar fat pad. As it was mentioned before, we are capable of replacing the malar fat pad by this technique. Maximum effects on lower face and neck can be achieved by creating a continuous SMAS-platysmal flap. The unnatural appearance of skin, which sometimes is seen in other facelift techniques, is prevented by reducing the tension of the skin flap due to separating the skin and SMAS flaps.

5.5.3. Disadvantages

The operation time of this technique is relatively longer than other modifications. This procedure is technically sensitive and needs a lot of experience to dissect the soft tissue of the face in two separate parts. The risk of facial nerve damage is relatively high is this method. Extensive dissection of the skin places is at a higher risk of necrosis. The compromised viability of the skin flap is a major concern in this technique. This procedure is not indicated in younger patients with mild aging changes and youthful lower face and neck. Less invasive procedures such as short scar facelift techniques are preferred in these patients.

5.6. Lateral SMASectomy

5.6.1. Procedure

Lateral SMASectomy was first described by Baker [29]. Lateral SMASectomy or limited SMAS procedure is a facelift modification in which the lateral portion of the SMAS located between the mobile and the fixed SMAS is removed.

Classical facelift procedure is begun at first until the SMAS layer is exposed. Superficial fascia covering the anterior border of parotid gland is excised and discarded. The anterior SMAS layer which is mobile is stretched in a superoposterior direction and fixed to the posterior fixed SMAS layer. The vector of tracing the SMAS layer is perpendicular to the nasolabial fold. Manipulating the SMAS layer is the key concept in determining the stability for satisfactory results (**Figure 5**).

This facelift method is indicated in patients younger than 50 with moderate skin laxity and moderate jowls. There should not be medial platysma bands present on normal animation although submental fat may be observed [30]. This technique can be performed in microgenia patients. This procedure is not indicated in the patients over 60 with severe skin laxity in the neck area.

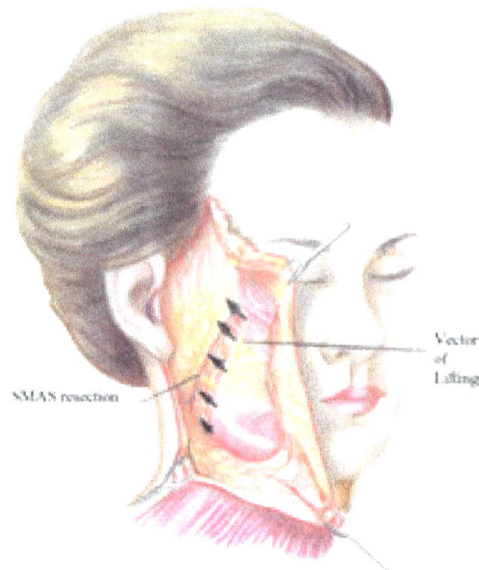

Figure 5. Vector of elevation in SMASectomy technique.

5.6.2. Advantages

The outcomes of this procedure continue much longer than SMAS plication technique due to the stronger fixation of SMAS layer. This technique is relatively easier than complicated procedures such as DPFL and composite facelift. It is a simple technique with minimal SMAS dissection and predictable postoperative results [31]. The postoperative pain may be more tolerable than MACS lift with similar short-term results [19].

5.6.3. Disadvantages

Manipulation of deep soft tissue is limited in this technique as in SMAS plication method. The intact facial ligaments after performing this surgery and limited advancement of deep facial tissues make the results less satisfactory [28]. The risk of facial nerve injury is relatively high in the current method. Preserving the integrity of SMAS layer after removing the indicated part is sensitive and needs experience [31]. The visible scar in this technique is a drawback compared to the short scar facelift modifications; the operation time is longer than MACS lift procedure [19].

5.7. Subperiosteal facelift

5.7.1. Procedure

Tessier proposed the subperiosteal facelift technique for the first time [32]. It is possible to lift the soft tissues of the face vertically and reposition them at the level of their bony origin. This technique rapidly developed and was accepted as a suitable procedure for lifting the upper two thirds of the face.

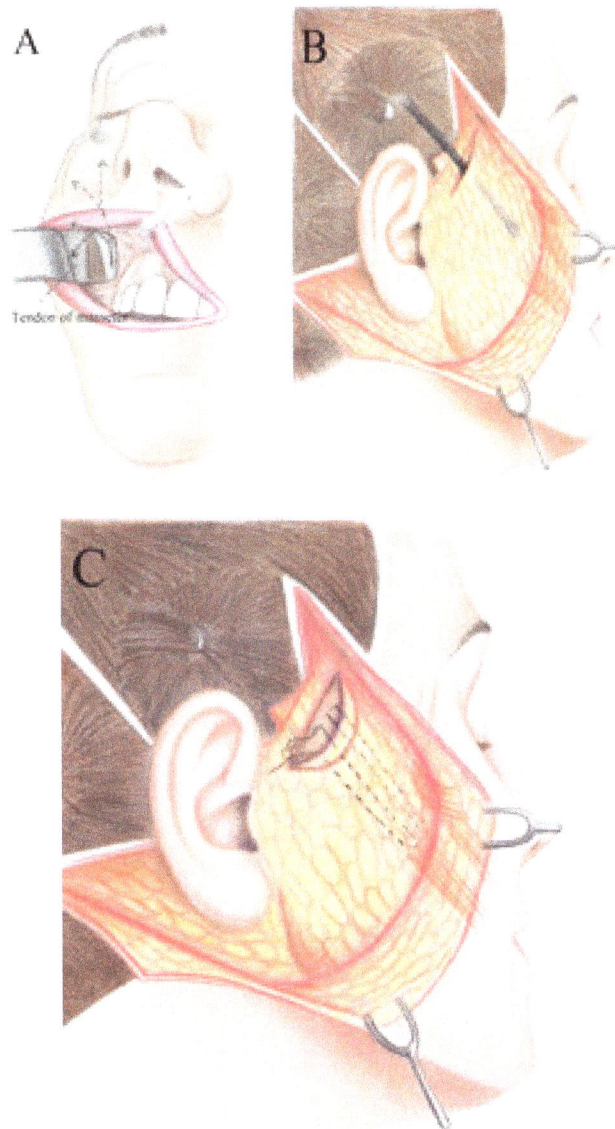

Figure 6. (A) Intraoral dissection to provide direct exposure of subperiosteal dissection. (B) Temporal incision to dissect zygomatic area subperiosteally. (C) Suturing the midface soft tissue to the temporalis fascia.

There are three main landmarks in subperiosteal facelift [33]:

The first is the SOOF [3]. This landmark is located at the cross point of two imaginary lines which pass through the lateral of the eyebrows and inferior orbital rims.

The malar fat pad is the second important landmark in this procedure. The location of this point is at the cross of a vertical line passing through the lateral canthus and the horizontal line passing through the superior margin of the nasal alae.

The last point is Bichat's fat pad, which is located at the cross point of the vertical line passing through the lateral canthus and the horizontal line passing through the nasal base.

---

[3] Suborbicularis oculi fat.

Subperiosteal dissection is performed through the incision in the temporal area (**Figure 6**). The three mentioned points are lifted and sutured to the deep temporalis fascia. The SOOF, malar fat pad, and Bichat's fat pad are sutured and suspended to the deep temporalis fascia laterally, centrally, and medially, respectively. Nowadays, intra-oral subperiosteal dissection is more popular due to decreased operation time and reduced nerve damage risk [34].

This procedure is indicated in the patients with significant aging changes. Endoscopic subperiosteal facelift is an appropriate approach in patients with good skin tone. The other indication of this technique is in the patient who needs other simultaneous cosmetic procedures like skin resurfacing and implant or fat transfer. This method is suitable in raising the eyebrows, eyelid lateral corners, forehead, glabella, cheeks, and nasolabial fold.

5.7.2. Advantages

This technique includes less incisions, use of endoscope, better fixation and allows for repositioning of the buccal and malar fat pads. Satisfactory results in correcting orbital festoons and brow ptosis are possible by this method. The risk of facial nerve damage is very low in this technique. Long lasting results of this method are expected due to manipulating deeper tissues and good fixation. The vascularity of the flap is maintained by minimal dissection and keeping whole layers together, which is an important advantage of this procedure in smokers. The face appears more natural comparing to SMAS lifting methods.

5.7.3. Disadvantages

This facelift technique is not suitable to use as the second facelift surgery. This procedure is relatively contraindicated in patients with a history of facial bone fractures. Irregularities of the face make the subperiosteal dissection much harder.

Prolonged operation time and recovery period are the major drawbacks of this technique. This technique is not suitable for correcting the aging changes of the lower third of the face and neck.

6. Post-operative care after facelift surgery

Facelift surgery is one of the most dramatic procedures for rejuvenation. The success rate of the surgery relies on the surgeon and the patient as well. The surgeon cannot gain satisfactory results unless the patients follow the post-operative care properly.

6.1. Immediately after surgery

The patient should be in complete bed rest for the first 24 hours after surgery. The patients will be wrapped in dressings that will not be removed until 24 hours later. The patient's head must be elevated for at least the first week after surgery. They should not sleep on the side of their face but rather sleep supine with the back of the head on the pillow for about 2 weeks. The surgeon should prescribe pain medications to prevent pain. The activities of the patient should be restricted the day of surgery and up to a week afterwards. The patient should place ice packs over the surgical site.

6.2. Bleeding

Mild bleeding from the surgical site is not unusual. Head elevation and applying an ice compress with mild pressure about the face and neck usually decrease the bleeding. Elevation of the patients' blood pressure by bending, sneezing, lifting, coughing, straining, straining on the toilet, and other strenuous activities are the main causes of bleeding. The patient should refrain absolutely from activities that may increase blood pressure for 10 days after the surgery to avoid complications from bleeding.

6.3. Swelling

Edema is a routine finding of any surgery. The amount of swelling is dependent on the looseness of the tissues and the amount of manipulation varies from person to person. Swelling around the eyes, cheeks, face, and down into the neck and chest are not uncommon. Swelling starts immediately following surgery and will reach its maximum 2 to 3 days post-operatively. Edema will decrease after the third day. The swelling will cause the skin of the face feel tight for a while. It may interfere with smiling before disappearing within a few weeks.

6.4. Pain

Acetaminophen may be taken every 4 hours for mild pain. NSAIDs are not recommended for the first several days after surgery because of the increased risk of bleeding and/or bruising. Narcotics are indicated in severe pain. The patients should avoid alcoholic beverages since it enhances the effect of the narcotics. Pain and discomfort usually decreased after the first 2 to 3 days. Persistent pain may need attention.

6.5. Diet

Clear liquids should be initially taken after general anesthesia or I.V. sedation. Over the next several days, a high calorie, high protein intake is very important. Supplements should be taken regularly. The patient should not be dehydrated by taking fluids regularly. Keeping well hydrated also prevents nausea and vomiting.

6.6. Wound care

The patients should start cleaning the skin incisions the day after surgery with soap and water three times per day very gently and pat dried (do not wipe). The incisions should be dried and cleaned with a 50% solution of 3% hydrogen peroxide. The hydrogen peroxide should be mixed with an equal amount of warm tap water and a Q-tip should be used to clean the incisions. The incisions should be covered with antibiotic ointment after that. Incisions should not be allowed to become dry or crust over.

6.7. Discoloration

Discoloration of the skin following swelling occurs in some cases. Blood spreading beneath the tissues leads to development of discoloration. This is a normal occurrence in most patients which occurs 2 to 3 days post-operatively. Applying moist heat to the area could speed up the removal of the discoloration. Bruising is rare in younger patients, and sometimes yields as a slight yellow discoloration. In older patients, bruising can be quite significant and is represented as black and blue discoloration. Bruising of large degree may take approximately 2 weeks to resolve.

6.8. Antibiotics

The patient should be prescribed the antibiotics on-time to prevent postoperative infection.

6.9. Nausea and vomiting

In the event of nausea and/or vomiting following surgery, do not give anything by mouth to the patient for at least an hour including the prescribed medicine. Anti-emetic drugs are useful to prevent nausea.

7. Complications of the facelift procedure

Some of the complications of facelift surgery are hematoma (the most common complication), pre- and postauricular scar hypertrophy, facial telangiectasia, stitch abscess, neck hyperpigmentation, pre- and postauricular skin necrosis, nerve damage, temporal alopecia cutaneous sloughing or necrosis, seroma, wound dehiscence, hypertrophic scarring, contour irregularities, dimpling, and infection [35–42].

The most dangerous complications include hematoma (rates 1.0–15%), infection (0.05–0.18%), nerve injury (0.07–2.5%), skin sloughing (1.0–1.85%), and systemic vascular complications like venous thromboembolism (VTE 0.1%) [37, 41, 43, 44]. It has been reported that the complication rate in patients with a high body mass index (BMI) over 25 was 9.5%, compared to 4.7% in normal weight patients undergoing a facelift [43].

7.1. Hematoma

Hematoma formation remains the most common major complication after facelift surgery [45–47]. Common themes in patients who may experience hematoma following facelift include male sex, hypertension, preoperative medications that affect coagulation such as aspirin use, smoking, BMI, pre- and post-surgical blood pressure spikes, retching vomiting, post-surgical activity, and nausea [46, 47].

Hematomas in face can cause tissue ischemia, long-term edema, hyperpigmentation, and patient complaint. The incidence of hematoma reported 0.2–8.1% (needs a space between reported and 0.2) in articles [35]. Studies that document the occurrence of hematoma formation following facelift surgery includes the use of drains in the surgical site which have some problems such as introducing infection into the wound, leakage, and being displaced [48, 49]. They create tracts at the site of removal, necessitate painful extraction, and risk injury to vessels on removal.

The incidence of hematoma following male rhytidectomy is lower than facelift in females although the incidence of hematoma in men remains higher than that in women in 30-year-old patients [49]. Meticulous perioperative blood pressure control significantly reduces the rate of postoperative hematoma formation [45]. Large hematomas can cause skin necrosis and need to be promptly evacuated.

7.2. Infection

Infection is the second most common major complication occurring in 0.3% facelifts. Combined procedures and high BMI are risk factors for developing major infection. A post-facelift infection is most commonly caused by *Staphylococcus aureus* [37, 38].

7.3. Nerve injury

Injury to the facial nerve during a face lift is a relatively rare but serious complication. Understanding of the anatomical course of the facial nerve and the relative danger zones can prevent this complication [50].

Two of the most feared complications of facelift surgery are motor and sensory nerve damage and flap necrosis [51]. Different injuries can result in frontal, buccal, zygomatic, marginal mandibular, and cervical nerve damage, including direct injury, neurapraxia, thermal injury from cautery, compression injury from sutures, edema, or hematoma. The greater auricular nerve is the most common sensory nerve that may be damaged during the facelift procedure.

7.4. Edema and ecchymosis

Although some degree of postsurgical edema can be seen in all patients undergoing a facelift procedure, some of them show impressive swelling. Patients undergoing multiple procedures, including brow lift, midface implant insertion, lip implants, and simultaneous laser resurfacing can swell to alarming proportions [52].

7.5. Skin slough

Skin slough is a rare occurrence following face lift. The skin flaps are monitored closely during the postoperative course. Usually, vascular compromise is noted in the preauricular region and may appear as a distinct area of ecchymosis [41].

7.6. Scarring

With a well-designed and well-executed facelift, noticeable scars are unusual, following a face lift procedure.

7.7. Alopecia

There is very little information associated with development of dermatological conditions after cosmetic surgical procedures, including hair transplantation and facelift surgery. Alopecia occurs following damage to the hair follicles from electrocautery, excess traction or tension on the skin flaps, and involuntary elevation or elimination of the temporal hair tuft [41].

7.8. Contour deformities

These temporary deformities are common immediately after rhytidectomy. The preauricular and submental regions are the usual regions of these deformities occurrence which are related to post-surgical edema or ecchymosis [41].

7.9. Flap necrosis

Flap necrosis following facial rhytidectomy is an irritating complication, both to the patient and to the surgeon [53]. Necrosis of the lipocutaneous flap may result in permanent scars and prolonged recovery. Causes vary from bandage compression, sleeping position of the patient, flap sutures under tension, inherent healing difficulties, and no detectable cause. Although smokers or patients with compromised health are more common to encounter this complication, flap necrosis may happen in the best conditions [52].

7.10. Systemic complications

Major complications included deep vein thrombosis (DVT), pulmonary embolism, blood transfusions, stroke, important anesthetic complications, and death [41].

8. New trends in non-surgical rejuvenation

Understanding the facial anatomy and its changes through aging has led to development of different facelift techniques that focus on being less invasive and less traumatic and also providing long-lasting results [54]. Numerous non-invasive face rejuvenation techniques have been investigated over the past decade to improve the results of the procedure and to avoid incisional surgery. Some of the treatment options are as follows: radiofrequency (RF) and ultrasound therapy that are useful in skin tightening/laxity. Also, there are numerous liposuction techniques/devices and injectable cytolytic drugs for submental fat reduction. Fractional lasers and RF devices, chemical peels, micro-needling, intense pulsed light (IPL), injectable fillers, pigment and vascular lasers, liquid nitrogen therapy are useful in superficial dyschromias and rhytides/crepe skin. Moreover, neuromodulators may enhance platysmal banding. Various types of fillers and volumizers including autologous fat, hyaluronic acid (HA), and injectable poly-L-lactic acid (PLLA) calcium or hydroxylapatite (CaHA) are used. A novel bimodal technique to restore volume loss facial structures for panfacial lipo-atrophy with PLLA has been introduced [55, 56].

A novel, minimally invasive, RF device employing a bipolar micro-needle electrode system is introduced, varying the pulse length allowed for fractional sparing of dermal tissue. In some studies, bipolar mode delivering energy directly within the dermis using five micro-needle electrode pairs is used with real-time feedback of tissue temperature for treatment control. Superficial cooling is achieved with a Peltier device [57].

The thermaCool TC (Thermage Inc.) is a RF device to induce tightening of the addressed skin problem via a uniform volumetric heating into the deep dermis tightening, resulting in a "nonsurgical facelift". RF produces a uniform volumetric heating into the deep dermis. Gradual tightening is produced by this technique in most patients with no adverse effects [58, 59].

Laser, light, and RF energy sources have succeeded in treating the second category of skin aging; however, the surgical facelift is still the gold standard in treatment of laxity associated with intrinsic aging [60].

Laser resurfacing was presented in the 1980s with continuous wave carbon dioxide (CO_2) lasers; however, because of many side effects, including scarring, short-pulse, high-peak power, and rapidly scanned, normal-mode erbium-doped yttrium aluminium garnet lasers and focused-beam CO_2 lasers were developed to remove skin in a precisely controlled manner [61]. Laser skin tightening is an FDA-approved method for the reduction of fine wrinkles and skin laxity. Laser skin tightening is a non-surgical, minimally invasive technique that uses an infrared light source to tighten skin through collagen heating under the skin's surface, causing the skin to contract [62]. Facial rejuvenation using polydioxanone (PDO) thread is a safe and effective procedure associated with only minor complications in cases of fine wrinkles, face sagging, and marked facial pores [63].

One important advance in facial rejuvenation is the use of fiber endoscopic video-assisted technique in aesthetic plastic surgery of the face. It substitutes the coronal incision with no skin resection and leads to a vertical reposition of the mobile soft tissue of the midface in indicated cases. It needs only a small incision of the scalp just behind the coronal incision and in the temporal area [64].

Pak et al. introduced a nonabsorbable polypropylene mesh as a newface lifting instrument, with the nasolabial fold as the main target area. Face lifting using a nonabsorbable mesh can improve nasolabial folds without serious adverse effects. So, this is a safe and effective technique in midface rejuvenation [65].

Incorporation of selective fat compartment volume restoration through SMAS manipulation allows for improved control in recontouring while addressing the problem of volume deflation in facial aging. Facial rejuvenation is described through merging two key important points based on lift-and-fill face lift: (1) lifting and tightening tissues in differential vectors according to original facial asymmetry and shape; and (2) precious facial contouring through selective fat compartment filling of malar locations (deep and high) and graft of nasolabial fold fat [66].

9. Summary

Cosmetic surgeries including facelift operation are becoming increasingly popular, and facial rejuvenation remains one of the most commonly requested aesthetic procedures. Many lifting procedures can be used in order to reduce sagging of skin and subcutaneous tissues and create a more youthful face. In the forehead and eyebrow region, the direct brow lift, temporal brow lift, transferable pharoplastic brow lift, coronal brow lift, and the endoscopic brow lift can be identified. The facelift is considered in the mid-face. Classic facelifts can be divided into the one layer, two layers, and the deep plane facelift (DPFL). The incidence of postoperative complications associated with lifting procedures is rare, but clinically important. Hematoma, skin necrosis of the wound edges, infection, nerve injuries are some of these complications. Today, the tendency toward minimally invasive procedures with smaller risk of complications and shorter recovery period are desired.

Author details

Fereydoun Pourdanesh[1], Mohammad Esmaeelinejad[1*], Seyed Mehrshad Jafari[1] and Zahra Nematollahi[2]

*Address all correspondence to: esmaeelnejad@gmail.com

1 Department of Oral and Maxillofacial Surgery, School of Dentistry, Shahid Beheshti University of Medical Sciences, Tehran, Iran

2 Dental Research Center, Research Institute of Dental Sciences, Shahid Beheshti University of Medical Sciences, Tehran, Iran and Craniomaxillofacial Research Center, Azad University, Dental Branch, Tehran, Iran

References

[1] Mitz V, Peyronie M. The superficial musculo-aponeurotic system (SMAS) in the parotid and cheek area. Plastic and reconstructive surgery 1976; 58:80–88.

[2] Hamra ST. The deep-plane rhytidectomy. Plastic and reconstructive surgery 1990; 86:53–61; discussion 62–53.

[3] Owsley JQ, Jr., Zweifler M. Midface lift of the malar fat pad: technical advances. Plastic and reconstructive surgery 2002; 110:674–685; discussion 686–677.

[4] Ramirez OM. The subperiosteal rhytidectomy: the third-generation face-lift. Annals of plastic surgery 1992; 28:218–232; discussion 233–214.

[5] Connell BF. Contouring the neck in rhytidectomy by lipectomy and a muscle sling. Plastic and reconstructive surgery 1978; 61:376–383.

[6] Dedo DD. "How I do it"—plastic surgery. Practical suggestions on facial plastic surgery. A preoperative classification of the neck for cervicofacial rhytidectomy. The Laryngoscope 1980; 90:1894–1896.

[7] Mang W, Verlag ÄGS, Neumann H, Einhorn-Presse G. Rhytidectomy. Facial plastic surgery 2007; 23:635.

[8] Marten E, Langevin CJ, Kaswan S, Zins JE. The safety of rhytidectomy in the elderly. Plastic and reconstructive surgery 2011; 127:2455–2463. DOI: 10.1097/PRS. 0b013e3182131da9

[9] Webster RC, Kazda G, Hamdan US, *et al.* Cigarette smoking and face lift: conservative versus wide undermining. Plastic and reconstructive surgery 1986; 77:596–604.

[10] Ellenbogen R. A 15-year follow-up study of the non-SMAS skin-tightening facelift with midface defatting. Equal or better than deeper plane procedures in result, duration, safety, and patient satisfaction. Clinics in plastic surgery 1997; 24:247–267.

[11] Rubin LR, Simpson RL. The new deep plane face lift dissections versus the old superficial techniques: a comparison of neurologic complications. Plastic and reconstructive surgery 1996; 97:1461–1465.

[12] Gamble WB, Manson PN, Smith GE, Hamra ST. Comparison of skin-tissue tensions using the composite and the subcutaneous rhytidectomy techniques. Annals of plastic surgery 1995; 35:447–453; discussion 453–444.

[13] Becker FF, Bassichis BA. Deep-plane face-lift vs superficial musculoaponeurotic system plication face-lift: a comparative study. Archives of facial plastic surgery 2004; 6:8–13. DOI: 10.1001/archfaci.6.1.8

[14] Mohammadi S, Ahmadi A, Salem MM, *et al.* A comparison between two methods of face-lift surgery in nine cadavers: SMAS (superficial musculo-aponeurotic system) versus MACS (minimal access cranial suspension). Aesthetic plastic surgery 2015; 39:680–685. DOI: 10.1007/s00266-015-0543-3

[15] Pitanguy I, Machado BH. Facial rejuvenation surgery: a retrospective study of 8788 cases. Aesthetic surgery journal/The American society for aesthetic plastic surgery 2012; 32:393–412. DOI: 10.1177/1090820x12438895

[16] Jacono AA, Parikh SS, Kennedy WA. Anatomical comparison of platysmal tightening using superficial musculoaponeurotic system plication vs deep-plane rhytidectomy techniques. Archives of facial plastic surgery 2011; 13:395–397. DOI: 10.1001/archfacial. 2011.69

[17] Verpaele A, Tonnard P, Gaia S, *et al.* The third suture in MACS-lifting: making midface-lifting simple and safe. Journal of plastic, reconstructive & aesthetic surgery 2007; 60:1287–1295. DOI: 10.1016/j.bjps.2006.12.012

[18] Verpaele A, Tonnard P. Lower third of the face: indications and limitations of the minimal access cranial suspension lift. Clinics in plastic surgery 2008; 35:645–659, vii. DOI: 10.1016/j.cps.2008.04.001

[19] Prado A, Andrades P, Danilla S, *et al.* A clinical retrospective study comparing two short-scar face lifts: minimal access cranial suspension versus lateral SMASectomy. Plastic and reconstructive surgery 2006; 117:1413–1425; discussion 1426–1417. DOI: 10.1097/01.prs.0000207402.53411.1e

[20] Tonnard PL, Verpaele A, Gaia S. Optimising results from minimal access cranial suspension lifting (MACS-lift). Aesthetic plastic surgery 2005; 29:213–220; discussion 221. DOI: 10.1007/s00266-005-0047-7

[21] Mast BA. Advantages and limitations of the MACS lift for facial rejuvenation. Annals of plastic surgery 2014; 72:S139–143. DOI: 10.1097/sap.0000000000000092

[22] Gordon NA, Adam SI, 3rd. Deep plane face lifting for midface rejuvenation. Clinics in plastic surgery 2015; 42:129–142. DOI: 10.1016/j.cps.2014.08.009

[23] Parikh SS, Jacono AA. Deep-plane face-lift as an alternative in the smoking patient. Archives of facial plastic surgery 2011; 13:283–285. DOI: 10.1001/archfacial.2011.39

[24] Marcus BC. Rhytidectomy: current concepts, controversies and the state of the art. Current opinion in otolaryngology & head and neck surgery 2012; 20:262–266. DOI: 10.1097/MOO.0b013e328355b175

[25] Lemmon ML. Color atlas of SMAS rhytidectomy. First ed. Michigan: Thieme Medical Publisher; 1993

[26] Stuzin JM, Baker TJ, Gordon HL, Baker TM. Extended SMAS dissection as an approach to midface rejuvenation. Clinics in plastic surgery 1995; 22:295–311.

[27] Lindsey JT. Five-year retrospective review of the extended SMAS: critical landmarks and technical refinements. Annals of plastic surgery 2009; 62:492–496. DOI: 10.1097/SAP.0b013e31818ba77d

[28] Ivy EJ, Lorenc ZP, Aston SJ. Is there a difference? A prospective study comparing lateral and standard SMAS face lifts with extended SMAS and composite rhytidectomies. Plastic and reconstructive surgery 1996; 98:1135–1143; discussion 1144–1137.

[29] Baker DC. Lateral SMASectomy. Plastic and reconstructive surgery 1997; 100:509–513.

[30] Baker DC. Lateral SMASectomy, plication and short scar facelifts: indications and techniques. Clinics in plastic surgery 2008; 35:533–550, vi. DOI: 10.1016/j.cps.2008.06.003

[31] Kim BJ, Choi JH, Lee Y. Development of facial rejuvenation procedures: thirty years of clinical experience with face lifts. Archives of plastic surgery 2015; 42:521–531. DOI: 10.5999/aps.2015.42.5.521

[32] Tessier P. Subperiosteal face-lift. Annales de chirurgie plastique et esthetique 1989; 34:193–197.

[33] Patrocinio LG, Patrocinio TG, Patrocinio JA. Subperiosteal midface-lift. Facial plastic surgery 2013; 29:206–213. DOI: 10.1055/s-0033-1347000

[34] Gentile RD. Subperiosteal deep plane rhytidectomy: the composite midface lift. Facial plastic surgery 2005; 21:286–295. DOI: 10.1055/s-2006-939507

[35] Griffin JE, Jo C. Complications after superficial plane cervicofacial rhytidectomy: a retrospective analysis of 178 consecutive facelifts and review of the literature. Journal of oral and maxillofacial surgery 2007; 65:2227–2234.

[36] De Cordier BC, de la Torre JI, Al-Hakeem MS *et al.* Rejuvenation of the midface by elevating the malar fat pad: review of technique, cases, and complications. Plastic and reconstructive surgery 2002; 110:1526–1536.

[37] Gupta V, Winocour J, Shi H, *et al.* Preoperative risk factors and complication rates in facelift: analysis of 11,300 patients. Aesthetic surgery journal 2015:sjv162. 2016 Jan;36(1): 1–13.

[38] Stuzin JM. MOC-PS (SM) CME article: face lifting. Plastic and reconstructive surgery 2008; 121:1–19.

[39] Mustoe TA, Park E. Evidence-based medicine: face lift. Plastic and reconstructive surgery 2014; 133:1206–1213.

[40] Matarasso A, Elkwood A, Rankin M, Elkowitz M. National plastic surgery survey: face lift techniques and complications. Plastic and reconstructive surgery 2000; 106:1185–1195.

[41] Chaffoo RA. Complications in facelift surgery: avoidance and management. Facial plastic surgery clinics of North America 2013; 21:551–558.

[42] Pitanguy I, Machado BH. Facial rejuvenation surgery: a retrospective study of 8788 cases. Aesthetic surgery journal 2012; 32:393–412.

[43] Abboushi N, Yezhelyev M, Symbas J, Nahai F. Facelift complications and the risk of venous thromboembolism: a single center's experience. Aesthetic surgery journal 2012; 32:413–420.

[44] Moyer JS, Baker SR. Complications of rhytidectomy. Facial plastic surgery clinics of North America 2005; 13:469–478.

[45] Ramanadham SR, Mapula S, Costa C, *et al.* Evolution of hypertension management in face lifting in 1089 patients: optimizing safety and outcomes. Plastic and reconstructive surgery 2015; 135:1037–1043.

[46] Maricevich MA, Adair MJ, Maricevich RL, *et al.* Facelift complications related to median and peak blood pressure evaluation. Aesthetic plastic surgery 2014; 38:641–647.

[47] Niamtu J. Expanding hematoma in face-lift surgery: literature review, case presentations, and caveats. Dermatologic surgery 2005; 31:1134–1144.

[48] Zoumalan R, Rizk SS. Hematoma rates in drainless deep-plane face-lift surgery with and without the use of fibrin glue. Archives of facial plastic surgery 2008; 10:103–107.

[49] Baker DC, Stefani WA, Chiu ES. Reducing the incidence of hematoma requiring surgical evacuation following male rhytidectomy: a 30-year review of 985 cases. Plastic and reconstructive surgery 2005; 116:1973–1985.

[50] Roostaeian J, Rohrich RJ, Stuzin JM. Anatomical considerations to prevent facial nerve injury. Plastic and reconstructive surgery 2015; 135:1318–1327.

[51] Baker DC, Conley J. Avoiding facial nerve injuries in rhytidectomy anatomical variations and pitfalls. Plastic and reconstructive surgery 1979; 64:781–795.

[52] Niamtu J. Complications in facelift surgery and their prevention. Oral and maxillofacial surgery clinics of North America 2009; 21:59–80.

[53] Weissman O, Farber N, Remer E, *et al.* Post-facelift flap necrosis treatment using charged polystyrene microspheres. The Canadian Journal of Plastic Surgery 2013; 21:45.

[54] Centurion P, Romero C, Olivencia C, *et al.* Short-scar facelift without temporal flap: a 10-year experience. Aesthetic plastic surgery 2014; 38:670–677.

[55] Weinkle A, Sofen B, Emer J. Synergistic approaches to neck rejuvenation and lifting. Journal of drugs in dermatology 2015; 14:1215–1228.

[56] Sadick NS, Manhas-Bhutani S, Krueger N. A novel approach to structural facial volume replacement. Aesthetic plastic surgery 2013; 37:266–276.

[57] Hantash BM, Renton B, Berkowitz RL, *et al.* Pilot clinical study of a novel minimally invasive bipolar microneedle radiofrequency device. Lasers in surgery and medicine 2009; 41:87–95.

[58] Ruiz-Esparza J, Gomez JB. The medical face lift: a noninvasive, nonsurgical approach to tissue tightening in facial skin using nonablative radiofrequency. Dermatologic surgery 2003; 29:325–332.

[59] Narins D, Narins R. Non-surgical radiofrequency facelift. Journal of drugs in dermatology 2003; 2:495–500.

[60]   Alexiades-Armenakas M, Rosenberg D, Renton B, *et al.* Blinded, randomized, quantitative grading comparison of minimally invasive, fractional radiofrequency and surgical face-lift to treat skin laxity. Archives of dermatology 2010; 146:396–405.

[61]   Alexiades-Armenakas MR, Dover JS, Arndt KA. The spectrum of laser skin resurfacing: nonablative, fractional, and ablative laser resurfacing. Journal of the American academy of dermatology 2008; 58:719–737.

[62]   Alexiades-Armenakas M. Laser skin tightening: non-surgical alternative to the face-lift. Journal of drugs dermatology 2006; 5:295–296.

[63]   Suh DH, Jang HW, Lee SJ, *et al.* Outcomes of polydioxanone knotless thread lifting for facial rejuvenation. Dermatologic surgery 2015; 41:720–725.

[64]   Hönig JF, Knutti D, Hasse FM. Centro-lateral subperiosteal vertical midface lift. GMS interdisciplinary plastic and reconstructive surgery DGPW 2014; 3: 1–12.

[65]   Pak CS, Chang LS, Lee H, *et al.* A multicenter noncomparative clinical study on midface rejuvenation using a nonabsorbable polypropylene mesh: evaluation of efficacy and safety. Archives of plastic surgery 2015; 42:572–579.

[66]   Rohrich RJ, Ghavami A, Constantine FC, *et al.* Lift-and-fill face lift: integrating the fat compartments. Plastic and reconstructive surgery 2014; 133:756e–767e.

4

Applications of the Buccal Fat Pad in Oral and Maxillofacial Surgery

Ali Hassani, Solaleh Shahmirzadi and Sarang Saadat

Abstract

The buccal fat pad (BFP) has become more and more popular in oral and maxillofacial surgery. Originally, it was described as an anatomic structure without any obvious function; it was even considered to be a surgical nuisance. Nowadays, the most reported application of the BFP is the closure of oroantral communications. In this chapter, different aspects of the BFP such as its applications, anatomy, physiology, and complications are explained.

Keywords: buccal fat pad, oral reconstruction, oroantral communication, oroantral fistula, cleft palate, surgical defects

1. Introduction

Although descriptions of the buccal fat pad (BFP) are typically very brief and lacking in detail in anatomical textbooks, they have recently received increased attention in the clinical literature [1]. After the first clinical use of the BFP by Egyedi in 1977, its use has increased rapidly during these years. The BFP has become more and more popular for closing oronasal and oroantral communications (OACs) and as a versatile pedicle graft for closing postsurgical maxillary defects [2].

The BFP initially believed to be an anatomic structure without any noticeable function was even considered to be a surgical nuisance [3–5]. However, with time, the use of the BFP as a pedicle graft has become more common; the relatively easy use and [6–8] the location of the BFP are anatomically favorable and minimal dissection allows it to be harvested and mobilized; good rate of epithelialization and low rate of failure have made it the preferred option for oral and maxillofacial applications [7]. The repair of oroantral and oronasal defects, the repair of pathological or traumatic defects (especially in the posterior maxilla and palate), the repair of congenital cleft palate defects, use as a biologic membrane for covering bone grafts, and its application in temporomandibular joint surgery are some of its common applications that are addressed here in this chapter.

2. History

Heister et al. introduced the BFP for the first time in 1732. They believed that the newly introduced structure was glandular and named it "glandula molaris" [9, 10]. Bichat in 1802 described this anatomic mass and realized its true nature. Therefore, it is commonly referred to as the boule de Bichat or bolle graisseusse in French; it is called "wangenfettpfropf" or "Wangenfettpolster" (Wangen means cheek, fett means fat, and polster means pad) in German, and the sucking pad, sucking cushion, masticatory fat pad, or BFP in English [10]. Samman was the first to explain the anatomy of the BFP and Goughram completed his description [11]. BFP's clinical importance was not discovered for years and due to its sudden egression during the surgical operations, it was known more as a nuisance factor [3, 4]. Egyedi for the first time in 1977 reported the use of the BFP in the regeneration of oral defects [2]. Neder introduced the use of the BFP as a pedicle and free graft in two patients with trauma of facial structures, but there were no reports available on the vascularization and functional anatomy of the BFP [12]. Tiedman et al. presented a complete report on anatomy, vascular supply, and operation method of the BFP for the first time [13]. Rapidis et al., Dean et al., and Hao used pedicle BFP for the reconstruction of medium-sized postsurgical oral defects of malignant lesions [11, 14, 15].

3. Anatomy, physiology, and embryology

3.1. General structures

The BFP is a simple lobulated mass described as consisting of a central body and four extensions: buccal, pterygoid, pterygopalatine, and temporal. The body consists of three independent lobes: anterior, intermediate, and posterior. Each lobe is encapsulated by an independent membrane and separated by a natural space [16] (**Figures 1–3**).

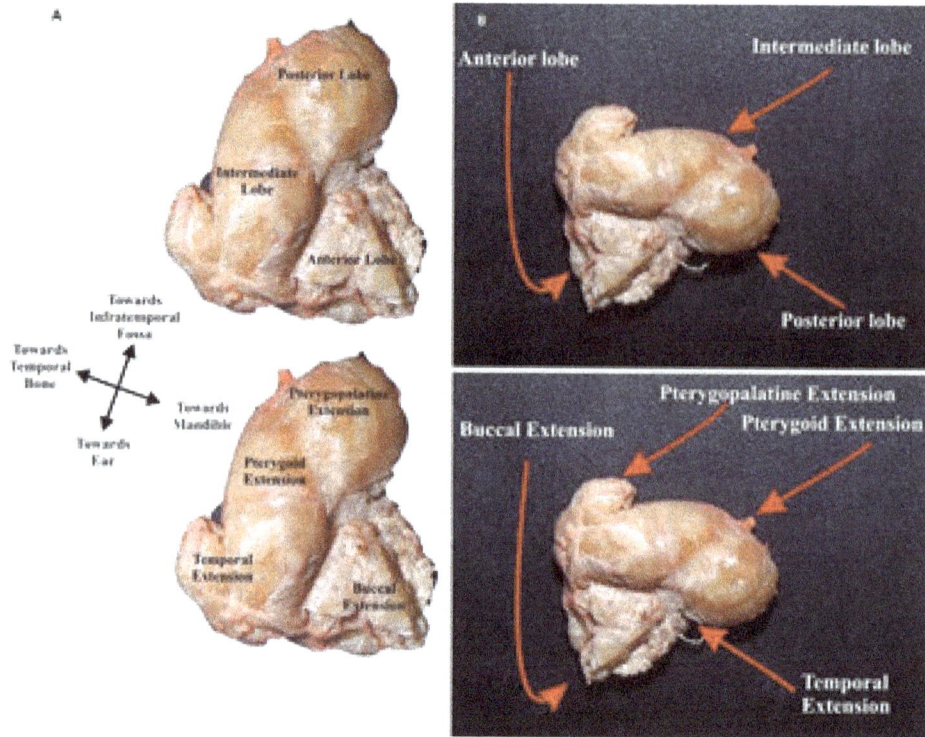

Figure 1. The BFP lobes and extensions (A, B) (Loukas M, et al. [1]).

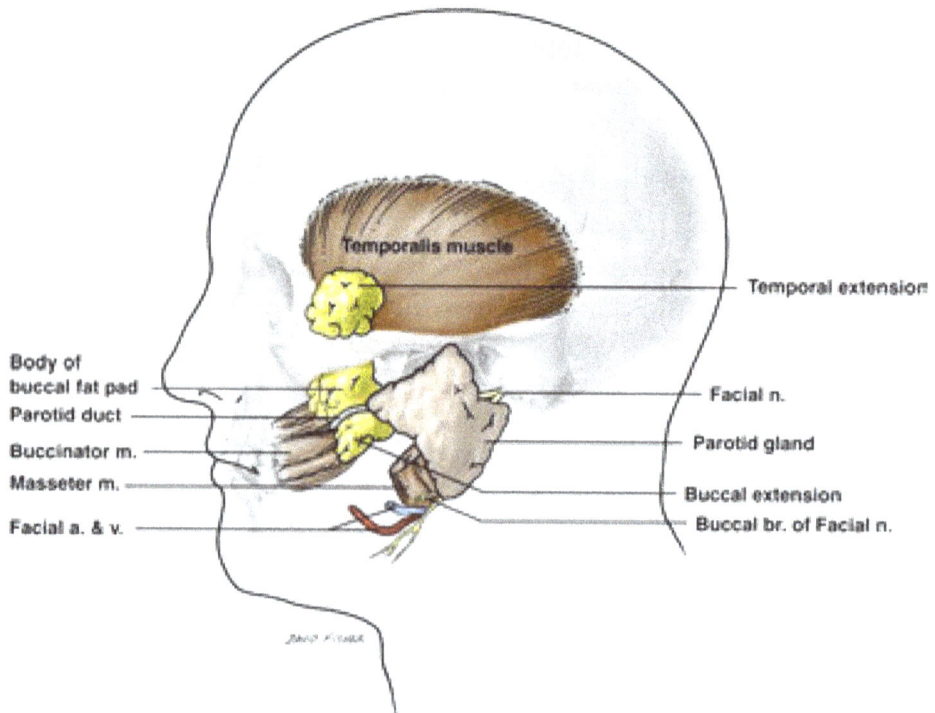

Figure 2. Anatomical relation of important adjacent structures (parotid duct, facial artery, parotid gland, and buccinator muscle) with the BFP, the temporal and buccal extensions of the BFP are present (Yousuf et al. [28]).

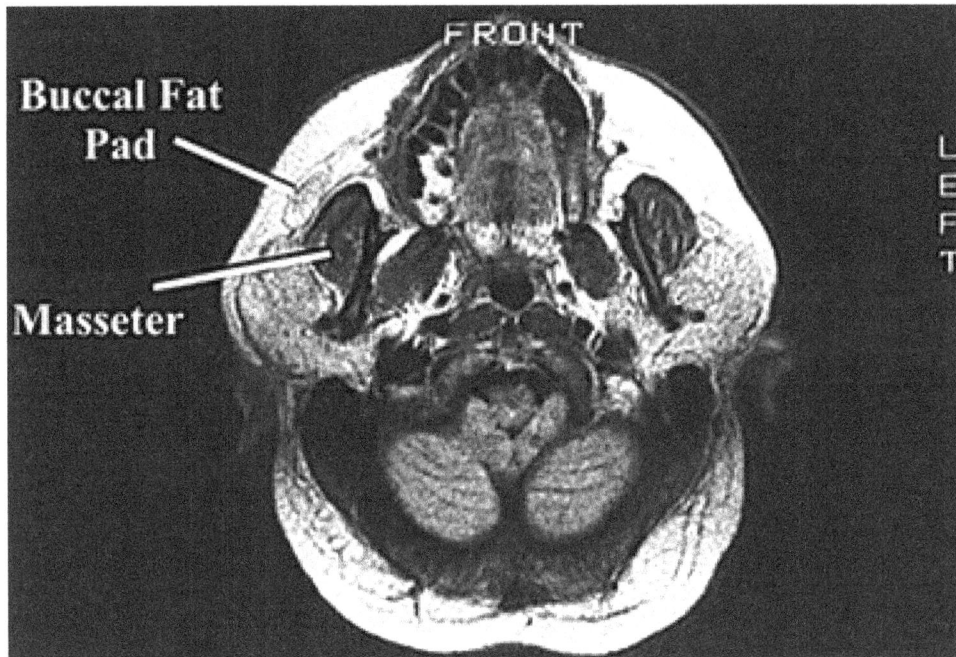

Figure 3. Cross-section of T1 MRI at the level of the oral cavity and the hard palate. The BFP is evident anteriorly to the masseter. Notice the volume of the BFP in relationship to the masseter (Yousuf et al. [28]).

The main body is situated deeply along the posterior maxilla and upper fibers of the buccinators, covered with a thin capsule.

The cheek contour is made generally by the buccal extension of the BFP, which is located superficially in the cheek. More than half of the total weight of the BFP mass is the body and the buccal extension together. Another extension of the BFP is pterygopalatine. It extends to the inferior orbital fissure and pterygopalatine fossa. The third extension is the pterygoid extension. It extends into the pterygomandibular space. The pterygoid extension packs the lingual nerve and mandibular neurovascular. The last extension of the BFP is the temporal extension. It has two parts, superficial and deep temporal extension. Actually, the superficial part is a distinct fat pad, its appearance is different, and has a different blood supply. Therefore, it is believed to be a distinct anatomical feature for the BFP.

A specific capsule covers each part of the BFP. Also, each part of the BFP is connected to the adjacent anatomical structures by ligaments. When the size of extensions is compared, the temporal, pterygopalatine, and pterygoid extensions are smaller and located deeper [1, 14, 16, 17].

3.2. Relation to the parotid duct and branches of the facial nerve

The parotid duct and zygomatic and buccal branches of the facial nerve cross the anterior and lateral surfaces of the BFP.

The parotid duct and zygomatic and buccal branches of the facial nerve cross the anterior and lateral surfaces of the BFP. The duct pierces the buccinators and presents in the oral cavity adjacent to the maxillary second molars [18]. It is established that the parotid duct either runs along the lateral surface of BFP or perforates the body of the posterior lobe before it comes up to the surface of the buccinators [19]. With respect to the BFP, the parotid duct is seen in three different situations. In 42% of cases, it travels over the buccal process (type A), in 26% of the cases, through the buccal process (type B), and 32% of the cases superior to the buccal process of the BFP (type C) (**Figure 4**).

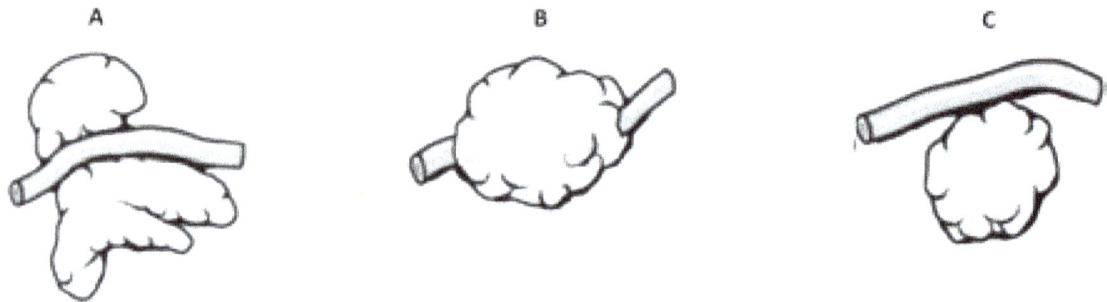

Figure 4. Relationship of the BFP with the parotid duct. (A) Type A: the parotid duct travels over the buccal extension. (B) Type B: the parotid duct travels through the buccal extension. (C) Type C: the parotid duct travels superior to the buccal extension of the BFP (Hwang et al. [18]).

The anterior surface of the BFP is covered by buccal branches of the facial nerve in 75% of cases, while the lateral border of the BFP is covered by the zygomatic branches in 90% of cases [1] (**Figure 5**).

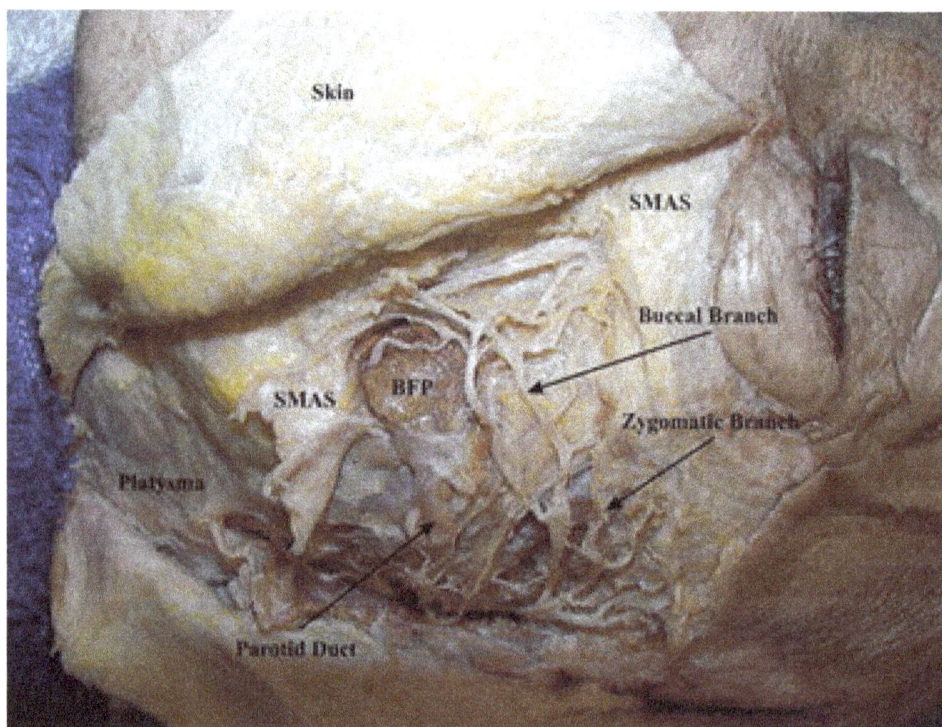

Figure 5. The relationship of the BFP with the branches of the facial nerve. Superficial musculoaponeurotic system (SMAS) (Loukas et al. [1]).

There are different types of the relations between the facial nerve and the BFP. Two different kinds of interrelations are present. First, in 73% of cases buccal branches of the facial nerve travel on the surface of the BFP (type one). Second, in 27% of cases the branches travel through into the buccal extension [18, 19].

3.3. Blood supply

There are three main sources of the BFP's blood supply. The maxillary artery (buccal and temporal branches), the superficial temporal artery (transverse facial branches), and the facial artery provide the blood supply for the BFP. These branches make a subcapsular plexus. Due to this rich blood supply, the BFP can be used as a pedicle graft. Also, it explains the great success rate of the BFP flap [17, 20–23]. The BFP has a very rich subcapsular capillary plexus. Arterioles go into the capsule, travel along the septa of the BFP, and finally make a capillary network among adipocytes. This circulation system is similar to the other white adipose tissues. However, the capillary plexus of the BFP is smaller and its capillaries are wider [19, 24]. The BFP venous system drains via the facial vein [23].

3.4. Volume and size

The mean volume of BFP is 10 cm^3 (average 9.6 ml, range 8.33–11.9 ml); weight is 9.3 g; if flattened, it can cover the surface of 10 cm^2, preserving a thickness of 6 mm [1, 2, 19, 25]. The size of the BFP is fairly constant among different individuals regardless of overall body weight and fat distribution; even cachectic patients have BFPs that are of normal weight and volume [10]. Investigation of age-related changes in BFP volume reveals that the most important alterations are found between two age groups namely 0–10 years and 21–50 years. Moderate decrease in volume after the age of 50 years is noted [25].

3.5. Embryology and physiology

Poissonnet et al. [26] reported that fat tissue differentiation begins in the second trimester of gestation. The size of fat lobules increases until the 29th week of gestation. However, the number of them is approximately constant. Cheek fat is the first fat that develops [26]. Like adults, the BFP has an important role in the cheek prominence of newborns. Among fetal adipose tissue, the BFP is one of the initial adipose tissues that develop.

Some functions were introduced for the BFP in newborns. First, the BFP prevents the negative pressure while a newborn is sucking. Second, it separates the masticator muscles from one another and nearby bony structures. Third, it protects the neurovascular bundles. Finally, it enhances the intermuscular movement; this function is performed by a specialized type of fat which is called syssarcosis [16, 17, 20, 22].

Bagdade and Hirsch are the first who measured and tabulated the fatty acid composition of the BFP. They used gas-liquid and thin-layer chromatography for this purpose [27]. Ranke claims that the amount of lipolysis of the BFP is different from subcutaneous fat. Like the periorbital fat, the BFP is constant during emaciation while subcutaneous fat is lost [8, 15, 20, 29, 30].

One of the desirable features of the BFP as a flap is its quick epithelialization property [10, 31, 32].

4. Surgical approach

The most direct access to the BFP is found at the distobuccal depth of the maxillary tuberosity, and it may be dissected through a vestibular incision if it has not been encountered during the resection [33]. Under either local or general anesthesia, an upper mucosal incision posterior to the area of the zygomatic buttress is made, followed by a simple incision through the periosteum and fascial envelope of the BFP [8]. After a single sharp scissor stab through the periosteum and scant buccinator muscle, the BFP extrudes into the operative site [33] (**Figure 6**).

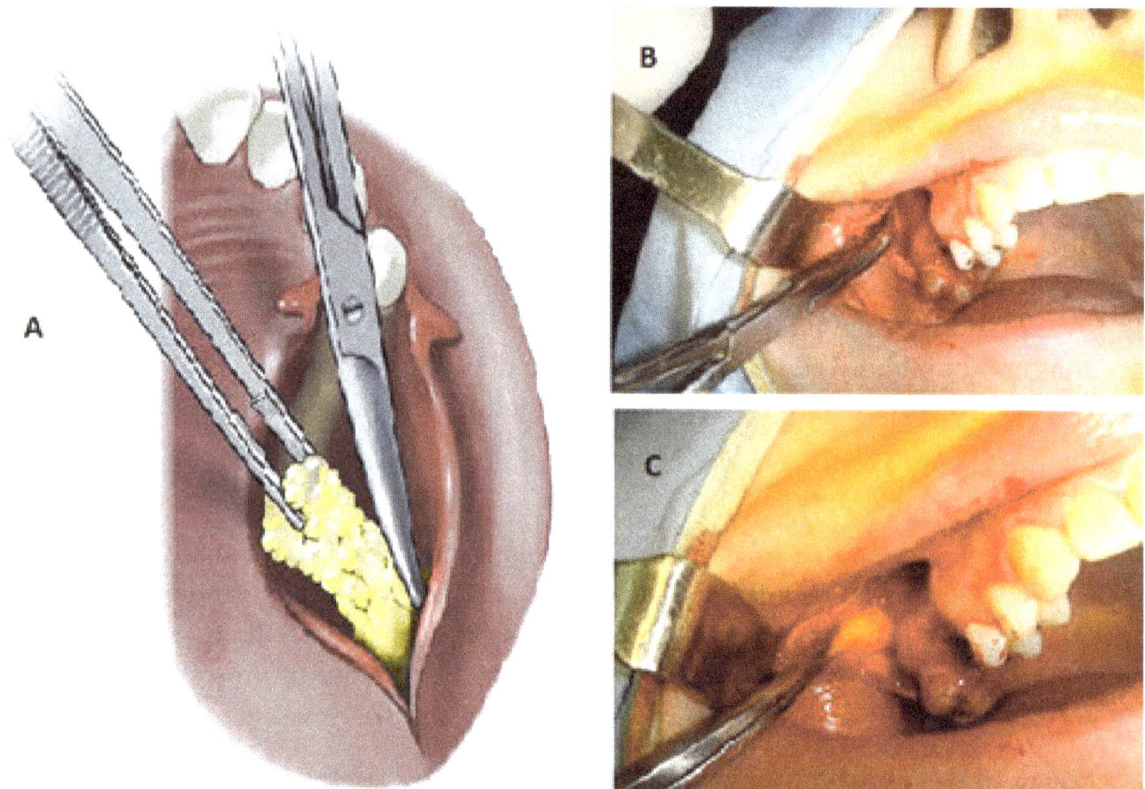

Figure 6. (A) Schematic view of the BFP intraoral approach (Arce [33]). Clinical view of intraoral approach. (B) The use of a hemostat to explore the site. (C) Pulling out the BFP very gently.

Mechanical suction must be avoided once the BFP is exposed. It easily herniates into the defect with a little teasing and is gently pulled out from its bed with a vascular clamp [8]. Since the main cause of sensory disturbances is the impairment of the metabolic supply due to the disturbed microvascular circulation of the nerve fibers by the mechanical trauma [34–36], surgeons should avoid the excessively and unnecessarily manipulating of the surgery site for finding the BFP. At this time, the external pressure helps the removal of the temporal extension of the BFP. Surgeons should evaluate the amount of fat required, then based on their need manipulate the site and extract various processes of the BFP [8].

Clinically, the color of the oral aspect of the exposed BFP changes to yellowish-white within three days; then, it changes to red within the first week. It is a consequence of the formation of granulation tissue. In the second week, the granulation tissue becomes firmer and completely epithelialized [9, 37].

5. Applications of the BFP

The BPF has different applications in oral and maxillofacial reconstruction. It has some physiological functions, such as filling deep tissue space, has a role of gliding pad for facial and masticatory muscles during contraction, and has a role of cushion for some structures from outer force impulsion [21]. Besides its physiological functions, it serves as a versatile flap in reconstructive procedures [38].

Applications of the BFP in oral and maxillofacial surgeries have increased rapidly [7], and nowadays, the BFP is used in different kinds of surgeries. Particularly in recent years, scientists have been working on regenerative properties of the BFP, which rely on adipose-derived stem cells.

5.1. OAC and oroantral fistula

The BFP flap, preferably pedicle type, has been used most commonly for the closure of OACs and oroantral fistula (OAF) [2, 8, 39–43].

There is no doubt that some characteristics of the BFP such as favorable anatomical position, perfect epithelialization outcome, simple dissection for harvesting, and low rate of failure make it a desirable alternative [9]. Dolanmaz et al. claimed that using the BFP flap for the management of OAC is a reliable alternative, and this method probably is the best treatment choice for recurrent OAF [32].

The choice of the BFP versus a buccal advancement flap closure must weigh the advantages and disadvantages, and other available techniques, in regard to location, height of alveolus, sinus membrane status, and obliteration of the vestibule. Using the BFP eliminates the needs for removal of additional alveolar bone and mobilizes a buccal advancement flap, which may obliterate the buccal vestibule. It is also helpful when traumatized surrounding attached gingiva or mucosa precludes the use of a buccal advancement flap for primary closure [33]. It has a favorable healing course after the operation, and the wounds become successfully epithelialized in 3–4 weeks after surgery [7].

There is the minimal obliteration of the vestibule in the closure of OAF with the BFP as compared to closure with buccal advancement flap. There are no differences in the level or color of the mucosa [37]. The majority of reports point out a perfect success rate of the BFP in the treatment of OAC or fistula. Most studies state a high success rate of BFP in the closure of

OAC/OAF [7]. Nevertheless, 7.5% complications were reported, for example, the elimination of vestibule and recurrence of OAF. The vestibular depth became normal in the due course of time resulting in no postoperative prosthodontics complications [8] (**Figure 7**).

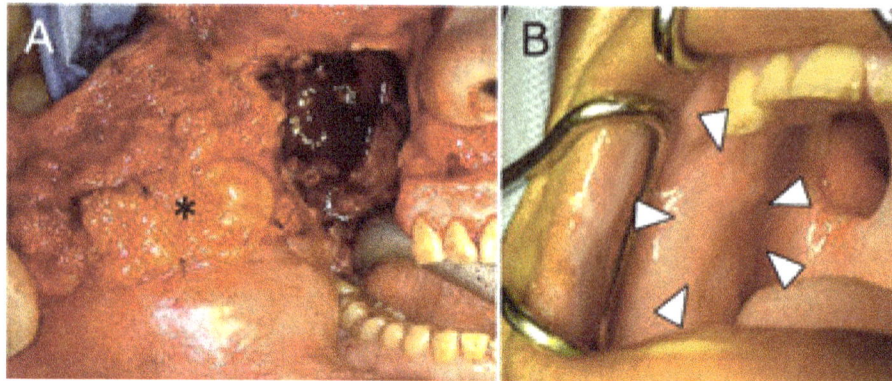

Figure 7. Reconstruction of the inner surface of a facial flap in a patient following resection of an ameloblastoma of the right upper gingiva. (A) BFP covers the inner surface of the facial flap (*). (B) At 1 year and 7 months postoperatively, cicatricial contracture is slight (arrowheads) (Toshihiro et al. [57]).

5.2. Regional defects

The other major use of the BFP is the closure of post-excision defects [9–11, 14, 29, 31, 39, 41, 44–48].

Different kinds of pathologies can cause a defect in the maxilla when resected. The applications of the BFP have been reported with a noted range of usage from the angle of the mouth to the retromolar trigone and palate [49]. The most used is for the reconstruction of the hard palate [44]. The most important consideration of using the BFP for reconstruction is the size of the defect. Most of the studies show a desirable result for closing defects up to 6 × 5 × 3 cm [8]. The authors have had successful experience in the treatment of nine patients with large hard palate defects as large as 7 × 5 cm.

The use of BFP in the reconstruction of defects is highly successful; however, some complications have been reported [7, 8, 29, 41, 44–48].

The application of the BFP for covering mucosal defects following ablation of the buccal cancer has been reported [50]. The result of epithelialization is acceptable after 4–6 weeks. The capability of the BFP in the treatment of mucosal defects is compared with radial free forearm flap and free split-thickness graft. Although the BFP epithelializes easily, due to the lack of lamina propria and submucosa in the dense fibrous connective tissue, the BFP restricts mouth opening [46].

Mehrotra et al. [51] performed a retrospective study of 100 patients and compared the BFP with nasolabial flap, tongue flap, and split-skin graft for the coverage of post-fibrotic band incision in oral submucous fibrosis with 25 patients in each group. They claimed that the BFP serves as the best substitute, providing excellent function without deteriorating esthetics. It offered the ease of surgery, little postoperative morbidity, and good patient acceptance [51].

5.3. Cleft palate

The use of BFP to repair primary cleft palate was first described by Zhao et al. [52] in 1998. Most researchers agree that the ease of harvesting and mobilization of the graft, an excellent blood supply, and minimal donor-site complications make the pedicle BFP graft a convenient and reliable method in cleft palate surgery [53] (**Figure 8**).

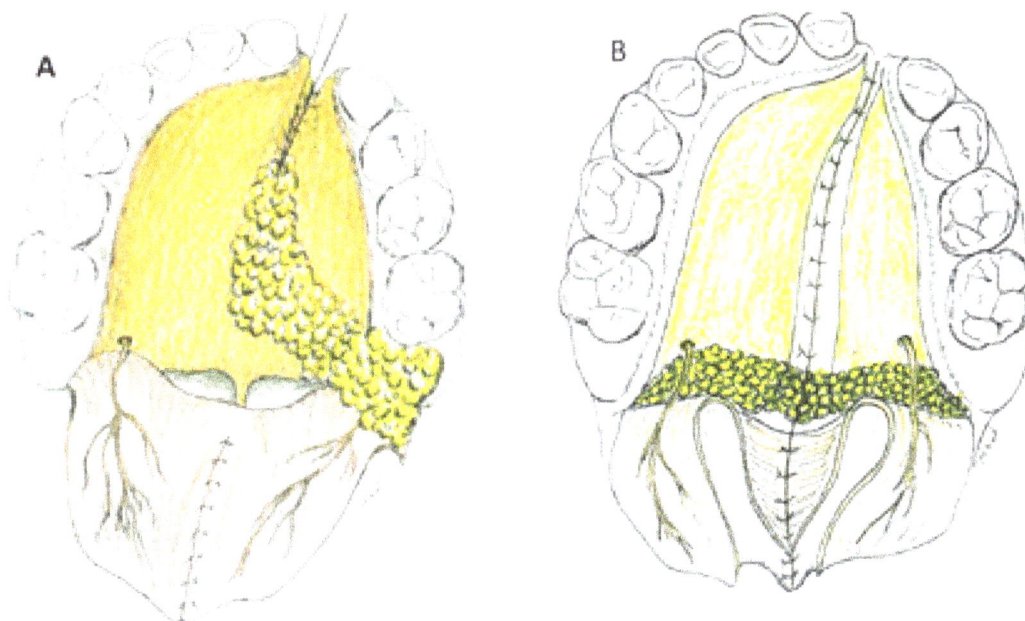

Figure 8. (A) The use of BFP for the closure of palatal fistulas. (B) The use of BFP to prevent type III fistulas between the hard and soft palate, minimizing scarring tension and obstructing the space of Ernst (Gröbe et al. [53]).

The transferred BFP was fully epithelialized with healthy-looking oral mucosa within 4 weeks, regardless of graft coverage with palatal mucosa or not. There is no significant impairment of palatal movement or any prevention of growth disturbances [54]. Levi et al. [54] suggests that the scar contraction and subsequent transverse maxillary growth restriction induced by the lateral hard palatal tissue defect decrease in this technique. Also, they believe that the hollowness of the child's cheek is unaffected.

Large, unlined, denuded palatal shelves serve as a key nidus of scar contraction as the palatal tissues attempt to fill the dead space [54]. Levi et al. state that adding the BFP to fill this open space causes an increase of vascularity in this area. Also, they believe that adding a layer of the BFP over the buccal mucosal flap decreases the time of surgery and needs less donor-site dissection [54, 55].

The combination of these two techniques, the BFP with pedicle mucosal flap, has some advantages: (1) the length of the soft palate increases without causing tension from the nasal side; (2) if the oral layer has failed and a perforation occurs, the graft serves as a bed for secondary granulation; (3) the flap also fills the secondary lateral defect; and (4) unlike buccal myomucosal flap, which is generated from another site, the BFP is easily accessible from the lateral incision [56].

5.4. Temporomandibular joint

Rattan used the BFP as a useful adjunct to autogenous or alloplastic temporomandibular joint (TMJ) reconstruction after TMJ ankylosis release. He claimed that the BFP can be used for TMJ reconstruction because of its local availability [16]. Toshihiro et al. used BFP graft in the TMJ region to repair the postoperative defect left by a synovial chondromatosis resected from the left condylar head in a 58-year-old female. The size of the defect was 20 × 25 mm and the size of the BFP was 30 × 30 mm. Although the tumor was resected via an extraoral approach, BFP grafting was prepared intraorally and tunneled to the TMJ region (**Figure 9**). There was no contraction of soft tissues or functional disorder of the TMJ during follow-up [57].

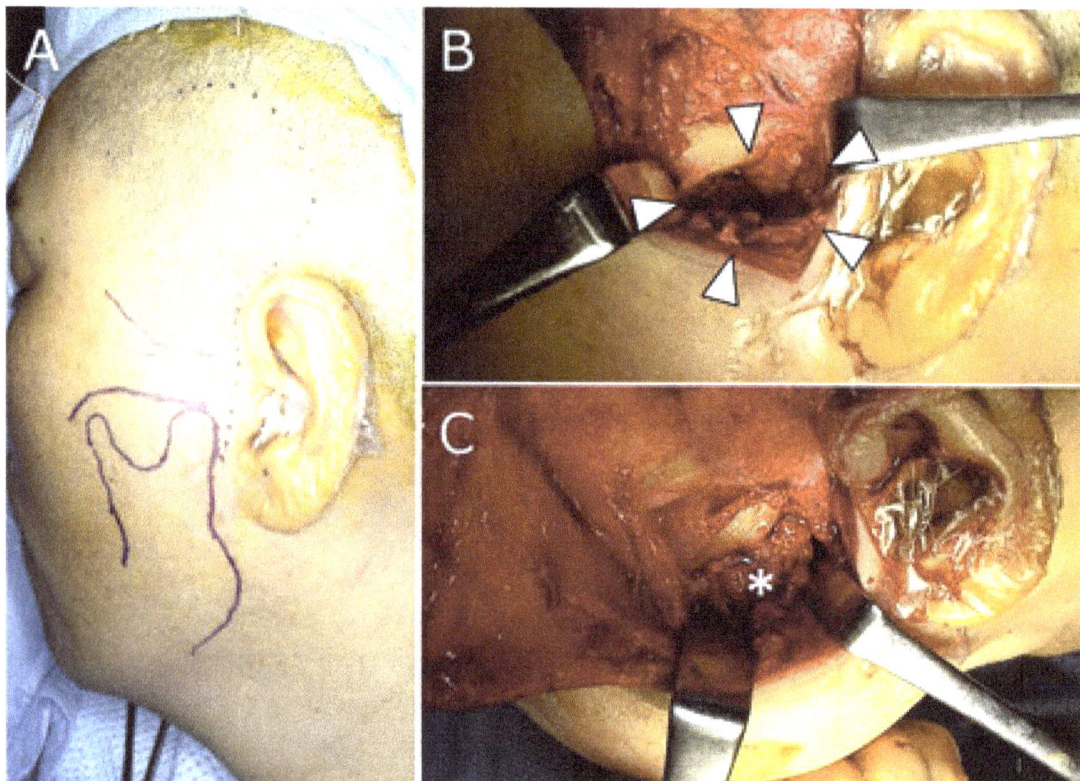

Figure 9. Reconstruction of a defect in the temporomandibular joint (TMJ) region in a patient following resection of a synovial chondromatosis of the left TMJ. (A) Preoperative view. (B) Resection of the mandibular condyle with the tumor (arrowheads). (C) Extension of the BFP to the surgical defect (*) (Toshihiro et al. [57]).

Singh et al. evaluated the feasibility and usefulness of BFP as an interposition graft in the treatment of TMJ ankylosis. Their findings showed the successful management of TMJ ankylosis using the BFP as an interposition graft. They assert that the mean of the maximum interincisal opening is 35.1 mm. Furthermore, the mean deviation to the affected side during opening the mouth is 1.6 mm. They claim that chewing function after this surgery satisfies the patients. Also, they believe that no major occlusal changes occur after this surgery and the intra-articular space is maintained well. Finally, they showed that using the BFP as an interposition graft is a desirable alternative to manage TMJ ankylosis, particularly in the short term [58].

Elimination of dead space is the main goal of using the BFP around the TMJ; the BFP prevents the hematoma around the joint. Also, due to the isolation of the joint by the BFP, the chance of the formation of fibrosis and bone decreases in the area [7].

5.5. Miscellaneous uses

Hassani et al. [59] reported the use of the BPF with a mixture of autogenous bone graft in sinus lifting procedure and covering the lateral wall of sinus for the first time. They believed that the BFP serves as both a physical barrier and a high vascularized bed for the bone graft. Tamura et al. used the BFP for augmentation of the vocal cord [60].

Khouw et al. reported the use of the BFP for palatal reconstruction when it is combined with a superiorly based pharyngeal flap. They used this technique to lengthen the soft palate in patients with extensive necrotizing defects [61].

El Haddad et al. reported the use of the pedicled BFP for covering of class IV Miller gingival defects. The BFP provides a significant amount of keratinized tissue for the gingival recession of the maxillary molars [62].

Also, some experts believe that the BFP can be used as a biologic membrane to cover bone grafts and in maxillary sinus lifting for implant placement. As mentioned before, the BFP can serve as a physical barrier. Also, it is well vascularized and contains adipose stem cells (ASCs), which have great potential to help bone regeneration in operation sites [59, 63, 64]. For these reasons and because the BFP is a source of stem cells, the BFP can be a great biologic membrane for covering the bone grafts.

Recently, researchers increased their focus of interest on adipose tissue-derived stem cells, and the BFP was introduced as a source of stem cells. Farré-Guasch et al. had claimed that the BFP is a source of stem cells. ASCs present in adipose tissue are able to differentiate into several lineages and express multiple growth factors, which makes them suitable for clinical application. The BFP represents an easy access source for dentists and oral surgeons. The stromal vascular fraction obtained from fresh BFP-derived adipose tissue and passaged ASCs were analyzed to detect and quantify the percentage of ASCs in this tissue. The BFP contains a huge amount of stem cells that has the capability to differentiate into the chondrogenic, adipogenic, and osteogenic lineages [65, 66].

6. BFP pathological conditions and complications

6.1. Pathological conditions

Kahn et al. explained that the continuity of fat tissue within the deep face makes it prone to pathological conditions such as cellulitis and abscess. The anaerobic organisms within the fat pad are responsible for it [67].

Although hemangioma in BFP is rare, some studies have reported the incidence of hemangioma with/without phleboliths inside the BFP mass [68] (**Figure 10**).

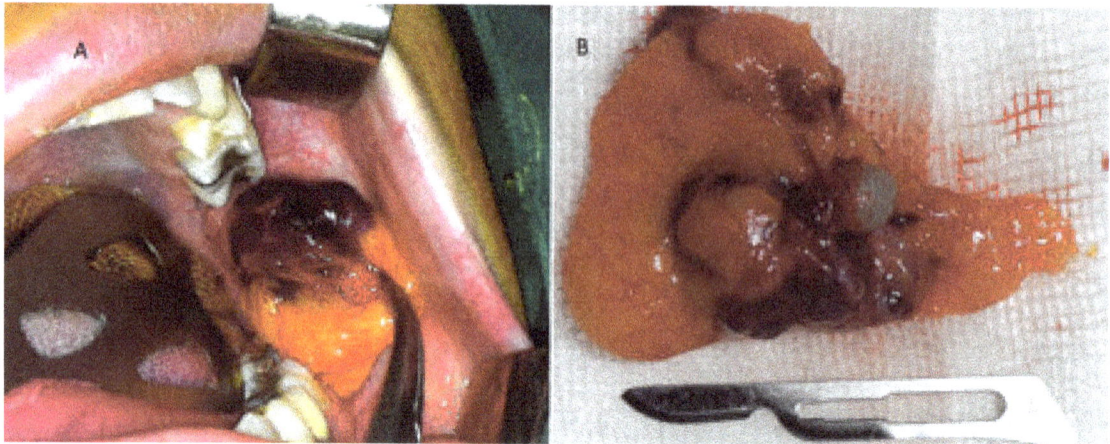

Figure 10. Hemangioma of the BFP. (A) Intraoperative view of the lesion. (B) View of the totally excised lesion showing hemangioma with phleboliths (Hassani et al. [68]).

BFP herniation is a common occurrence, particularly in infants and children. The BFP can pierce the oral mucosa and buccinators to the oral cavity [12]. Also, it may enter into the maxillary sinus after herniation [10].

A review of the literature shows that most cases of the BFP herniation involve children less than 5 years of age [28]. This fact can be due to some reasons. First, the BFP prominency is more in children. Second, because children put foreign objects into their mouth, they are more prone to the BFP herniation via rupturing the oral mucosa. Third, neonates and infant have a suckling activity which makes them prone to the BFP herniation [69].

6.2. Complications

Complications due to the mobilization of BFP are rare, and the BFP in the reconstruction of defects is highly successful [7, 19].

Partial necrosis accounted for the majority of failures involving the use of the BFP. A small dehiscence can be treated conservatively to see if spontaneous closure occurs. Reattempts at closure involve contralateral buccal fat flaps, palatal flaps, or buccal flaps. Rarely can the same flap be mobilized again, unless the defect was small and the reason for failure is easily identified. Trismus from scarring has been reported mainly when the BFP is used for the reconstruction of retromolar trigone or buccal mucosa defects. The range of motion should be noted in the few weeks after the use of the flap so that physical therapy, if necessary, is activated as soon as possible. A rarely visible change in facial contour has been reported in patients only when the BFP is used for the reconstruction of large defects. A surgeon might consider a contralateral buccal lipectomy to correct this alteration. The low morbidity and failure rate associated with the use of the BFP in maxillary reconstruction allows this simple reconstructive option to be used in carefully selected defects [33].

Different complications following application of the BFP have been reported. Although the complications are usually rare, it is a fact that it could be partial or complete loss of flap, limitation in mouth opening [44], hematoma, hemorrhage [45], postoperative infection [29,

47], and depressed cheek [8, 29, 46]. If a clinician harvests a large amount of the BFP for reconstruction purpose, the cheek may be depressed.

7. Summary

Generally, extraction of the BFP from the deep facial region is a safe procedure with minimal risk of unhazardous complications [19].

Due to the unique features of the BFP, such as its location, easy accessibility, rich blood supply, a rich source of ASCs, and high rate of epithelialization, using the term "versatile flap" is truly fitting. The BFP can be used in different directions. It can displace anteriorly up to the canine region, not beyond the midline, posteriorly in the hard palate tuberosity region, retromolar region, the soft palate, and to the anterior tonsillar pillar (**Figure 11**) [45].

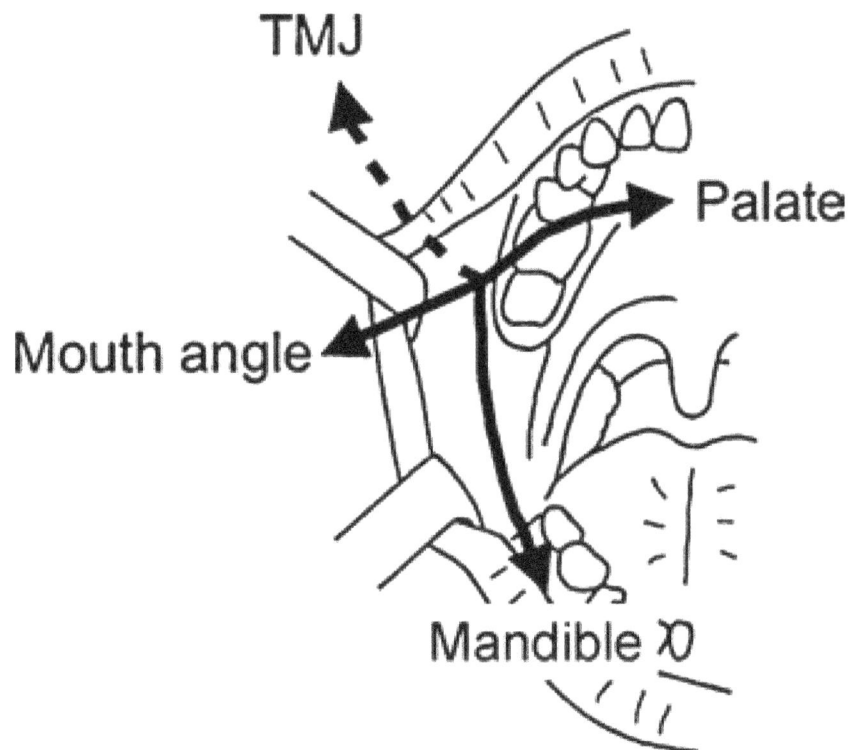

Figure 11. Applicability of the BFP. The graft could be extended in four directions to the palate via the maxilla, mandible, mouth angle, and TMJ region (Toshihiro et al. [57]).

The BFP has a variety of applications in oral and maxillofacial surgery. Among different applications, using it for the closure of OAC is the most common application reported. Although most of the time the BFP flap is used solely, it can be used in conjunction with other flaps, such as the pedicle temporalis muscle myocutaneous flap [31]. The success of the BFP has been attributed to its rich vascular supply, less donor-site morbidity, ease of harvest, and a lower rate of complications [39].

Author details

Ali Hassani[1*], Solaleh Shahmirzadi[2] and Sarang Saadat[2]

*Address all correspondence to: drhassani.omfs@gmail.com

1 Department of Oral and Maxillofacial Surgery, Implant Department, Dental Implant Research Center, Tehran Dental Branch, Islamic Azad University, Tehran, Iran

2 Dental Implant Research Center, Tehran Dental Branch, Islamic Azad University, Tehran, Iran

References

[1] Loukas M, Kapos T, Louis RG Jr, Wartman C, Jones A, Hallner B. Gross anatomical, CT and MRI analyses of the buccal fat pad with special emphasis on volumetric variations. Surg Radiol Anat. 2006;28(3):254–60.

[2] Egyedi P. Utilization of the buccal fat pad for closure of oro-antral and/or oro-nasal communications. J Maxillofac Surg. 1977;5(4):241–4.

[3] Messenger K, Cloyd W. Traumatic herniation of the buccal fat pad: Report of a case. Oral Surg Oral Med Oral Pathol. 1977;43(1):41–3.

[4] Wolford DG, Stapleford RG, Forte RA, Heath M. Traumatic herniation of the buccal fat pad: Report of case. J Am Dent Assoc. 1981;103(4):593–4.

[5] Scott P, Fabbroni G, Mitchell D. The buccal fat pad in the closure of oro-antral communications: An illustrated guide. Dent Update. 2004;31(6):363–4, 366.

[6] Allais M, Maurette PE, Cortez AL, Laureano Filho JR, Mazzonetto R. The buccal fat pad graft in the closure of oroantral communications. Braz J Otorhinolaryngol. 2008;74(5): 799.

[7] Singh J, Prasad K, Lalitha RM, Ranganath K. Buccal pad of fat and its applications in oral and maxillofacial surgery: A review of published literature (February) 2004 to (July) 2009. Oral Surg Oral Med Oral Pathol Oral Radiol Endod. 2010;110(6):698–705.

[8] Poeschl PW, Baumann A, Russmueller G, Poeschl E, Klug C, Ewers R. Closure of oroantral communications with Bichat's buccal fat pad. J Oral Maxillofac Surg. 2009;67(7):1460–6.

[9] Marzano UG. Lorenz Heister's "molar gland". Plast Reconstr Surg. 200515;115(5):1389–93.

[10] Baumann A, Ewers R. Application of the buccal fat pad in oral reconstruction. J Oral Maxillofac Surg. 2000;58(4):389–92; discussion 392–3.

[11] Rapidis AD, Alexandridis CA, Eleftheriadis E, Angelopoulos AP. The use of the buccal fat pad for reconstruction of oral defects: Review of the literature and report of 15 cases. J Oral Maxillofac Surg. 2000;58(2):158–63.

[12] Neder A. Use of buccal fat pad for grafts. Oral Surg Oral Med Oral Pathol. 1983;55(4): 349–50.

[13] Tideman H, Bosanquet A, Scott J. Use of the buccal fat pad as a pedicled graft.

[14] Dean A, Alamillos F, García-López A. The buccal fat pad flap in oral reconstruction. Head Neck. 2001;23(5):383–8.

[15] Hao SP. Reconstruction of oral defects with the pedicle buccal fat pad flap. Otolaryngol Head Neck Surg. 2000;122(6):863–7.

[16] Rattan V. A simple technique for use of buccal pad of fat in temporomandibular joint reconstruction. J Oral Maxillofac Surg. 2006;64(9):1447–51.

[17] Matarasso A. Buccal fat pad excision: aesthetic improvement of the midface. Ann Plast Surg. 1991;26(5):413–8.

[18] Hwang K, Cho H, Battuvshin D. Interrelated buccal fat pad with facial buccal branches and parotid duct. J Craniofac Surg. 2005;16(4):658–60.

[19] Cherekaev V, Golbin D, Belov A. Translocated pedicle buccal fat pad: closure of anterior and middle skull base defects after tumor resection. J Craniofac Surg. 2012;23(1):98–104.

[20] Dubin B, Jackson I, Halim A, Triplett WW, Ferreira M. Anatomy of the buccal fat pad and its clinical significance Plast Reconstr Surg. 1989;83(2):257–64.

[21] Zhang HM, Yan YP, Qi KM, Wang JQ, Liu ZF. Anatomical structure of the buccal fat pad and its clinical adaptations. Plast Reconstr Surg. 2002;109(7):2509–18; discussion 2519–20.

[22] Jackson I. Anatomy of the buccal fat pad and its clinical significance. Plast Reconstr Surg. 1999;103(7):2059–60; discussion 2061–3.

[23] Tostevin P, Ellis H. The buccal pad of fat: A review. Clin Anat. 1995;8(6):403–6.

[24] Kahn JL, Sick H, Laude M, Koritke JG. Vascularization of the adipose body of the cheek. Arch Anat Histol Embryol. 1990;73:3–20.

[25] Xiao H, Bayramicli M, Jackson IT. Volumetric analysis of the buccal fat pad. Eur J Plast Surg. 1999;22(4):177–80.

[26] Poissonnet C, Burdi A, Bookstein F. Growth and development of human adipose tissue during early gestation. Early Hum Dev. 1983;8(1):1–11.

[27] Bagdade J, Hirsch J. Gestational and dietary influences on the lipid content of the infant buccal fat pad. Proc Soc Exp Biol Med. 1966;122(2):616–9.

[28] Yousuf S, Tubbs RS, Wartmann CT, Kapos T, Cohen-Gadol AA, Loukas M. A review of the gross anatomy, functions, pathology, and clinical uses of the buccal fat pad. Surg Radiol Anat. 2010;32(5):427–36.

[29] Amin M, Bailey B, Swinson B, Witherow H. Use of the buccal fat pad in the reconstruction and prosthetic rehabilitation of oncological maxillary defects. Br J Oral Maxillofac Surg. 2005;43(2):148–54.

[30] Stuzin JM, Wagstrom L, Kawamoto HK, Baker TJ, Wolfe SA. The anatomy and clinical applications of the buccal fat pad. Plast Reconstr Surg. 1990;85(1):29–37.

[31] Samman N, Cheung L, Tideman H. The buccal fat pad in oral reconstruction. Int J Oral Maxillofac Surg. 1993;22(1):2–6.

[32] Dolanmaz D, Tuz H, Bayraktar S, Metin M, Erdem E, Baykul T. Use of pedicle buccal fat pad in the closure of oroantral communication: Analysis of 75 cases. Quintessence Int. 2004;35(3):241–6.

[33] Arce K. Buccal fat pad in maxillary reconstruction. Atlas Oral Maxillofac Surg Clin North Am. 2007;15(1):23–32.

[34] Hassani A, Saadat S, Moshiri R, Shahmirzad S, Hassani A. Nerve retraction during inferior alveolar nerve repositioning procedure: A new simple method and review of the literature. J Oral Implantol. 2015;41 Spec No: 391–4. doi: 10.1563/AAID-JOI-D-13-00108. Epub 2013 Dec 17.

[35] Hassani A, Saadat S. Nerve repositioning injuries of the trigeminal nerve. In: Miloro M, editor.Trigeminal Nerve Injuries. 1st ed. Berlin: Springer; 2013. p. 109–135. DOI: 10.1007/978-3-642-35539-4_7

[36] Hassani A, Motamedi MH, Saadat S. Inferior alveolar nerve transpositioning for implant placement. In: Motamedi MH, editor. A Textbook of Advanced Oral and Maxillofacial Surgery. 1st ed. Rijeka: InTech; 2013. p. 659–93). DOI: 10.5772/52317

[37] Haraji A, Zare RE. The use of buccal fat pad for oro-antral communication closure. J Mashhad Dent Sch Mashhad Univ Med Sci. 2007;31:9–11.

[38] Yousif NJ, Gosain A, Sanger JR, Larson DL, Matloub HS. The nasolabial fold: A photogrammetric analysis. Plast Reconstr Surg. 1994;93(1):70–7.

[39] Adeyemo WL, Ogunlewe MO, Ladeinde AL, James O. Closure of oro-antral fistula with pedicle buccal fat pad. A case report and review of literature. African Journal of Oral Health. 2004;1(1):42–6.

[40] Dolanmaz D, Tuz H, Bayraktar S, Metin M, Erdem E, Baykul T. Use of pedicle buccal fat pad in the closure of oroantral communication: analysis of 75 cases. Quintessence Int. 2004;35(3):241–46.

[41] Hassani A, Motamedi M, Saadat S, Moshiri R, Shahmirzadi S. Novel technique to repair maxillary sinus membrane perforations during sinus lifting. J Oral Maxillofac Surg. 2012;70(11):e592–7. doi: 10.1016/j.joms.2012.06.191.

[42] Kim Y, Hwang J, Yun P. Closure of large perforation of sinus membrane using pedicle buccal fat pad graft: A case report. Int J Oral Maxillofac Implants. 2008;23(6):1139–42.

[43] Hanazawa Y, Itoh K, Mabashi T, Sato K. Closure of oroantral communications using a pedicle buccal fat pad graft. J Oral Maxillofac Surg. 1995;53(7):771–5.

[44] Colella G, Tartaro G, Giudice A. The buccal fat pad in oral reconstruction. Br J Plast Surg. 2004;57(4):326–9.

[45] Chakrabarti J, Tekriwal R, Ganguli A, Ghosh S, Mishra PK. Pedicled buccal fat pad flap for intraoral malignant defects: A series of 29 cases. Indian J Plast Surg. 2009;42(1):36–42.

[46] Chien CY, Hwang CF, Chuang HC, Jeng SF, Su CY. Comparison of radial forearm free flap, pedicle buccal fat pad flap and split-thickness skin graft in reconstruction of buccal mucosal defect. Oral Oncol. 2005;41(7):694–7.

[47] Liu YM, Chen GF, Yan JL, Zhao SF, Zhang WM, Zhao S, Chen L. Functional reconstruction of maxilla with pedicle buccal fat pad flap, prefabricated titanium mesh and autologous bone grafts Int J Oral Maxillofac Surg. 2006;35(12):1108–13.

[48] Zhong LP, Chen GF, Fan LJ, Zhao SF. Immediate reconstruction of maxilla with bone grafts supported by pedicle buccal fat pad graft. Oral Surg Oral Med Oral Pathol Oral Radiol Endod. 2004;97(2):147–54.

[49] Alkan A, Dolanmaz D, Uzun E, Erdem E. The reconstruction of oral defects with buccal fat pad. Swiss Med Wkly. 2003;133(33/34):465–70.

[50] Ferrari S, Ferri A, Bianchi B, Copelli C, Magri AS, Sesenna E. A novel technique for cheek mucosa defect reconstruction using a pedicle buccal fat pad and buccinator myomucosal island flap. Oral Oncol. 2009;45(1):59–62.

[51] Mehrotra D, Pradhan R, Gupta S. Retrospective comparison of surgical treatment modalities in 100 patients with oral submucous fibrosis. Oral Surg Oral Med Oral Pathol Oral Radiol Endod. 2009;107(3):e1–10.

[52] Zhao Z, Li S, Li Y. The application of the pedicle buccal fat pad graft in cleft palate repair. Zhonghua Zheng Xing Shao Shang Wai Ke Za Zhi. 1998;14(3):182–5.

[53] Gröbe A, Eichhorn W, Hanken H, Precht C, Schmelzle R, Heiland M, et al. The use of buccal fat pad (BFP) as a pedicle graft in cleft palate surgery. Int J Oral Maxillofac Surg. 2011;40(7):685–9.

[54] Levi B, Kasten SJ, Buchman SR. Utilization of the buccal fat pad flap for congenital cleft palate repair. Plast Reconstr Surg. 2009;123(3):1018–21.

[55] Cole P, Horn T, Thaller S. The use of decellularized dermal grafting (AlloDerm) in persistent oro-nasal fistulas after tertiary cleft palate repair. J Craniofac Surg. 2006;17(4): 636–41.

[56] Pappachan B, Vasant R. Application of bilateral pedicle buccal fat pad in wide primary cleft palate. Br J Oral Maxillofac Surg. 2008;46(4):310–2.

[57] Toshihiro Y, Nariai Y, Takamura Y, Yoshimura H, Tobita T, Yoshino A, et al. Applicability of buccal fat pad grafting for oral reconstruction. Int J Oral Maxillofac Surg. 2013;42(5):604–10.

[58] Singh V, Dhingra R, Sharma B, Bhagol A, Kumar P. Retrospective analysis of use of buccal fat pad as an interpositional graft in temporomandibular joint ankylosis: Preliminary study. J Oral Maxillofac Surg. 2011;69(10):2530–6.

[59] Hassani A, Khojasteh A, Alikhasi M, Vaziri H. Measurement of volume changes of sinus floor augmentation covered with buccal fat pad: A case series study. Oral Surg Oral Med Oral Pathol Oral Radiol Endod. 2009;107(3):369–74.

[60] Tamura E, Fukuda H, Tabata Y, Nishimura M. Use of the buccal fad pad for vocal cord augmentation. Acta Otolaryngol. 2008;128(2):219–24.

[61] Khouw YL, van der Wal KG, Bartels F, van der Biezen JJ. Bilateral palatal reconstruction using 2 pedicle buccal fat pads in rhinolalea aperta after extensive necrotizing tonsillitis: A case report. J Oral Maxillofac Surg. 2004;62(6):749–51.

[62] El Haddad SA, Abd El Razzak MY, El Shall M. Use of pedicle buccal fat pad in root coverage of severe gingival recession defect. J Periodontol. 2008;79(7):1271–9.

[63] Hudson JW, Anderson JG, Russell RM Jr, Anderson N, Chambers K. Use of pedicle fat pad graft as an adjunct in the reconstruction of palatal cleft defects. Oral Surg Oral Med Oral Pathol Oral Radiol Endod. 1995;80(1):24–7.

[64] Khojasteh A, Hassani A, Motamedian SR, Saadat S, Alikhasi M. Cortical bone augmentation versus nerve lateralization for treatment of atrophic posterior mandible: A retrospective study and review of literature. Clin Implant Dent Relat Res. 2016;18(2): 342–59. DOI: 10.1111/cid.12317

[65] Farré-Guasch E, Martí-Pagè C, Hernádez-Alfaro F, Klein-Nulend J, Casals N. Buccal fat pad, an oral access source of human adipose stem cells with potential for osteo-chondral tissue engineering: An in vitro study Tissue Eng Part C Methods. 2010;16(5): 1083–94.

[66] Broccaioli E Niada S, Rasperini G, Ferreira LM, Arrigoni E, Yenagi V, et al. Mesenchymal stem cells from Bichat's fat pad: In vitro comparison with adipose-derived stem cells from subcutaneous tissue. Biores Open Access. 2013;2(2):107–17.

[67] Kahn JL, Wolfram-Gabel R, Bourjat P. Anatomy and imaging of the deep fat of the face. Clin Anat. 2000;13(5):373–82.

[68] Hassani A, Saadat S, Moshiri R, Shahmirzadi S. Hemangioma of the buccal fat pad. Contemp Clin Dent. 2014;5(2):243–6. doi: 10.4103/0976-237X.132368.

[69] Matarasso A. Pseudoherniation of the buccal fat pad: A new clinical syndrome. Plast Reconstr Surg. 1997;100(3):723–30.

5

Shared Medical and Virtual Surgical Appointments in Oral Surgery

Alexandra Radu and Michael P. Horan

Abstract

Access to care and patient satisfaction are primary objectives in most, if not all, surgical practices. With current healthcare reform and implementation of The Affordable Care Act of 2010, surgeons are more frequently being challenged by their administrative counterparts to improve clinical efficiency and quality of care while maintaining current profit margins. This chapter describes two non-traditional, innovative concepts that can be incorporated into full scope, oral and maxillofacial surgery practices in order to allow more efficient delivery of care while maintaining quality. The two programs outlined herein are shared medical appointments (SMAs) and virtual surgical appointments (VSAs). These programs, when implemented in a busy academic or group private practice, have the potential to allow for efficient delivery of care while simultaneously improving patient satisfaction.

Keywords: shared medical appointments, virtual surgical appointments, telemedicine, third molar surgery, cost-effective medicine

1. Shared medical appointments

1.1. Introduction

An SMA can be defined as a medical appointment where multiple patients with similar medical conditions or needs are seen in a group setting. The appointment is moderated by the physician, surgeon, or medical team. Being in a group setting allows patients to share experiences, voice concerns, and receive feedback from others with similar conditions as well as with their provider. Whereas individual medical appointments are typically 15–20 minutes long, SMA can last up to 90 minutes. Patients are allotted more time to their provider and medical team, and most often indicate increased satisfaction relative to individual appointments.

The concept of the SMA was first established by Dr. John Scott, a Kaiser Permanente staff internist and geriatrician, in 1991. Dr. Scott's cooperative healthcare clinic model for geriatric patients helped to shape early SMAs. At that time of its inceptions, Dr. Scott's model focused on 15–20 patients with a chronic medical condition. The appointment was staffed by a physician, nurse, and medical assistant [1]. Even though medical SMAs geared toward chronic illnesses have maintained this basic structure over the years, this model is currently being adopted by medical specialists in an attempt to provide knowledge to a larger group of patients in an environment that is more welcoming and nurturing for patients [2]. In addition, several surgical specialties have adopted this model as a pre-operative consultation or informational session, as in the case of breast [3] or dermatological surgery [4]. SMAs are also currently being utilized for post-operative monitoring of patients who have undergone bariatric [5] or cardiac surgery [6].

Participating in SMAs provides patients with the benefit of a longer visit with their physician and other members of the healthcare team, including nurses, physician's assistants, or health educators. Studies by Prescott et al. and Bartley et al. have both demonstrated that SMAs improved patient access to care, enhanced outcomes, and patient understanding by offering the same information at varied levels of literacy, and promoted patient satisfaction, while at the same time providing education for self-management in a more efficient manner for practitioners and patients [7, 8]. Giladi and co-workers showed that patients also benefit from developing a sense of camaraderie, peer support, and group education [3]. In the case of patients with morbid conditions undergoing cardiac surgery, Harris demonstrated that SMAs can reduce depression, anxiety, or the sense of isolation related to the severity of the patients' medical condition and the post-operative course [6].

Utilization of SMAs has not yet taken hold in the field of oral and maxillofacial surgery despite its potential to improve the accessibility and efficiency of care. Although SMAs were initially developed to manage patients with chronic diseases, the format is easily adaptable to meet the needs of patients who require minor oral surgical procedures, such as third molar surgery, or in patients with chronic conditions treated by oral and maxillofacial surgeons (e.g., temporomandibular joint disease, obstructive sleep apnea).

1.2. Economics of SMAs

The cost-effectiveness of SMAs has been shown in several studies since the beginning of the 1990s. Not only is the physician's productivity increased, but SMAs also provide many other economic and patient care benefits, while reducing the costs by leveraging staff [9]. In a case study performed by Caballero at Sutter Medical Foundation in California, the productivity among primary care physicians improved by 200% and specialty clinics by 300% [10]. When this model was introduced in the management of diabetic patients in Australia, it was calculated that the lifetime cost reduction of diabetes was estimated at over $126,000 per person. In addition, by reducing one individual appointment for the diabetic population in

Australia (~2 million diabetic patients nationwide), the annual cost reduction would be an estimated $100 million, considering one individual appointment to cost $50 per patient [11].

When discussing about SMAs, it is also important to understand the billing aspect of the process. In general, medical insurance companies do not reimburse for group visits. However, an SMA is not a class or seminar but an actual office visit. Because the same documentation for individual appointments is required for SMA (e.g., history, physical examination, vital signs, laboratory testing, plan), it is possible to bill each patient according to the current procedural terminology (CPT) code based on the level of care provided. It is not advisable, however, to bill according to the time spent with patients [7].

1.3. Measuring patient satisfaction

Since the model of SMA is fairly new and not commonly used, there is a perceived skepticism on the patients' side that the medical team should consider and address at the time the appointment is made. In a controlled study done for patients undergoing post-operative bariatric surgery, 47 patients were asked to complete the same 13-question survey before and after the SMA. The patient's opinion of the SMA improved from baseline levels after taking part in one, and patients were generally happy with the level of confidentiality relative to individual appointments [5].

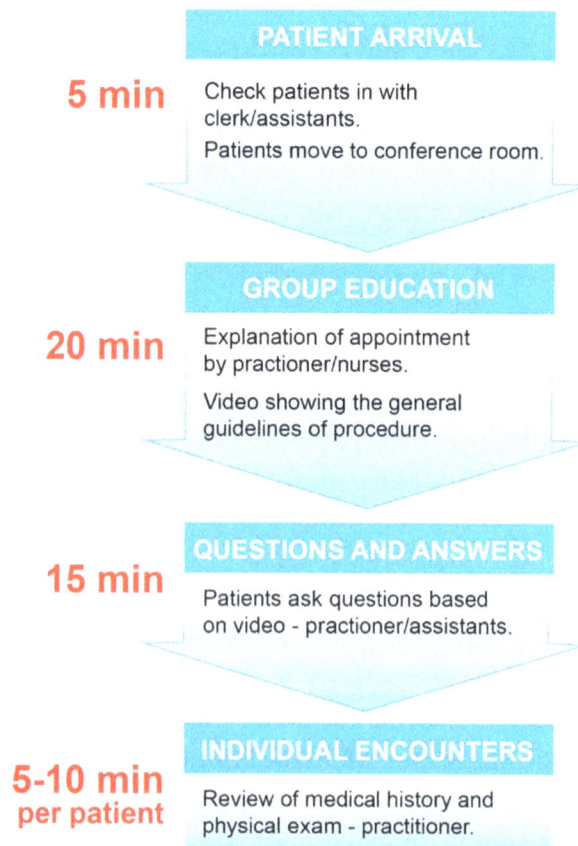

5 min

PATIENT ARRIVAL
Check patients in with clerk/assistants.
Patients move to conference room.

20 min

GROUP EDUCATION
Explanation of appointment by practioner/nurses.
Video showing the general guidelines of procedure.

15 min

QUESTIONS AND ANSWERS
Patients ask questions based on video - practioner/assistants.

5-10 min per patient

INDIVIDUAL ENCOUNTERS
Review of medical history and physical exam - practitioner.

Figure 1. Structure and flow of the SMA.

We have implemented the concept of shared medical appointments over the past year in our Oral and Maxillofacial Surgery clinic for patients who needed third molar surgery. The patients are briefly explained the SMA model at the time that the appointments are made. **Figure 1** shows the flow of events and the approximate time allotted for each step in our SMA model.

Eighteen surveys were collected from the patients who participated in such appointments throughout this period. The surveys asked 7 questions that were graded by the participants on a scale of 1 to 5 (1-Strongly Disagree, 2-Disagree, 3-Neutral, 4-Agree, 5-Strongly Agree). Additionally, there were two questions asking the patient to provide qualitative short answers (questions 8 and 9). The questions in the survey are shown below:

1. Scheduling my shared medical appointment was easy

2. I gained valuable information from responses to other patient's questions

3. There was adequate time for my questions

4. I gained a sense of group support

5. I would participate in a shared medical appointment again

6. I would recommend shared medical appointments to other patients

7. I feel my medical information is secure in the group setting

8. How would you compare an SMA to a one-on-one appointment?

9. Do you have any further comments about the SMA?

After data collection was finalized, the survey results were analyzed by calculating averages, standard deviations, and standard errors for the first seven questions (**Table 1**).

Question	Average	Standard deviation	Standard error
1	4.33	1.08	0.25
2	4.11	0.83	0.19
3	4.50	0.98	0.23
4	3.94	1.05	0.24
5	4.55	0.75	0.17
6	4.44	0.51	0.12
7	4.61	0.50	0.11

1—Strongly disagree, 2—Disagree, 3—Neutral, 4—Agree, 5—Strongly agree.

Table 1. Summary of the data collected for the seven questions that had numerical quantification.

For Questions 8 and 9, there were no numerical data to analyze. The answers were generally favorable, with six neutral (i.e., the SMA was the same as a typical one-on-one appointment) and two negative responses (i.e., the one-on-one appointment was a better fit). One positive recurrent answer found in the surveys was that SMAs benefited the patients in learning about the condition and treatment while benefiting from questions and concerns raised by others.

The data presented in **Table 1** indicate that SMAs were predominantly received well by patients, with respondents strongly agreeing that they would participate in a shared medical appointment again. With the exception of Question 4, all other question ranked in the 4–5 range. One of the main goals of SMAs in oral and maxillofacial surgery is to increase accessibility, and based on the answers received for Question 1, the patients had scheduled their appointments with ease in a timely manner.

2. Virtual surgical appointments

Telemedicine is the use of telecommunication technology to provide clinical care at a remote location. Telemedicine was first adopted in the 1990s. With the low cost and wide availability of mobile devices, the field continues to grow. Virtual appointments can aid practitioners by fostering the patient–doctor relationship and improve practice efficiency. Virtual appointments have the potential to reduce the wait times by offering more online services, such as virtual consultation (VCA) and post-operative appointments (VPAs). Telemedicine has been successfully employed in various medical and surgical fields, including primary care, psychiatry, dermatology, oncology, otolaryngology, and orthopedics, resulting in increased patient satisfaction while providing high-quality care [12]. Virtual patient–doctor relationships have been used for several purposes, such as scheduling of appointments, referrals to other doctors, the writing of prescriptions, discussion of test results, and certificates of health [13].

VSA can be effectively incorporated into oral and maxillofacial surgery practices in the form of VCAs and VPAs. VCAs allow surgeons to meet and screen potential surgical candidates whom otherwise may need to travel nationally or internationally, to be evaluated. The patient's medical history can be reviewed and bidirectional communication can be established to determine the patient's chief complaint and history of present illness. With the use of image exchange servers, previous clinical photographs, radiographs, and virtual surgical plans can be reviewed. A determination can then be made as to whether or not this patient would be an appropriate candidate for treatment in the surgeons practice. The use of virtual appointments for post-operative monitoring has not been greatly explored, most likely due to the potential oversight of surgical complications and the perceived importance of performing a "hands on" physical examination. However, VPAs are ideal for monitoring outcomes of minor surgical procedures performed on an outpatient basis (e.g., dentoalveolar surgery, third molar surgery, implant surgery, minor bone grafting procedures) that have a low risk for post-operative complications.

As defined by the American Dental Association (ADA), teledentistry is the electronic exchange of dental patient information from one geographic location to another for interpretation and/ or consultation among authorized healthcare professionals [14]. Teledentistry employs both information and communication technologies to accomplish the electronic exchange of diagnostic image files, such as radiographs, photographs, video, or optical impressions. The

ADA released a policy on teledentistry in 2012. However, the policy was resolved in November 2015, explaining the scope of teledentistry and encouraging dentists to consider conformance with the Digital Imaging and Communications in Medicine (DICOM) standards when selecting and using imaging systems [14]. The 2015 resolution included more detailed guidelines addressing licensure of practitioners providing teledentistry, patient privacy, and billing issues. More specifically, the resolution states that dental benefit plans, and other paying public and private programs, should cover services provided through teledentistry at the same level as if the services were delivered in a traditional in-person encounter [15]. The ADA has encouraged both practitioners and patients alike to take advantage of teledentistry, as it greatly improves efficiency and access to care, respectively.

Teledentistry is a growing field that is currently utilized to virtually supervise the oral health care of patients in skilled nursing facilities, residents in rural areas, or others who do not have immediate access to a dentist [15]. According to the 2015 resolution, teledentistry can take multiple forms namely:

- Live video, which is a two-way interaction between patients and dental providers using audiovisual technology, such as smart phones, tablets, and computers equipped with webcams. This could include VPAs.

- Store and forward, which takes advantage of recorded health information that is transmitted through a secure electronic communications system to a practitioner at a distant site. The practitioner can then use the information to evaluate the patient's condition and render a consulting service outside of a real-time or live interaction. The health information communicated through this method includes radiographs, photographs, video, digital impressions, or photomicrographs.

- Remote patient monitoring is a method that could be used in the setting of a nursing home facility. It is the collection of personal health and medical information from an individual in one location and electronic transmission to another provider in a different location. This procedure differs from "store and forwards" in that it implies long-term monitoring.

- Mobile health, which involves the use of mobile communication devices to perform education projects in public health. This could include apps that monitor patient brushing (**Figure 2**).

In the field of oral and maxillofacial surgery, VPAs can be used to effectively and efficiently follow up patients who have undergone minor surgical procedures. These procedures include third molar surgical extraction, dental implant placement, allogenic bone grafting for ridge augmentation, adjunct implant procedures, and biopsies, and minimally invasive temporomandibular joint (TMJ) surgical procedures (e.g., arthroscopy, arthrocentesis, and intra-articular injections). Using a camera-equipped mobile device (e.g., cell phone, tablet, laptop, etc.) or desktop computer, patients can participate with their clinician in video conferences that are compliant with the Health Insurance Portability and Accountability Act (HIPAA). The clinician is able to do everything that would normally be done during a traditional post-operative appointment, except for a "hands-on" clinical examination. If the clinician has any concern about the patient's recovery, an in-office visit can be scheduled.

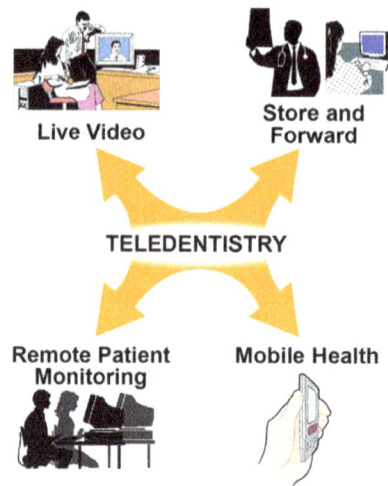

Figure 2. Four major practices employed through teledentistry [15].

Author details

Alexandra Radu[1] and Michael P. Horan[2*]

*Address all correspondence to: horanm@ccf.org

1 Case Western Reserve University School of Dental Medicine, Department of Oral and Maxillofacial Surgery, Cleveland, OH, USA

2 The Cleveland Clinic Head and Neck Institute, Section of Oral and Maxillofacial Surgery, Cleveland, OH, USA

References

[1] Kaidar-Person O, Swartz EW, Lefkowitz M, Conigliaro K, Fritz N, Birne J, Alexander C, Szomstein S, Rosenthal R. 2006. *Shared medical appointments: new concept of high volume follow-up for bariatric patients.* Surg Obesity Relat Dis. 2:509–512.

[2] Kirsh S, Watts S, Pascuzzi K, O'Day ME, Davidson D, Strauss S, Kern EO, Aron DC. 2007. *Shared medical appointments based on the chronic care model: a quality improvement project to address the challenges of patients with diabetes with cardiovascular risk.* Qual Saf Health Care 16:349–353.

[3] Giladi AM, Brown DL, Alderman AK. 2014. *Shared medical appointments for preoperative evaluation of symptomatic macromastia.* Plastic Reconstruct Surgery. 134(6):1108–1115.

[4] Knackstedt TJ, Samie FH. 2015. *Shared medical appointments for the preoperative consultation visit of Mohs micrographic surgery.* J Am Acad Dermatol. 72(2):340–344.

[5] Seager MJ, Egan RJ, Meredith HE, Bates SE, Norton SA, Morgan JDT. 2012. *Shared medical appointments for bariatric surgery follow-up: a patient satisfaction questionnaire.* Obes Surg. 22:641–645.

[6] Harris MD. 2010. *Shared medical appointments after cardiac surgery - The process of implementing a novel pilot paradigm to enhance comprehensive post discharge care.* J Cardiovasc Nurs. 25(2):124–129.

[7] Bartley KB, Haney R. 2010. *Shared medical appointments: improving access, outcomes, and satisfaction for patients with chronic cardiac diseases.* J Cardiovasc Nurs. 25(1):13–19.

[8] Prescott LS, Dickens AS, Guerra SL, Tanha JM, Phillips DG, Patel KT, Umberson KM, Lozano MA, Lowe KB, Brown AJ, Taylor JS, Soliman PT, Garcia EA, Levenback CF, Bodurka DC. 2015. *Fighting cancer together: development and implementation of shared medical appointments to standardize and improve chemotherapy education.* Gynecol Oncol. Retrieved October 18, 2015 from http://dx.doi.org/10.1016/j.ygyno.2015.11.0006.

[9] Caballero CA. 2015. *Shared medical appointments: an innovative approach to care.* The Nurse Practitioner. Retrieved online from Wolters Kluwer Health, Inc. DOI: 10.1097/01.NPR. 0000470357.85590.46

[10] Noffsinger EB, Atkns TN. 2001. *Assessing a group medical appointment program: a case study at Sutter Medical Foundation.* Group Pract J. 50(4):42–49.

[11] Egger G, Dixon J, Meldrum H, Binna A, Cole MA, Ewald D, Stevens J. 2015. *Patients' and providers' satisfaction with shared medical appointments.* Australian Family Physician. 44(9):674–679.

[12] Mair F, Whitten P. 2000. *Systematic review of studies of patient satisfaction with telemedicine.* BMJ 320:1517.

[13] Bidmon S, Terlutter R. 2015. *Gender differences in searching for health information on the internet and the virtual patient-physician relationship in Germany: exploratory results on how men and women differ and why.* J Med Internet Res. 17(6):e156.

[14] American Dental Association. 2012. *Current policies.* Retrieved December 20, 2015 from http://www.ada.org/~/media/ADA/Member%20Center/FIles/2013%20Current %20Policies%20Final.ashx.

[15] ADA News. 2015. House passes guidelines on teledentistry. American Dental Association. Retrieved December 15, 2015 from http://www.ada.org/en/publications/ada-news/2015-archive/december/house-passes-guidelines-on-teledentistry.

6

Complications of Antibiotic Therapy and Introduction of Nanoantibiotics

Esshagh Lasemi, Fina Navi, Reza Lasemi and
Niusha Lasemi

Abstract

Oral and maxillofacial surgeons play a major role in therapy, preventing morbidity, mortality from odontogenic and non-odontogenic maxillofacial infections; therefore, it is essential to have knowledge of current advancements in microbiological diagnosis and antibiotic therapy for odontogenic maxillofacial infections. Fortunately, we live in an era where antibiotics are readily available to prevent and treat against infections. The exact cause should be determined once the specific antibiotic is prescribed; additionally, the empirical, definitive treatments, side effects, pharmacokinetics and pharmacodynamics of antibacterial agents have to be considered.

Nowadays, antimicrobial resistance which is spreading rapidly is of great concern, because it is common in hospitals where acquired infections can be perilous. This situation compels scientists to synthesize new antibiotics and treatment modalities. The reason of microbial resistance can be due to increased misuse of antibiotics in foods (livestock, poultry and agriculture). A number of significant factors, such as organism identification, antibiotic sensitivity testing and host factor situations, should be taken into account in order to treat various infections effectively.

Currently, investigations are ongoing to impede antibacterial resistance by nanoscience technology seeking new chemotherapeutic agents. Scientists focusing on microbiological investigations aim to invent novel nanoantibiotic agents with high efficiency, low toxicity and low percentage of resistance. In recent years, nanoantibiotics have been applied against infections intelligently. The average size, polydispersity and composition of generated nanomaterials can be controlled by various methods in order to make them appropriate for biomedical applications.

The goal of this chapter is to provide an overview of the complications of various antibiotics used for therapeutic and prophylactic purposes in the oral and maxillofacial regions; furthermore, some essential nanoantbiotics are introduced and discussed.

Keywords: antibiotics, complications, nanoantibiotics, resistance, adverse effect

1. Introduction

Antibiotics can improve cell defense effectively; some key factors should be considered in antibiotic therapy, including the health of the host, identity of the organism and the antibiotic susceptibility; moreover, adverse reactions, interactions, resistance and other complications should be taken into account. The origin of most orofacial infections is odontogenic. The major relevant organisms of dental origin infections are aerobic and anaerobic Gram-positive cocci and anaerobic Gram-negative rods. The predominant aerobic bacteria in odontogenic infections are *Streptococcus milleri* genus [1]. Oral Gram-negative anaerobic rods are cultured in three quarters of the infections; however, several Gram-positives and Gram-negatives play more important pathogenic roles [1, 6]. Pure aerobic infections are less common (5%) [7]. Brook et al. detected that 50% of odontogenic deep facial infections yielded anaerobes, and only 44% of infections are a combination of aerobic and anaerobic flora [8]. Most sinus infections are viral, and only a small proportion develop a secondary bacterial infection in which the most common bacteria are Gram-positive and anaerobic bacteria [7, 9]. It is reasonable to use narrow-spectrum antibiotics for simple infections and broad-spectrum for complex infections to prevent resistance. Penicillin, clindamycin, metronidazole are narrow-spectrum, while amoxicillin+clavulanic acid, ampicillin+sulbactam, azithromycin, tetracycline, cephalosporin, moxifloxacin, ciprofloxacin and co-trimoxazol are broad-spectrum antibiotics [10]. Recently, there has been an alarming increase in the incidence of resistant bacterial isolates in odontogenic infections. Many anaerobic bacteria have developed resistance to beta-lactam antibiotics via beta-lactamase [7]. Inappropriate use of antibiotics causes the emergence of resistant bacteria. Today, many common and life-threatening infections are becoming difficult or impossible to treat and sometimes turning a common infection into a life-threatening one [11]. The antibiotic resistance is facilitated by repeated exposure of bacteria to antibiotics and access of bacteria to a large antimicrobial pool. Pathogenic and nonpathogenic bacteria are becoming increasingly resistant to conventional antibiotics. The focus has now shifted to multi-drug-resistant Gram-negative bacteria, while initial studies were investigated on antibiotic resistance such as methicillin-resistant *Staphylococcus aureus* and vancomycin-resistant Enterococcus spp. [12]. Gram-negative pathogens are particularly troublesome as they are becoming resistant to nearly all drugs. Bear in mind that resistance occurs for the Gram-positive infections (Staphylococcus and Enterococcus) but not on the same scale [13].

Nanoantibiotic drug delivery with low toxicity and extended release would be an appropriate alternative to reduce antibiotic resistance. When an antibiotic is administered, strains of resistant organisms may proliferate; therefore, the antibiotic becomes ineffective. An antibiotic can act as an antigenic stimulus and produce an allergic reaction. They can kill or halt the proliferation of sensitive bacteria. This may include normal flora. Thus, an antibiotic may cause diarrhea, increased risk of bleeding especially in patients taking warfarin. Once the susceptible bacteria are killed, they may be replaced by more resilient organisms such as *Candida albicans* and *Clostridium difficile*; moreover, hepatobiliary dysfunctions and nephrotoxicity are the other complications that may occur [14].

2. Mechanisms of resistance

- Mutations of bacterial genes (chromosomal) leading to cross-resistance.

- Gene transfer from one microorganism to other by plasmids, transpositions (conjugation), integrons and bacteriophages (transduction). After these, they can use various biochemical types of resisting mechanisms (**Figures 1** and **2**).

- Antibiotic inactivation (with cell wall synthesis by beta-lactams and glycopeptide).

- Target alteration (inhibition of protein synthesis for tetracyclines and macrolides).

- Interfering with nucleic acid synthesis for rifampin and fluoroquinolones.

- Altered permeability (modifications of the cell surface for aminoglycosides).

- Bypass metabolic pathway (metabolic route inhibition for co-trimoxazole) [2–4].

- In recent studies, Lee et al. recommended that not all interactions of bacteria with antibiotics can be clarified within the standard theory; however, the new Kin selection hypothesis

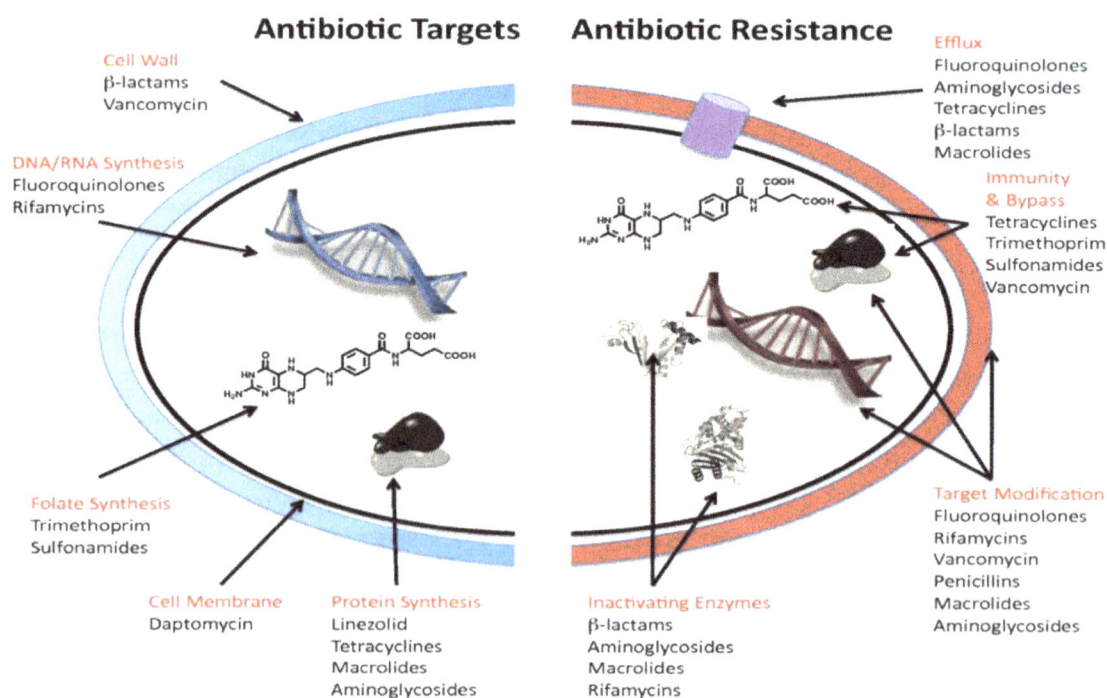

Figure 1. Gerard D Wright. Antibiotic targets and mechanisms of resistance. BMC Biology 2010 8:123.

proposed by W.D. Hamilton in 1964 suggested if one group of microorganisms is going to be resistant or destroyed, then others with similar genes have an opportunity to resist and mutate [15, 16].

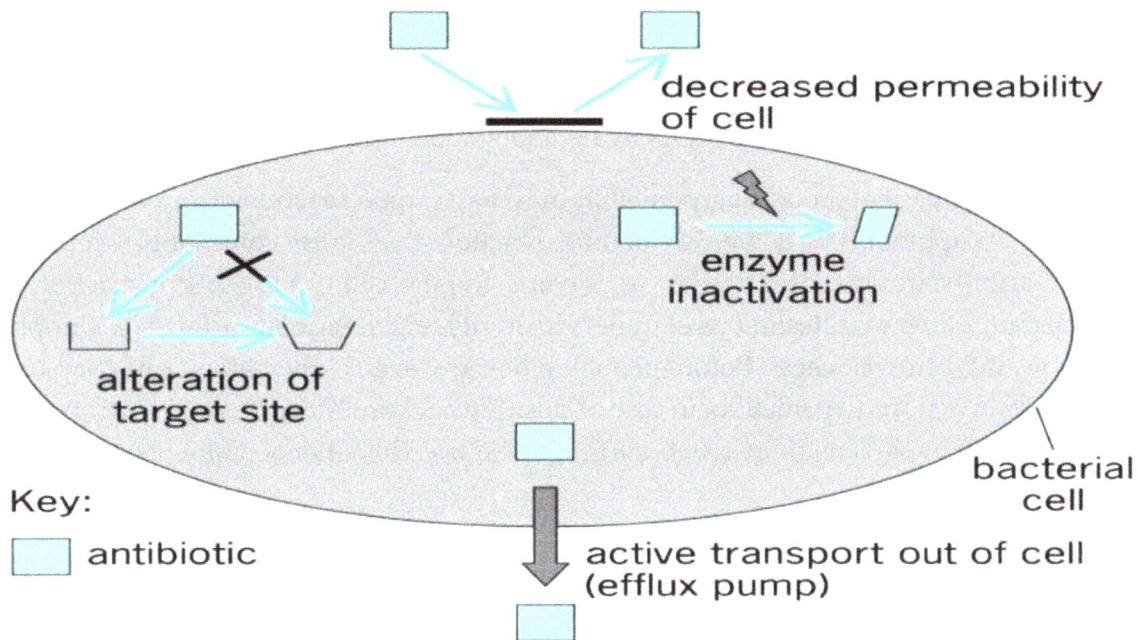

Figure 2. Four common mechanisms of antibiotics resistance. McGraw-Hill Concise Encyclopedia of Bioscience. 2002 by the McGraw-Hill Companies, Inc.

Resistance is formed by the lack of proper diagnosis, the widespread use of antibiotics in hospital, wrong use for patients with a viral infection or still undiagnosed illness and livestock farming and exploiting antibiotics in poultry and food industry (may cause some resistance in the long term) [11]. Clinical signs of resistance include prolonged and chronic infections, increasing disease manifestations and outbreaks, distributing diseases to other organs and increasing the probability of other diseases due to immune system weakening, malnutrition and organ failure. Adverse effects include hypersensitivity reactions to agents, that is, interaction between drugs, cells, organ functions and normal electrolyte concentration. In addition, the presence of background diseases, organ disorders, and physiologic factors such as old age and pregnancy may increase side effects [17].

3. The adverse effects and resistance of the several common antibiotics which are used in oral and maxillofacial surgery

3.1. Penicillins

The base structure of penicillins is a thiazolidine ring which is adherent to the beta-lactam and carries the subordinate amino group (RNH), and in fact, substituents can attach to the amino chain [3]. Natural penicillins are beta-lactam antibiotics and the most important ones are as follows [18]:

- Penicillins (penicillin G) have little activity against Gram-negative rods, and they are susceptible to hydrolysis by beta-lactamases.

- Anti-staphylococcal penicillins (nafcillin) are resistant to staphylococcal beta-lactamases. They are active against staphylococci and streptococci but not against anaerobic bacteria, Gram-negative cocci or rods.

- Extended-spectrum penicillins (aminopenicillins and antipseudomonal penicillins). They are relatively susceptible to hydrolysis by beta-lactamases [3].

More than 10% of patients receiving penicillin may have some reactions from a mild rash to anaphylaxis. Anaphylaxis is a life-threatening reaction that most commonly occurs with parenteral administration. It appears as severe hypotension, bronchoconstriction and abdominal pain. Other manifestations of hypersensitivity reactions include fever, eosinophilia, angioedema and serum sickness. Before penicillin therapy begins, the patient's history should be assessed for reactions to penicillin, in case of positive background, alternative drugs should be used; however, hypersensitivity reactions may occur even in patients with a negative history [18].

3.1.1. Adverse effects

Penicillins are bactericidal and act by interfering with bacterial cell wall synthesis. They infiltrate well into body tissues and fluids. Penetration into the cerebrospinal fluid is poor except when the meninges are inflamed. Allergic situations happen in 1–10% of patients, but anaphylactic reactions occur in less than 0.05% of treated patients. Patients with a history of atopic allergy are at higher risk of anaphylactic reactions to penicillins. Patients who are allergic to one penicillin will be allergic to all. Patients with the background of immediate hypersensitivity to penicillin may also have a reaction to cephalosporin and other beta-lactam antibiotics. Individuals with a history of a minor rash (non-confluent, non-pruritic) or a rash that occurs more than 72 hours after penicillin administration are probably not allergic to penicillin, and penicillin should not be withheld unnecessarily for serious infections [19]. Other side effects are rare, but serious toxic effects of the penicillins are encephalopathy due to intrathecal injection. In renal failure, the accumulation of electrolytes may occur due to either sodium or potassium content in injection. Diarrhea frequently occurs during oral penicillin therapy, and it can also cause antibiotic-associated colitis in a prolonged case [19]. Penicillins are classified as category B. Penicillin is excreted into breast milk in low concentrations and is considered safe to use in breastfeeding women [20, 21]. Exfoliating dermatitis and Stevens-Johnson syndrome are the most severe dermatologic signs. Gastrointestinal adverse effects are most common in response to ampicillin [22]. Aqueous crystalline penicillin G and procaine penicillin G have been implicated in neurological reactions including seizures, neuromuscular instability, confusion and hallucinations [21]. Rarely, penicillin G causes hemolytic anemia [23, 24]. Candidiasis is more common in patients taking broad-spectrum aminopenicillins. Other side effects of natural penicillins include bone marrow suppression, and with high-dose therapy, seizures may occur [18].

3.1.2. Significant interactions

Probenecid increases blood levels of penicillins and may be given alongside for this purpose. Antibiotic antagonism occurs when erythromycin, tetracycline or chloramphenicol is given within an hour after taking penicillin. Prolonged reactions may arise in utilizing penicillin G procaine and benzathine. Penicillin G procaine should not be injected into or near an artery or nerve due to possible permanent neurological damage [3, 18].

Penicillinase-resistant penicillin is not hydrolyzed by beta-lactamases. These agents include methicillin, nafcillin, the isoxazolyl penicillin, dicloxacillin and oxacillin. The penicillinase-resistant group can cause hypersensitivity reactions. Methicillin may cause nephrotoxicity and interstitial nephritis. Oxacillin may be hepatotoxic. The most dangerous situation is methicillin-resistant *Staphylococcus aureus* (MRSA). This bacterium resists numerous antibiotics including methicillin, amoxicillin, penicillin and oxacillin [25]. Wide-ranging cross-resistance exists among the penicillinase-resistant penicillins. Methicillin sodium and nafcillin have been reported to be incompatible with aminoglycosides, acidic and alkaline drugs [26]. Aminopenicillins, because of their broader range, are identified as broad-spectrum penicillins. The incompatibility of ampicillin sodium and aminoglycosides appears to be more evident at higher concentrations and with glucose-containing solutions [26].

Extended-spectrum penicillins have the extensive antibacterial spectrum of all penicillins. Also called antipseudomonal penicillins, this group includes the carboxypenicillin and ureidopenicillin [18]. Hypersensitivity reactions are the other penicillins. Ticarcillin may cause hypokalemia. The high sodium content of ticarcillin can pose a danger to patients with heart failure (HF) and inhibits platelet aggregation [26].

3.1.3. Resistance

Modification of drug penicillin-binding proteins (PBPs) impairs penetration of drug to target PBPs and efflux. Beta-lactamase production is the most common mechanism of resistance. Altered target PBPs are the basis of methicillin resistance in staphylococci and penicillin resistance in pneumococci. These resistant organisms produce PBPs which have low affinity for binding beta-lactam antibiotics. PBP targeting is decreased only in Gram-negative species because of their water-resistant outer cell membrane. Reduced penetration is not sufficient to confer resistance because enough antibiotic ultimately enters the cells. However, this barrier can become important in the presence of the beta-lactamase as long as hydrolyzing the drug is faster than entering the cells. Gram-negative organisms may produce an efflux pump that efficiently transports some beta-lactam antibiotics from the periplasm back across the outer membrane [27].

3.2. Cephalosporins

The cephalosporins are a class of beta-lactam antibiotics originally derived from the fungus Acremonium, and they also constitute a subgroup of beta-lactam antibiotics called cephems, and both are based upon the cephem nucleus. Unlike most cephalosporins, cephamycins are a very effective antibiotic group against anaerobic microbes. Cephamycins include cefoxitin, cefotetan and cefmetazole which are often grouped with the second-generation cephalosporins. The structure of most of the cephalosporins contains N-methylthiotetrazole side chain, and when it becomes metabolized in the body, it releases free N-methyl-thiotetrazole which can cause hypoprothrombinemia (due to the inhibition of vitamin K enzyme, epoxide reductase) and a reaction with ethanol similar to performing by disulfiram, due to inhibition of aldehyde dehydrogenase [3]. Cephalosporins are similar to penicillins but more stable to many bacterial beta-lactamases; therefore, they have a broader spectrum of activity.

3.2.1. First generation

They are very active against Gram-positive cocci; however, they are not active against methicillin-resistant strains of staphylococci. Oral therapy should not be relied on in serious systemic infections.

3.2.2. Second generation

They have extended Gram-negative efficacy. Cephamycins have activity against anaerobes. The oral second-generation cephalosporins are active against beta-lactamase-producing organisms [3].

3.2.3. Third generation

They have an expanded Gram-negative coverage, and some of them are able to cross the blood-brain barrier. Third generation acts against beta-lactamases; however, they should be avoided in enterobacter infections because of the emergence of resistance [3, 5].

3.2.4. Fourth generation

They are more resistant to hydrolysis by chromosomal beta-lactamases (those produced by Enterobacter) [3].

3.2.5. Fifth generation

Beta-lactam antibiotics with activity against methicillin-resistant staphylococci are currently under progress, for instance ceftaroline fosamil is the first drug to be approved for clinical use. Ceftaroline has better binding to penicillin-binding protein 2a which facilitates methicillin resistance in staphylococci. It is not active against AmpC or extended spectrum beta-lactamase-producing organisms [3].

3.2.6. Adverse effects

Reactions can be allergic or toxic or both [3]. Common adverse drug reactions (>1%) include rash, diarrhea, electrolyte instabilities, nausea, pain and inflammation at injection site. Rare side effects (0.1–1%) include vomiting, headache, dizziness, oral candidiasis, pseudomembranous colitis, eosinophilia, neutropenia, hemolytic anemia, nephrotoxicity, thrombocytopenia and fever. Some other adverse reactions are pruritus, Stevens-Johnson syndrome, vaginitis, increased hepatic transaminases, thrombocytosis, phlebitis, increased BUN and creatinine, renal failure and anaphylaxis. Some cephalosporins have reactions when they are combined and utilized such as encephalopathy, asterixis neuromuscular excitability, seizure, aplastic anemia, interstitial nephritis, PT prolonged, agranulocytosis, cholestasis and erythema multiform [5]. A potentially life-threatening arrhythmia has been reported in patients who received a rapid bolus cefotaxime injection via central line, and granulocytopenia and more rarely agranulocytosis may develop through long treatment (>10 days) [3, 5]. Secondary to biliary obstruction possibly due to ceftriaxone-calcium precipitates, pancreatitis has been reported rarely by using ceftriaxone [3, 5]. Cross-allergenicity appears to be most common among penicillins, carbapenems, aminopenicillins and early-generation (group I and II) cephalosporins due to sharing the same R-1 side chains. Patients with documented penicillin anaphylaxis have an increased risk to cephalosporins. Previously, extensive warnings of 10% cross-reactivity had been given, but nowadays, in the absence of proper alternatives, oral cefixime or cefuroxime, injectable cefotaxime, ceftazidime and ceftriaxone are used with precaution [4]. Local irritation can produce pain after intramuscular injection and thrombophlebitis after intravenous injection [3, 5, 28]. Cephalosporins may cause increased international normalized ratio (INR) particularly in nutritional-deficient patients, extended treatment, hepatic and renal disease. Long usage may result in fungal or bacterial superinfection particularly with renal impairment [5]. The pregnancy risk factor is B. Small amounts of cephalosporins are excreted in breast milk but most are not harmful, however, have influence on bowel flora [5].

3.2.7. Drug interactions

Uricosuric agents may decrease the excretion of cephalosporins. Cephalosporins may increase the anticoagulant effect of vitamin K antagonists. Tablets containing sodium caseinate can cause allergic reactions in patients with milk protein hypersensitivity. Cephalexin may increase the serum concentration of metformin. Antacids, H2-antagonists and food may decrease the absorption of cephalosporin [5]. Calcium salts (intravenous) and every fluid containing calcium may enhance the adverse/toxic effect of ceftriaxone due to the formation of an insoluble precipitate. Some test interactions might be changed such as positive direct Coombs, false-positive urinary glucose, false-positive serum or urine creatinine [5, 16].

Resistance to cephalosporin antibiotics can involve either reduced affinity of existing PBP components or the acquisition of a supplementary beta-lactam-insensitive PBP. Currently, some *Citrobacter freundii*, *Enterobacter cloacae*, *Neisseria gonorrhea* and *Escherichia coli* strains are resistant [3, 28]. Other beta-lactam drugs such as monobactams and aztreonam are drugs with a monocyclic beta-lactam ring; their spectrum of activity is limited to aerobic Gram-negative rods. Their Gram-negative spectrum is similar to the third-generation cephalosporins.

3.3. Beta-lactamase inhibitors (clavulanic acid, sulbactam and tazobactam)

These substances look like beta-lactam molecules and have weak antiseptic action. They can protect hydrolysable penicillins from inactivation. Beta-lactamase inhibitors are available only in fixed combinations with specific penicillins [5].

Carbapenems are structurally related to other beta-lactam antibiotics. It is resistant to most beta-lactamases but not carbapenemases or metallo-beta-lactamases. Methicillin-resistant strains of staphylococci are resistant. The dosage must be reduced in the case of renal insufficiency [3]. The most common adverse effects of carbapenems as imipenem are gastrointestinal signs, skin rashes and reactions at the infusion sites. Patients allergic to penicillins may be allergic to carbapenems, but the incidence is low [5].

3.4. Glycopeptide antibiotics

Vancomycin is an antibiotic produced by Streptococcus and *Amycolatopsis orientalis*. It is active only against Gram positives [3]. Resistance to vancomycin is due to reform of the D-Ala-D-Ala binding site of the peptidoglycan building block with conversion to D-lactate and thickened cell wall with increased numbers of D-Ala-D-Ala which serve as dead-end binding sites for vancomycin. Vancomycin is effective against staphylococci, including those producing beta-lactamase and those resistant to nafcillin and methicillin [5, 6, 29].

Adverse reactions take place in almost 10% of cases. Most reactions are rather slight and reversible. Vancomycin is an irritant to tissue because of phlebitis at the site of injection. Chills and fever may occur. Ototoxicity is rare, and nephrotoxicity is uncommon. However, prescribing another ototoxic or nephrotoxic drug increases the risk of these toxicities. Ototoxicity can be minimized by maintaining peak serum concentrations below 60 mcg/ml. The more common reaction is "red man" syndrome which is caused by the release of histamines. It can be prevented by prolonging the infusion period to 1–2 hours or pretreatment with an antihistamine [3]. Other side effects include tinnitus or vertigo which can be the symptoms of vestibular injury and future bilateral irreversible damage. Elongated therapy or total doses above 25 g may increase the risk of neutropenia. Oral vancomycin is only specified for pseudomembranous colitis due to *C. difficile* and enterocolitis due to *S. aureus* and is not effective for systemic infections. Pregnancy risk factor is B for the oral type and C for intravenous type. Vancomycin may develop the neuromuscular-blocking effect. Nonsteroidal anti-inflammatory drugs (NSAIDs) may decrease the elimination of vancomycin [5].

3.5. Other glycopeptides

Teicoplanin is very similar to vancomycin in the mechanism of action and antibacterial spectrum; telavancin is active with Gram-positive bacteria and potentially teratogenic; hence, it must be avoided in pregnant women. Daptomycin is a new cyclic lipopeptide fermentation creation of *Streptomyces roseosporus*. It may be active against vancomycin-resistant strains of enterococci and *S. aureus*. It should be used with care in renal impairment [3, 29].

3.6. Tetracyclines (tetracycline, doxycycline, minocycline, tigecycline)

Tetracyclines chelate divalent metal ions which can restrict their absorption and activity. Tetracyclines are broad-spectrum bacteriostatic antibiotics that inhibit protein synthesis.

3.6.1. Resistance

Three mechanisms of resistance to tetracycline analogs have been described: 1) impaired influx or increased efflux, 2) ribosome shield due to the production of proteins that interfere with tetracycline binding to the ribosome regularly by Gram positives and 3) enzymatic inactivation. The most important of these is the formation of an efflux pump and ribosomal protection [3, 30].

3.6.2. Adverse reactions

Hypersensitivity reactions to tetracyclines are uncommon. Most adverse effects take place due to direct drug toxicity or modification of microbial flora; moreover, gastrointestinal adverse effects are the most common symptoms. Tetracyclines are readily bound to the calcium deposited in newly formed bone or teeth in young children under 8 years and in the fetus. It can accumulate in fetal teeth, leading to fluorescence, discoloration and enamel dysplasia; therefore, tetracyclines are avoided in pregnancy (category D). Tetracyclines in breast milk can chelate with calcium and interferes with growing teeth. Hepatic necrosis has been reported with daily doses of 4 g or more with intravenous injection. Renal tubular acidosis and Fanconi syndrome have been attributed to the administration of outdated tetracycline; if it is given along with diuretics it may cause nephrotoxicity. Intravenous injection can lead to venous thrombosis. Intramuscular injection produces painful local irritation and should be avoided. Demeclocycline can induce sensitivity to sunlight or ultraviolet light mainly in fair-skinned people [3]. An erythematous rash in sun-exposed parts of the body has been reported to appear in 7–21% of people taking doxycycline. Unlike some other members of the tetracycline group, it may be used in those with renal impairment. Doxycycline is contraindicated in the pediatric treatment of acute bacterial rhinosinusitis. Other reactions of doxycycline are similar to other tetracyclines [3, 5, 17]. Oral tetracyclines should be given in an empty stomach. Meals containing aluminum and magnesium may reduce tetracycline absorption. Other side effects include pericarditis, intracranial pressure increase, bulging fontanels in infants, pseudotumor cerebri, paresthesia, pigmentation of nails, exfoliative dermatitis, insipidus syndrome, discoloration of teeth enamel hypoplasia (young children) and anaphylaxis [5].

3.6.3. Drug interactions

Antacids, bile acid, bismuth, iron, magnesium and zinc salts may decrease the absorption of tetracyclines. Tetracycline derivatives can boost the neuromuscular-blocking effect and may diminish the therapeutic effect of penicillin and increase the toxic effect of retinoic acid and the anticoagulant effect of vitamin K antagonists [3, 5].

3.7. Macrolides (azithromycin, erythromycin)

The macrolides are categorized by a macrocyclic lactone ring to which deoxy sugars are attached. Erythromycin loses activity rapidly at 20°C and at acidic pH. Its activity is enhanced at alkaline pH [3, 17].

Clarithromycin is derived from erythromycin by the addition of a methyl group and has an improved acid stability, but erythromycin-resistant streptococci and staphylococci are also resistant to clarithromycin. The advantages of clarithromycin are lower incidence of gastro-intestinal intolerance and less regular dosing [3].

Macrolides resistance to erythromycin is usually plasmid encoded. Three mechanisms have been recognized: 1) Reduced permeability of the cell membrane, 2) production of esterases that hydrolyze macrolides and modification of the ribosomal binding site and 3) efflux and methylase production are the most important resistance mechanisms in Gram-positive organisms. Fundamental methylase construction confers resistance to structurally unrelated but systematically similar compounds such as clindamycin which share the same ribosomal binding site. However, constitutive mutants which are resistant can be selected and emerge during therapy with clindamycin [3, 17].

3.7.1. Adverse reactions

Anorexia and gastrointestinal signs are common, and they occur due to a direct stimulation of gut motility, and it is the most common reason for discontinuing erythromycin and substituting another antibiotic. Erythromycins, particularly the estolate type, can produce acute cholestatic hepatitis probably as hypersensitivity reaction but is reversible. Macrolides have been associated with rare (QTc) = QT Interval of the electrocardiogram prolongation and ventricular arrhythmias, including torsade de pointes; extensive use may result in fungal or bacterial superinfection [3, 5].

3.7.2. Disease-related concerns

Macrolides should be used with caution in coronary artery disease (CAD), in the elderly, myasthenia gravis, with narrowing of the gastrointestinal (GI) tract (may cause obstruction) and severe renal impairment. Pregnancy risk factor is B for erythromycin and C for clarithro-mycin. Macrolides can decline the metabolism of benzodiazepines, calcium channel blockers, carbamazepine, cisapride, antifungal agents, clozapine, colchicine, corticosteroids, cyclospor-ine, theophylline derivatives and vitamin K antagonists and may increase the serum concen-tration of alosetron, cardiac glycosides, fentanyl, salmeterol and tacrolimus. Macrolides may diminish the therapeutic effect of clopidogrel, the metabolism of HMG-CoA reductase inhibitors and some SSRIs [3, 5, 17].

Azithromycin is derived from erythromycin by the addition of methylated nitrogen into the lactone ring and different from clarithromycin mainly in pharmacokinetic properties. How-ever, azithromycin penetrates into most tissues (except cerebrospinal fluid) and phagocytic cells extremely well. Antacids do not alter the bioavailability but delay absorption and reduce peak serum concentrations. Because they have a 15-element (not 14) lactone ring, they do not inactivate cytochrome P450 enzymes [3]. Other reactions are similar to macrolides [5, 17].

Ketolides are semisynthetic 14-membered-ring macrolides, differing from erythromycin by substitution of a 3-keto group for the neutral sugar L-cladinose which is permitted for limited clinical use. It is active in vitro against *Streptococcus pyogenes*, *S. pneumonia* and *S. aureus*. Many macrolide-resistant strains are susceptible to ketolides because the basic modifications of these compounds change as poor substrates for efflux pump-mediated resistance, and they bind to ribosomes of some bacterial species with higher affinity than macrolides. It may slightly prolong the QTc interval. The use of ketolides can cause hepatitis and liver failure and are also contraindicated in patients with myasthenia gravis [3, 17].

3.8. Lincosamides

Clindamycin is a chlorine-substituted derivative of lincomycin, an antibiotic that is produced by *Streptomyces lincolnensis* [3]. Clindamycin, like erythromycin, inhibits protein synthesis by interfering with the formation of initiation complexes and with aminoacyl translocation reactions. The binding site for clindamycin is on the 50S subunit. It is often active against community-acquired strains of methicillin-resistant *S. aureus* [5, 17]. Ordinary adverse effects are diarrhea, nausea and skin rashes. Impaired liver function and neutropenia occur occasionally [3]. Physicians must use clindamycin carefully in patients with hepatic impairment. Some products may contain benzyl alcohol which has been related to "gasping syndrome" in neonates, and some others may have tartrazine which causes allergic reactions in certain persons. Elderly patients have a higher risk of developing severe colitis. Clindamycin is excreted in breast milk, and thus it is suggested to suspend drug intake. Lincosamide may diminish the therapeutic effect potential of erythromycin [3, 5, 17].

3.9. Streptogramins

They share the same ribosomal binding site as macrolides and clindamycin, and it is active against Gram-positive cocci, multidrug-resistant strains of streptococci, penicillin-resistant strains of *S. pneumoniae*, methicillin-susceptible and resistant strains of staphylococci. Resistance may occur due to alteration of the quinupristin binding site (MLS-B type resistance), enzymatic inactivation of dalfopristin or efflux. Quinupristin-dalfopristin is permitted for the treatment of infections caused by staphylococci or by vancomycin-resistant strains of *E. faecium*. The major toxicities are infusion-related events, such as pain at the infusion site and an arthralgia-myalgia syndrome [3, 31].

3.10. Oxazolidinones

Linezolid is an affiliate of the oxazolidinones, a novel class of synthetic antimicrobials. It is active against Gram-positive organisms. Its resistance is caused by the mutation of linezolid binding site on 23S ribosomal RNA. Linezolid is confirmed for use in vancomycin-resistant *E. faecium* infections, health care-associated pneumonia and community-acquired pneumonia. Tedizolid is a next-generation oxazolidinone with high potency against Gram-positive bacteria such as methicillin-resistant *S. aureus*. Possible benefits over linezolid include bigger impact against staphylococci and one daily dosing [3, 6]. The main toxicity of linezolid is hematologic which is reversible and commonly minor. Thrombocytopenia is the most common sign when the drug is ordered for use more than 2 weeks. Optic and peripheral neuropathy and lactic acidosis have been reported with long courses of linezolid. There are reports of serotonin syndrome arising when linezolid is co-participated with serotonergic drugs [3, 5].

3.11. Aminoglycosides

They are used broadly in combination with a beta-lactam antibiotic in serious infections with Gram-negative bacteria and with vancomycin or a beta-lactam antibiotic for Gram-positive endocarditis. Acidic pH and anaerobic conditions inhibit the passage across the cell membrane into the cytoplasm by reducing the gradient. Transport may be improved by cell wall-active drugs such as penicillin or vancomycin [3, 32]. Aminoglycosides are absorbed very poorly from the intact gastrointestinal tract.

3.11.1. Adverse effects

The threshold is not precisely defined for the beginning of toxicity, but concentrations above 2 µg/mL are perilous [5]. All aminoglycosides are ototoxic and nephrotoxic, and they are more likely to emerge when therapy is persistent for more than 5 days, with higher doses, in the elderly and in renal failure. Parallel consumption with loop diuretics or other nephrotoxic antimicrobial agents (vancomycin or amphotericin) can create nephrotoxicity. Ototoxicity can appear as auditory damage (tinnitus and high frequency hearing loss) or as vestibular impairment (vertigo, ataxia, loss of balance). Neomycin, kanamycin and amikacin are the most ototoxic drugs. Streptomycin and gentamicin are the most vestibulotoxic. Neomycin, tobramycin and gentamicin are the most nephrotoxic. Aminoglycosides can produce a curare-like effect, in high doses, with neuromuscular blockade. This reaction is usually reversible by calcium gluconate or neostigmine. Hypersensitivity occurs intermittently [3, 5].

Gentamicin is effective against both Gram-positive and Gram-negative organisms and has no activity against anaerobes. Resistance emerges in staphylococci during monotherapy. Gram-negative bacteria resistance is most commonly due to plasmid-encoded aminoglycoside-modifying enzymes. Gram negatives which are gentamicin-resistant generally are vulnerable to amikacin. Low pH and low oxygen pressure create poor environment for drug activity [5, 32].

3.11.2. Gentamicin adverse reactions

Nephrotoxicity is usually reversible. It occurs in 5–25% of patients consuming gentamicin for longer than 3–5 days. Ototoxicity, which is permanent, shows itself as vestibular dysfunction. Gentamicin has a rare hypersensitivity reaction. Pregnancy risk factor is C (ophthalmic, topical) and D (injection).The nephrotoxic effect of aminoglycosides may be enriched with amphotericin B, cisplatin, cyclosporine, colistimethate, loop diuretics and vancomycin. Aminoglycosides may increase the hypocalcemic effect of bisphosphonate derivatives and the neuromuscular-blocking effect of Botulinum toxin type A and Botulinum toxin type B. Some penicillins may accelerate the degradation of aminoglycosides in vitro. This may be clinically significant for certain penicillin (ticarcillin, piperacillin, carbenicillin) and aminoglycoside combination therapy in patients with significant renal impairment. Close monitoring of aminoglycoside levels is warranted [5, 32].

Tobramycin, like other aminoglycosides, is ototoxic and nephrotoxic. Nephrotoxicity of tobramycin may be slightly less than that of gentamicin.

Amikacin is semisynthetically derived from kanamycin; it is less toxic than the near relative molecule. It is resistant to many enzymes that inactivate gentamicin and tobramycin; therefore, it can be used against some resistant microorganisms. Similar to all aminoglycosides, amikacin is nephrotoxic and ototoxic [3, 5, 17].

3.12. Sulfonamides

The basic structure of the sulfonamides has similarity to p-amino benzoic acid (PABA). Sulfonamides are more soluble in alkalosis than in acidosis. It can be prepared with sodium salts which are utilized for intravenous injection. Sulfonamides deter Gram-positive and Gram-negative bacteria. Its activity is reduced against anaerobes. *Pseudomonas aeruginosa* is certainly resistant to sulfonamide antibiotics. A mixture of a sulfonamide with an inhibitor of dihydrofolate reductase (trimethoprim) is synergistic due to sequential inhibition of folate synthesis [3, 5].

3.12.1. Resistance

Several bacteria, like mammal cells, do not have the crucial enzymes for folate synthesis from PABA and depend on exogenous sources; therefore, they are not vulnerable to sulfonamides. Sulfonamide resistance may take place by mutations that cause high production of PABA and production of a folic acid-synthesizing enzyme that has low affinity for sulfonamides or impermeability to the sulfonamide. In significant renal failure, the dosage must be reduced. The previous susceptible species such as meningococci, pneumococci, streptococci, staphylococci and gonococci are now resistant [3, 5, 32].

3.12.2. Adverse reactions

Traditionally, drugs with the basic structure of sulfonamide including antimicrobial sulfas, diuretics, diazoxide and the sulfonylurea hypoglycemic drugs are measured to be cross-allergenic. The most common adverse effects are fever, skin rashes, exfoliative dermatitis, photosensitivity, gastrointestinal signs and difficulties due to urinary tract problems. Stevens-Johnson syndrome is uncommon, and potentially fatal type of skin or mucous membrane eruption may be appeared. They may precipitate in acidic urine producing crystalluria or obstruction. This is rarely a problem with the more soluble sulfonamides such as sulfisoxazole. Sulfonamides have also been associated in various types of nephrosis. They can cause hemolytic or aplastic anemia and may incite hemolysis in patients with G6PD. Sulfonamides taken near the end of pregnancy increase the risk of kernicterus [3, 5].

3.13. Trimethoprim and trimethoprim-sulfamethoxazole

Trimethoprim selectively inhibits bacterial dihydrofolic acid reductase for repelling the synthesis of purines and DNA. Trimethoprim or pyrimethamine by merging with a sulfonamide can block folate synthesis (synergism). It is active against most *Staphylococcus aureus* strains, both methicillin-susceptible and methicillin-resistant and against respiratory tract pathogens.

Resistance to trimethoprim results from reduced cell permeability, overproduction of dihydrofolate reductase or production of an altered reductase with reduced binding. Mutation due to plasmid-encoded causes rapid and widespread trimethoprim resistance.

3.13.1. Adverse effects

Anti-folate activity causes megaloblastic anemia, leukopenia and granulocytopenia, and with the trimethoprim-sulfamethoxazole mixture, all reactions connected to sulfonamides may occur. Patients with AIDS and pneumocystis pneumonia have a particularly high frequency of reactions to this mixture (fever, rashes, leukopenia, diarrhea, hepatic enzymes rising, hypoglycemia, hyperkalemia, hyponatremia) [3, 5, 29]. It should be used with cautiousness in patients with allergies or asthma, hepatic and renal impairment, thyroid dysfunction, in the elderly, G6PD deficiency and folate deficiency. Trimethoprim can increase the hyperkalemic effect of ACE Inhibitors and the adverse effect of amantadine. It may decrease the metabolism of thiazolidinedione, repaglinide, procainamide and the excretion of lamivudine. Sulfamethoxazole can boost the myelosuppressive effect of azathioprine and cyclosporine. Procaine may reduce the activity of trimethoprim. Sulfonamides and trimethoprim may decrease the metabolism of phenytoin [5, 29].

3.14. Fluoroquinolones—DNA gyrase inhibitors

Quinolones are synthetic fluorinated analogs of nalidixic acid. They are active against Gram-positive and Gram-negative bacteria. Methicillin-resistant strains of staphylococci are often resistant [3, 33]. Quinolones as whole are divided into three groups including nalidixic acid, the first generation with better effect on Gram negatives, ciprofloxacin as the second and moxifloxacin as the third generation. In some references they are divided into two groups based on antimicrobial spectrum and pharmacology [3, 34]. Gemifloxacin and moxifloxacin have better action against Gram-positive organisms while older fluroquinolones have moderate effects on Gram positive as well as Gram negative [3, 34].

Resistance appears in around one of every 107–109 bacteria, especially staphylococci, *P. aeruginosa* and *Serratia marcescens*. Resistance will be appeared in the quinolone-binding region of the target enzyme with mutations or by changing the permeability; recently, two forms of plasmid-mediated resistance have been defined. The first utilizes Qnr proteins which protect DNA gyrase from the fluoroquinolones; the second is an aminoglycoside acetyltransferase capable of modifying ciprofloxacin. Resistance to one fluoroquinolone normally confers cross-resistance to all of this class [3, 34].

3.14.1. Adverse effects

Fluoroquinolones are typically well tolerated. The most common side effects are nausea, vomiting and diarrhea. Intermittently, some interactions are headache, dizziness, insomnia, skin rash and high liver function tests. Prolongation of the QTc interval may occur with levofloxacin, gemifloxacin and moxifloxacin; therefore, it must be used with care to QTc interval prolongation and hypokalemia. Due to impaired cartilage growth and arthropathy by fluoroquinolones, they are not prescribed for patients under 18 years. Nevertheless, if arthropathy is reversible, it may be feasible for the treatment of pseudomonal infections in some patients with cystic fibrosis. Fluoroquinolones should be suspended during pregnancy due to lack of data verifying their safety. Neuropathy can appear and may continue for several months or years during and after treatment; in some cases it may be perpetual [3]. Fluoroquinolones have been related to serious and occasionally fatal hypoglycemia especially in elderly patients with diabetes, but it has been reported in cases without a previous history of diabetes [5, 33].

3.15. Moxifloxacin

It is effective on Gram-positive bacteria. Side effects include tremor, restlessness, confusion and rarely hallucinations or seizures; must be used with caution in cases with known or suspected CNS disorders [5]. Reactions may present as typical allergic symptoms or can present as severe idiosyncratic dermatologic disorder (Stevens-Johnson, toxic epidermal necrolysis, vasculitis). Pneumonitis, nephritis, hepatic failure or necrosis and cytopenias are frequently seen after multiple doses. Patients must avoid excessive sunlight because of moderate-to-severe phototoxicity reactions [5, 6]. Prolonged use can produce fungal or bacterial superinfection. It should be used carefully in patients with significant bradycardia or acute myocardial ischemia, hepatic impairment, myasthenia gravis, rheumatoid arthritis, elderly and G6PD deficiency. Safety and efficacy of moxifloxacin have not been established in children, but in pregnancy, the risk factor is category C [5]. All these adverse effects are rare or about 1–2%, and it may also have some other reactions less than 1% such as hyperlipidemia, hyper or hypotension, hypoesthesia, laryngeal edema, nightmares, paresthesia, pelvic pain, peripheral neuropathy, decreased prothrombin time, speech disorder, taste loss, abnormal thinking, tinnitus, tongue discoloration, arrhythmia and vision abnormalities [3, 5]. It may increase the QTc-prolonging effect. Antacids, magnesium, iron and zinc salts may decrease the absorption of quinolone antibiotics (oral tables), but it is not affected by taking with a high-fat meal, yogurt or sodium bicarbonate. Quinolone antibiotics may expand the toxic effect of corticosteroids (systemic) and the effect of vitamin K antagonists. Insulin and sulfonylureas may increase the hyperglycemic or hypoglycemic effects. The neurotoxicity or seizure-potentiating effect might increase with NSAIDs [5, 33].

3.16. Ciprofloxacin

It has moderate effects on both Gram-negative and Gram-positive bacteria. In consequence of its extensive usage even for minor infections which are curable with older and narrower spectrum antibiotics, many bacteria have developed resistance in recent years. Numerous pathogens, including enterococci, *Streptococcus pyogenes* and *Klebsiella pneumonia*, have become resistant [33]. Most side effects are similar to other fluoroquinolone drugs above. Alkaline urine may escalate the risk of crystalluria. In patients over 60 years, rupture of the Achilles' tendon may take place. Due to secretion in breast milk and because of damage to joint cartilage, it should be avoided during breast feeding; the pregnancy risk factor is C [3, 5, 17]. Intravenous injection must be slow to avoid the risk of venous irritation. Oral tablets should be taken with food to minimize GI distress. Consuming large quantities of caffeinated drinks may pose a danger due to cardiac or CNS reactions. Ciprofloxacin can reduce the serum concentration of phenytoin and theophylline derivatives [3, 5].

3.17. Metronidazole

It is a nitroimidazole antibiotic and antiprotozoal drug. Metronidazole is absorbed selectively by anaerobic bacteria and sensitive protozoa and does not affect any human cells directly or aerobic bacteria [3, 17].

3.17.1. Adverse reactions

It has been found to be carcinogenic in rats [35]. Chronic treatment causes seizures and neuropathies; if this occurs, therapy must be withdrawn. It should be used with restriction in patients with a history of seizure disorder and CNS disease. Metronidazole should be utilized carefully in patients with blood dyscrasias, the elderly, heart failure or other sodium-retaining states, liver impairment and severe renal failure (creatinine clearance less than 10 mL/min). The pregnancy risk factor is B and should be avoided in the first trimester. Other reactions include flattening the T-wave, flushing, ataxia, dizziness, fever, headache, insomnia, irritability, seizure, vertigo, erythematous rash, Disulfiram-like reaction, dysmenorrhea, nausea (very common), abdominal cramping, constipation, diarrhea, furry tongue, stomatitis, metallic taste, xerostomia, cystitis, darkened urine (rare), incontinence, neutropenia (reversible), thrombocytopenia (reversible), peripheral neuropathy, nasal congestion, rhinitis, sinusitis, pharyngitis, flu-like syndrome and moniliasis [3, 5, 35].

Metronidazole can increase the toxic effect of alcohol (ethyl). It may augment the toxic effect of amprenavir, tipranavir, disulfiram and mebendazole (risk for Stevens-Johnson syndrome). It may increase the serum level of busulfan, fentanyl and salmeterol. This drug may reduce the metabolism of calcineurin inhibitors and vitamin K antagonists. It may affect the enzymes aspartate transaminase (AST), and alanine transaminase (ALT) for Liver function test, triglycerides, glucose and LDH tests. Metronidazole may possibly cause mood fluctuation [36].

4. Nanoantibiotics

4.1. Introduction

Nanoscience in association with medicine can bring new opportunities for scientists to introduce novel solutions against medical complications. In recent years, the development of innovative drugs to combat multi-drug resistant (MDR) bacteria is growing strongly [28–30, 32, 37–40]. The advantage of nanoantibiotic therapy is to proficiently decrease a variety of side effects which originate from conventional antibiotics; furthermore, a specific nanostructure can be synthesized for a distinctive goal since the production process is safe, inexpensive and innovative.

As biocompatibility, low toxicity and noticeable purity of antibacterial nanoparticles are vital for medical treatments, in the near future the conventional methods of nanoantibiotic assembly such as sonication [41–43] and chemical routes [44] will be replaced by laser-assisted generation of nanoparticles (NPs) in liquids since no chemical precursors are required [45–49]. Shape and size of the nanoparticles play an essential role in the antibacterial behavior of nanoparticles, as a case in point the average size of 1–10 nm demonstrated a dominant antibacterial activity [50]; therefore, laser ablation in particular liquids along with controlled laser parameters can design nanomaterials with desired shape, size and composition in a very strategic mechanism without using surface active agents which can trigger surface impurity and toxicity. The large surface area to volume ratio is a main property of nanomaterial which increases the antibacterial activity. Co-delivery process of two or more drugs can be efficiently achievable by using nanomaterials [51]; antibiotic resistance is significantly avoided since nanoparticles do not enter the bacterial cell, and its mechanism of killing bacteria is fundamentally done via direct contact with the bacterial cell wall [52]. There are critical procedures which occur during nanoantibiotic therapy; as nanomaterials electrostatically bind to the bacterial cell wall, they can induce membrane destruction and depolarization which initiate cell death [53–55]. Nanomaterials with extremely high surface area can catalyze the production of reactive oxygen species (ROS) which have a critical potential to damage bacterial cells [56].

4.2. Essential nanocarriers for drug delivery

Antibacterial drugs due to their fast degradation, low water-solubility, cytotoxicity to healthy tissues and weak membrane transportation are fairly hard to manage; nanoparticles including dendrimers, liposomes and polymer-based nanoparticles can simplify drug delivery against infectious diseases. Dendrimers as a tree-like structure with many branches with typical size of 10 nm were used in drug delivery and diagnostic systems. Liposome nanoparticles in the size range of 50–200 nm were broadly used for drug delivery system initially proposed in the 1970s [57]. Liposomes with a distinctive bilayer lipid structure are able to transfer hydrophobic and hydrophilic compounds without any chemical alteration; they can proficiently combine with bacterial membranes and release antibacterial agents to their cell membranes. In order to extend liposome longevity and stability in the blood stream, they can easily be functionalized with biocompatible polyethylene glycol (PEG) by forming a stealth layer on the liposome surface [58, 59]. Biocompatible chitosan nanoparticles with nontoxic nature, high antibacterial activity and high stability can encapsulate or embed drugs in the polymeric network. Hydrogels with biocompatible hydrophilic networks allow delivery of hydrophilic and small-molecule drugs. Highly porous silica nanoparticles are well known for local drug delivery to reduce cytotoxicity and side effects [60–62].

Metal-based nanoparticles including nickel, tungsten, gadolinium, gold, silver, zinc oxide, titanium dioxide and iron oxide nanoparticles were commonly used for diagnosis and delivery. A critical disadvantage is toxicity from the accumulation of metal nanoparticles in the human body after treatment; therefore, drug delivery process should be performed in a very strategic way.

Zinc oxide nanoparticles (ZnO NPs) with potent antibacterial activity were designed as enzyme-nanoparticle conjugates in order to improve mono-dispersity and stability of nano-antibiotics during treatment; extremely greater antibacterial behavior was obtained by using positively charged lysozyme enzyme covalently bonded to ZnO nanoparticles [63].

Interestingly not only nanoparticles but also ions can demonstrate very strong antibacterial activity. Researchers at Rice University discovered that only silver ions behave destructively to the bacteria. Delivered silver ions can stimulate lysis in which the membrane of the bacterial cell breaks down and causes bacterial cell death [64].

The release of antibiotics can be prolonged by using nanocarriers for drug delivery systems to reduce extremely antibiotic resistance. Gold nanoparticles capped with glutathione can bring a higher rate of gentamicin loading; these capped gold nanoparticles which were covalently attached to gentamicin revealed strong antimicrobial activity with extended release of antibiotic over several days [65].

4.3. Antibacterial activity of core-shell nanoparticles

Recently, scientists were accentuated over designing of biocompatible core-shell nanoparticles for antibacterial activity, controlled drug release and targeted drug delivery [66]. Core-shell nanoparticles are advantageous in contrast to single nanoparticles because of their advanced properties such as high stability, great dispersity and efficient functionality.

Silver-titanium dioxide (Ag-TiO$_2$) core-shell nanoparticles presented strong antibacterial activity against infectious diseases as a result of releasing silver ions from silver cores through the porous matrix of titanium dioxide shells; one can assume in such a core/shell assembly is the extension of the release time of silver ions which can be beneficial for a persistent antibacterial effect [67].

Gold-copper sulfide (Au-CuS) core-shell nanoparticles demonstrated extreme capability to deactivate *B. anthracis* cells by disordering and damaging its cell membrane; furthermore, antibacterial activity depends on nanoparticle concentration and treatment time [68]. The antimicrobial activity of nanoparticles and microbial cell death can be related to the electrostatic interaction between negatively charged bacterial cells and positively charged nanoparticles which stimulates the loss of membrane integrity [69]. The negatively charged bacterial cell wall composition has a thick layer of peptidoglycan which is linked to teichoic acid. Osmotic imbalance and cytoplasmic content leakage of the damaged membrane probably initiate the cell disintegration.

Alumina-coated iron oxide magnetic nanoparticles (Fe$_3$O$_4$-alumina core-shell MNPs) as a photothermal factor under near-infrared (NIR) illumination were used to selectively destroy bacteria. Alumina coating triggers the targeting ability of Fe$_3$O$_4$ magnetic nanoparticles in the direction of bacteria. The magnetic behavior of Fe$_3$O$_4$/alumina nanoparticles allows them to accumulate in the desired region under a magnetic field and photothermally destroys them by NIR irradiation at the populated region. Remarkably, the cell growth of nosocomial bacteria (Gram positive, Gram negative) and antibiotic resistance can be efficiently avoided in over

95% by applying 10 minutes irradiation via NIR laser beam at the accumulated region of core/shell Fe3O4-alumina MNPs [70].

Core-shell silica-gold nanoparticles were represented loading a significant amount of gentamycin about 87 µg/mg for drug targeting process. Silica core particles were prepared by Stober's method and functionalized with amine groups. Amine group of gentamycin was attached to the gold nano shell surface, and the drug releasing from core-shell nanoparticles was simply prepared by breaking the gold-gentamycin coordinate linkers [71].

Core-shell silica-polyrhodanine nanoparticles were synthesized by chemical oxidation polymerization; they revealed brilliant antimicrobial activity against Gram-positive *Staphylococcus aureus*. In fact, biocidal activity of these nanoparticles was improved by increasing the surface area to volume ratio; core/shell NP size can be experimentally modified by changing the silica core diameter [72].

Novel mesoporous silica nanoparticles were efficiently loaded with chlorhexidine (CHX) which is generally used as antimicrobial agent in dentistry; they were synthesized with an average particle diameter of 140 nm and pore size of around 2.5 nm. Nano-CHX core-shell nanoparticles exhibited promising antimicrobial activity against critical oral pathogens including *S. mutans, S. sobrinus, F. nucleatum, A. actinomycetem comitans* and *E. faecalis* [73].

Hybrid core-shell zinc oxide-silver (ZnO-Ag) nanorods presented remarkable antibacterial activity against *Staphylococcus aureus* and *Pseudomonas aeruginosa*. Silver nanoparticles with an average size of about 7 nm were designed on heterojunctions at the surface of the ZnO nanorods. The probable mechanism derives from the generation of reactive oxygen species due to electron transfer between zinc oxide nanorods and silver nanoclusters which triggers physical destruction of the bacterial cell wall [74].

5. Conclusion

The normal human body has an intrinsic order which is known as physiology; when a bacterial infection occurs, human cells occasionally need help to defend themselves; therefore, various antibiotics have roles to assist cells, and at the same time, some interactions may take place among antibiotics and human cells then side effects appear. Adverse reactions can be predicted by recognizing the normal situation, background diseases, spectrum of antibiotic effects and mechanism of action. Nowadays, due to extensive use of antibiotics in many fields such as veterinary, agriculture, farming, food industries, and exaggerative prophylaxis, bacteria have a greater chance to resist with mutation, selection and gene transferring; therefore, action against bacterial infection should be with caution, proper drug doses, good background hygiene, adequate therapy, synergism, novelty in treatment and enhanced diagnosis should be considered; one of these innovative treatments is nanoantibacterial therapy. Nanoantibiotics revealed innovative mechanisms against infectious diseases in comparison with conventional drug delivery procedures. Biocompatibility, low toxicity and pronounced purity of antibacterial nanomaterials have prepared them appropriately for therapeutic processes as an auspicious alternative in medicine to decrease antibiotic resistance and cytotoxicity in a very efficient way.

Author details

Esshagh Lasemi[1], Fina Navi[1*], Reza Lasemi[2] and Niusha Lasemi[3]

*Address all correspondence to: fina_navi@yahoo.com

1 Department of Oral and Maxillofacial Surgery, Dental Branch, Islamic Azad University, Tehran, Iran

2 Department of Public Health, Medical University of Vienna, Vienna, Austria

3 Department of Physical Chemistry, Vienna University, Vienna, Austria

References

[1] Hupp, J. R., M. R. Tucker, et al. (2014). Contemporary Oral and Maxillofacial Surgery, 6th Edition, Elsevier. 3251 Riverport Lane St. Louis, Missouri 63043 CONTEMPORARY ORAL AND MAXILLOFACIAL SURGERY, SIXTH EDITION: ISBN: 978-0-323-09177-0 Copyright © 2014 by Mosby, an affiliate of Elsevier Inc. Copyright © 2008, 2003, 1998, 1993, 1988 by Mosby, Inc.

[2] Giedraitienė, A., A. Vitkauskienė, et al. (2011). "Antibiotic resistance mechanisms of clinically important bacteria." Medicina (Kaunas) 47(3): 137–146.

[3] Katzung, B. G., S. B. Masters, et al. (2015). Basic & Clinical Pharmacology, Thirteenth Edition Copyright © 2015 by McGraw-Hill Education. Printed in the United States of America.

[4] Cephalosporins and Other Beta-Lactams (2008). British National Formulary, 56 Edition, London: BMJ Publishing Group Limited and Royal Pharmacentical Society Publishing. p. 295.

[5] American Pharmacists Association. Editors: Judith A. Aberg, Kenneth A. Bachmann, Verna L. Baughman, Matthew M. Cooney, Amy Van Orman et al.Meagan McCord Lexi-Comp, Inc.1100 Terex Road Hudson, Ohio 44224

[6] Miloro, M., G. Ghali, et al. (2012). Peterson's Principles of Oral and Maxillofacial Surgery, 3rd Edition, Publisher: PMPH - USA (People's Medical Publishing House), 2011

[7] Brook, I. (2005). "Microbiology of Acute and Chronic Maxillary Sinusitis Associated with an Odontogenic Origin." The Laryngoscope 115(5): 823–825.

[8] Brook, I. (2002). "Antibiotic resistance of oral anaerobic bacteria and their effect on the management of upper respiratory tract and head and neck infections." Semin Respir Infect 17(3): 195–203.

[9] Brook, I. (1981). "Aerobic and anaerobic bacterial flora of normal maxillary sinuses." The Laryngoscope 91(3): 372–376.

[10] Leekha, S., C. L. Terrell, et al. (2011). "General principles of antimicrobial therapy." Mayo Clin Proc 86(2): 156–167.

[11] The Evolving Threat of Antimicrobial Resistance – Options for Action, World Health Organization (2012), Authors:World Health Organization. WHO Press, World Health Organization, 20 Avenue Appia, 1211 Geneva 27,Switzerland.

[12] Pana, M. (2012). Antibiotic Resistant Bacteria – A Continuous Challenge in the New Millennium, Published by InTech Janeza Trdine 9, 51000 Rijeka, Croatia

[13] Frieden, T. R. (2013). Meeting the Challenge of Drug-Resistant Diseases in Developing Countries, Centers for Disease Control and Prevention CDC. National Antimicrobial Resistance Monitoring 1600 Clifton Road Atlanta, GA 30329-4027 USA 800-CDC-INFO (800-232-4636), TTY: 888-232-6348.

[14] Montazem, A. (1998). "Antibiotic Prophylaxis in Dentistry." Mount Sinai School of Medicine 65: 388–392.

[15] Lee, H. H., M. N. Molla, et al. (2010). "Bacterial charity work leads to population-wide resistance." Nature 467(7311): 82–85.

[16] West, S. A., A. S. Griffin, et al. (2006). "Social evolution theory for microorganisms." Nat Rev Micro 4(8): 597–607.

[17] Ritter, J., L. Lewis, et al. (2008). A Textbook of Clinical Pharmacology and Therapeutics, This fifth edition published in Great Britain in 2008 by Hodder Arnold, an imprint of Hodden Education, part of Hachette Livre UK, 338 Euston Road, London NW1 3BH

[18] Shargel, L., A. H. Mutnick, et al. (2013). Comprehensive Pharmacy Review for NA-PLEX, 8th Edition, Lippincott Williams & Wilkins, New York, USA: 2013

[19] Joint Formulary Committee (2014–2015). British National Formulary BNF, Royal Pharmaceutical Society, 66-68 East Smithfield, London, E1W 1AW

[20] Hale, T. W. (2000). Medication and Mothers' Milk. A Manual of Lactational Pharmacology, 9th Edition, Amarillo (TX): Pharmasoft Publishers.

[21] Wright, A. J. (1999). "The Penicillins." Mayo Clinic Proceedings 74(3): 290–307.

[22] Holten, K. and E. Onusko (2000). "Appropriate prescribing of oral beta-lactam antibiotics." Am Fam Physician 62(3): 611–620.

[23] Kuhn, M. Pharmacotherapeutics: A Nursing Process Approach, 3rd Edition. Pharma-cotherapeutics: A Nursing Process Approach.Edited by Merrily Mathewson - Daemen College, Amherst, New York. New edition of Brandon, USA.

[24] Gleckman, R. and J. Czachor (2000). "Antibiotic side effects." Sem Resp Crit Care Med 21: 53–60.

[25] Methicillin-resistant Staphylococcus aureus (MRSA) Infections, CDC, Last updated 28 May 2014, this publication belong to Centers for Disease Control and Prevention, 1600 Clifton Rd, Atlanta, GA 30333, United States. http://www.cdc.gov/. Accessed 11 June 2014.

[26] Sweetman, S. (2009). Martindale: The Complete Drug Reference, 36th Edition, Martindale: The Complete Drug Reference, London, UK.

[27] Katzung, B. G., S. B. Masters, et al. (2012). Basic and Clinical Pharmacology, 12th Edition, Chapter 43, McGraw-Hill Education. Printed in the United States of America.

[28] Botnarciuc, M., I. Stan, et al. (2015). "Cephalosporin resistant bacterial strains isolated from respiratory infections." ARS Medica Tomitana 21: 7.

[29] Paul, M., J. Bishara, et al. (2015). "Trimethoprim-sulfamethoxazole versus vancomycin for severe infections caused by meticillin resistant *Staphylococcus aureus*: randomised controlled trial." BMJ 2015; Vol: 350 doi: http://dx.doi.org/10.1136/bmj.h2219.

[30] Peng, S., Y. Wang, et al. (2015). "Long-term application of fresh and composted manure increase tetracycline resistance in the arable soil of eastern China." Sci Total Environ 506–507: 279–286.

[31] Gurk-Turner, C. (2000). "Quinupristin/dalfopristin: the first available macrolide-lincosamide-streptogramin antibiotic." Proceedings (Baylor University. Medical Center) 13(1): 83–86.

[32] Wanxiang, L., L. Jing, et al. (2015). "Characterization of aminoglycoside resistance and virulence genes among Enterococcus spp. isolated from a hospital in China." Int J Environ Res Public Health 12(3): 3014.

[33] Jacoby, G. A. (2005). "Mechanisms of Resistance to Quinolones." Clinical Infectious Diseases 41(Supplement 2): S120–S126.

[34] O'Neil, M., P. Heckelman, et al. (2007). The Merck Index, 14th Edition, Merck & Co., Inc., Whitehouse Station, NJ, USA.

[35] The American Society of Health-System Pharmacists. AHFS DI Monographs, AHFS DI from the American Society of Health-System Pharmacists'(ASHP) is the most comprehensive source of unbiased and authoritative drug information available to health professionals today. A wholly independent staff of drug information pharmacists and other professional editorial and analytical staff thoroughly research AHFS DI content. Authors incorporate clinical research findings, therapeutic guidelines, and Food and

Drug Administration (FDA) approved labeling to ensure that monographs include an evidence-based foundation for safe and effective drug therapy. Retrieved 31 July 2015.

[36] Karamanakos, P., P. Pappas, et al. (2007). "Pharmaceutical agents known to produce disulfiram-like reaction: effects on hepatic ethanol metabolism and brain monoamines." Int J Toxicol 26(5): 423–432.

[37] World Health Organization, 20 Avenue Appia,1211 Geneva 27, Switzerland - Design and Layout: www.paprika-annecy.com Reprinted June 2014, Printed in France.

[38] Gelband, H., M. Miller-Petrie, et al. (2015). The State of the World's Antibiotics, Chapter 1, 14–24. 1400 Eye Street, CENTER FOR DISEASE DYNAMICS, ECONOMICS 0026 POLICY 1400 Eye Street, NW Suite 500 Washington, DC 20005 USA

[39] Neu, H. C. (1992). "The crisis in antibiotic-resistance." Science 257: 1064–1073.

[40] Alanis, A. J. (2005). "Resistance to antibiotics: are we in the post-antibiotic era?" Arch Med Res 36: 697–705.

[41] Moradi, S., P. A. Azar, et al. (2008). "Preparation of nickel nanoparticles under ultrasonic irradiation." J Appl Chem Res (2008) 2(2): 43-51.

[42] Kasap, S., H. Tel, et al. (2011). "Preparation of TiO2 nanoparticles by sonochemical method, isotherm, thermodynamic and kinetic studies on the sorption of strontium." J Radioanalytical Nucl Chem 289(2): 489–495.

[43] Elsupikhe, R., K. Shameli, et al. (2015). "Green sonochemical synthesis of silver nanoparticles at varying concentrations of k-carrageenan." Nanoscale Res Lett 10(1): 916.

[44] Rajput, N. (2015). "Methods of preparation of nanoparticles – a review." Int J Adv Eng Technol 7(4): 1806–1811.

[45] Patil, P. P., D. M. Phase, et al. (1987). "Pulsed-laser-induced reactive quenching at liquid-solid interface: aqueous oxidation of iron." Phys Rev Lett 58(3): 238–241.

[46] Mafune, F., J. Y. Kohno, et al. (2000). "Formation and size control of silver nanoparticles by laser ablation in aqueous solution." J Phys Chem B 104(39): 9111–9117.

[47] Kabashin, A. V. and M. Meunier (2003). "Synthesis of colloidal nanoparticles during femtosecond laser ablation of gold in water." J Appl Phys 94(12): 7941–7943.

[48] Barcikowski, S. and G. Compagnini (2012). "Advanced nanoparticle generation and excitation by lasers in liquids." Phys Chem Chem Phys 15(9): 3022–3026.

[49] Lasemi, N., O. Bomati-Miguela, et al. (2015). Laser Ablation Synthesis of Colloidal Dispersions of Nickel Nanoparticles. 16th Austrian Chemistry Days, Joint Meeting of the Italian and Austrian Chemical Societies, University of Innsbruck, Gesellschaft Österreichischer Chemiker: GÖCH.

[50] Subramani, K., W. Ahmed, et al. (2012). Nanobiomaterials in Clinical Dentistry, Elsevier, 225 Wyman Street, Waltham,02451,USA

[51] Emeje, M. O., O. I. C, et al. (2012). Nanotechnology in Drug Delivery.

[52] Beyth, N., Y. Houri-Haddad, et al. (2015). "Alternative antimicrobial approach: nano-antimicrobial materials." Evidence-Based Complementary and Alternative Medicine 2015: 16.

[53] Pelgrift, R. Y. and A. J. Friedman (2013). "Nanotechnology as a therapeutic tool to combat microbial resistance." Adv Drug Deliv Rev 65(13–14): 1803–1815.

[54] Huh, A. J. and Y. Kwon, J. (2011). "Nanoantibiotics: a new paradigm for treating infectious diseases using nanomaterials in the antibiotics resistant era." J Control Release 156(2): 128–145.

[55] Blecher, K., A. Nasir, et al. (2011). "The growing role of nanotechnology in combating infectious disease." Virulence 2(5): 395–401.

[56] Slauch, J. M. (2011). "How does the oxidative burst of macrophages kill bacteria? Still an open question." Mol Microbiol 80(3): 580–583.

[57] Bangham, A. D. (1983). Liposome Letters, London: Academic Press.

[58] Zhang, L., D. Pornpattananangku, et al. (2010). "Development of nanoparticles for antimicrobial drug delivery." Curr Med Chem 17(6): 585–594.

[59] Nikalje, A. P. (2015). "Nanotechnology and its applications in medicine." Med Chem 5(2): 081–089.

[60] Tripathy, N., R. Ahmad, et al. (2014). "Tailored lysozyme-ZnO nanoparticle conjugates as nanoantibiotics." Chem Commun 50(66): 9298–9301.

[61] Salouti, M. and A. Ahangari (2014). Nanoparticle Based Drug Delivery Systems for Treatment of Infectious Diseases.

[62] Rabea, E., M. Badawy, et al. (2003). "Chitosan as antimicrobial agent: applications and mode of action." Biomacromolecules 4(6): 1457–1465.

[63] Tripathy, N., R. Ahmad, et al. (2014). "Tailored lysozyme-ZnO nanoparticle conjugates as nanoantibiotics." Chem Commun 50(66): 9298–9301.

[64] Xiu, Z. M., Q. B. Zhang, et al. (2012). "Negligible particle-specific antibacterial activity of silver nanoparticles." Nano Lett 12(8): 4271–4275.

[65] Perniab, S. and P. Prokopovich (2014). "Continuous release of gentamicin from gold nanocarriers." RSC Adv 4: 51904–51910.

[66] Ghosh Chaudhuri, R. and S. Paria (2012). "Core/shell nanoparticles: classes, properties, synthesis mechanisms, characterization, and applications." Chem Rev 112(4): 2373–2433.

[67] Lin, Y., W. Qiqiang, et al. (2011). "Synthesis of Ag/TiO2 core/shell nanoparticles with antibacterial properties." Bull. Korean Chem. Soc. 2011, Vol. 32, No.8 page: 2607-2610.

[68] Addae, E., X. Dong, et al. (2014). "Investigation of antimicrobial activity of photothermal therapeutic gold/copper sulfide core/shell nanoparticles to bacterial spores and cells." J Biol Eng 8(11): 1–11 DOI: 10.1186/1754-1611-8-11.

[69] Hamouda, T. and J. R. Baker Jr (2000). "Antimicrobial mechanism of action of surfactant lipid preparations in enteric Gram-negative bacilli." J Appl Microbiol 89(3): 397–403.

[70] Yu, T. J., P. H. Li, et al. (2011). "Multifunctional Fe_3O_4/alumina core/shell MNPs as photothermal agents for targeted hyperthermia of nosocomial and antibiotic-resistant bacteria." Nanomedicine 6(8): 1353–1363.

[71] Amirthalingam, T., J. Kalirajan, et al. (2011). "Use of silica-gold core shell structured nanoparticles for targeted drug delivery system." J Nanomedic Nanotechnol 2(119): 1–5, doi: 10.4172/2157-7439.1000119.

[72] Song, J., H. Song, et al. (2011). "Fabrication of silica/polyrhodanine core/shell nanoparticles and their antibacterial properties." J Mater Chem 21(48): 19317–19323.

[73] Seneviratne, C. J., K. C. F. Leung, et al. (2014). "Nanoparticle-encapsulated chlorhexidine against oral bacterial biofilms." PLoS ONE 9(8): e103234.

[74] Ponnuvelu, D. V., S. P. Suriyaraj, et al. (2015). "Enhanced cell-wall damage mediated, antibacterial activity of core–shell ZnO@Ag heterojunction nanorods against *Staphylococcus aureus* and *Pseudomonas aeruginosa*." J Mater Sci Mater Med 26(7): 1–12.

7

Management of the Oroantral Fistula

Guhan Dergin, Yusuf Emes, Cagrı Delilbası and
Gokhan Gurler

Abstract

Communication between the maxillary sinus and oral cavity is a common complication in oral surgery. It results mainly from maxillary premolar and molar extractions when the sinus floor is close to the tooth apex. It can also occur after an infection involving the maxillary teeth, invasion of the sinus cavity by a cyst or carcinoma, trauma, the Caldwell-Luc operation, or other dentoalveolar or implant procedures. Openings smaller than 2 mm may heal spontaneously, whereas larger openings require surgical treatment. An oroantral fistula (OAF) may develop as a complication of dental extractions, as a result of infection, or as sequelae of radiation therapy, trauma, and removal of maxillary cysts or tumors. Various techniques have been examined for the closure of oroantral communications. However, the most common question is how to provide better healing of the defect area and the donor site. In this chapter, etiology, clinical features, medical and surgical managements of OAFs, and advantages and disadvantages of different closure methods of closure techniques are discussed in this chapter.

Keywords: oroantral fistulas, maxillary sinus, flaps, oral surgery, oral cavity

1. Introduction

An abnormal connection between the oral and antral cavities is defined as an oroantral communication (OAC). OAC between the maxillary sinus and oral cavity is a common complication in oral surgery, resulting mainly from premolar and molar extractions when the sinus floor is close to the tooth apex and separated by a thin bony lamella [1–3]. In physiologic circumstances, maxillary sinus mucosa thickness ranges from 1 to 7 mm [4, 5] but in some cases, when the bony floor of the antrum is resorbed by periapical infections or cysts the risk of an

OAC increases. It can also occur after an invasion of the sinus cavity by cysts and tumors, maxillofacial surgical procedures such as indirect or direct sinus lifts, dentoalveolar-grafting operations or corrective surgery such as orthognathic surgeries. OACs can also occur due to trauma [1, 3]. Epithelialization of a communication between the oral cavity and the maxillary sinus forms a pathologic tract, which is called an oroantral fistula (OAF). Various techniques have been described for the closure of OAFs. However, the question is how to provide better healing of the defect area and the donor site. In this chapter, etiology, clinical features, and medical and surgical management methods of OAFs are discussed.

2. Etiology

The most common cause of the OACs is the extraction of the posterior teeth, which have their roots in close relationship to the maxillary sinus. Even though earlier studies have pointed to the second premolars as the highest risk of OAC during extraction [6], later studies have reported that the molar teeth have their roots in the closest proximity to the sinus floor [7–10]; Güven [11] has stated that in his study, second molar extraction followed by first molar had the highest risk. OACs as a result of tooth extraction are the most common in the third decade of life and encountered mostly in adults with few posterior teeth, in which the maxillary sinuses are enlarged. Due to their underdeveloped small maxillary sinuses, the risk of OAC during extraction is very low in children. General consensus is that the OACs must be closed within 24–48 h to prevent fistula and sinusitis [12, 13].

Infections, cyst-, and tumor-removal operations performed in the posterior maxilla and trauma can also lead to the formation of an OAC. OACs can be encountered following a sinus augmentation procedure due to infection of graft material or an improper incision during the operation. Nedir et al. [14] reported the formation of an OAC after the failure of a dental implant in the second molar region. The implant, which was placed 10 years after a sinus-lift procedure and the loss of osseointegration, led to the removal of the implant, causing an OAC. Maxillary osteonecrosis due to the use of bisphosphonates can cause sinusitis and OAF, and when indicated in these patients, the removal of the necrotic bone may cause an OAC [15].

3. Clinical findings and diagnosis

Air and fluids passing into the nose and mouth are the main clinical findings following the formation of an OAC. The clinician may see blood bubbles in the defect or the patient may sense the leakage of air when blowing while nostrils are closed. Usually, patients complain of an unpleasant salty discharge into the mouth from the opening, odor, and reflux of fluids and foods into the nose from the mouth or leakage of air, which sometimes makes it difficult to smoke. Patients may also experience resonance of their sound and speech problems if the defect is large. Suctioning of the socket may create a hollow sound that shows communication. Sinus membrane can be sometimes intact. Therefore, great attention should be paid during the exploration of the perforation with probing or suctioning methods that may lacerate the sinus membrane, which may sometimes be intact [16, 17].

The presence of one or more of these mentioned symptoms could be the indicator of an OAC or a fistula, while some patients may not show any of these findings if the passage is too small or closed by a large polyp. To validate clinical findings, the clinician needs to radiologically examine the site via a panoramic radiograph or a computed tomography (CT). Dental tomography gives clear data about the perforation and its size if the defect is closed by a polyposis or a granulation tissue [18].

4. Management of OACs/fistula

As almost all of posterior teeth have the risk of OAC, the clinician must evaluate the patient thoroughly prior to extraction. The relationship between the maxillary teeth apices and the maxillary sinus, cortical thickness of the sinus floor, apical granulomas, and cysts, which may have caused the sinus floor resorption, should be evaluated radiographically. After the extraction, it is safer if wound edges are well approximated and stabilized with sutures if the surgeon suspects a small perforation. Larger perforations may be closed with local flaps [1, 19, 20].

An accidental small perforation during a dentoalveolar surgical intervention, such as drilling in implant surgery, apicoectomy of maxillary teeth, and excision of cysts and tumors, can be repaired intraoperatively if the sinus is not infected. The surgeon should be careful not to close the defect with the excessive tension of the tissues, which may enhance the risk of postoperative wound dehiscence [21].

The main goal of the clinician in the management of OAC/fistula is the closure of the defect and prevention of oral bacteria and food debris penetrating the sinus. These oral contaminants may infect the sinus or induce inflammation, which may cause impaired ciliary function, problems of sinus areolation, congestion, and sinusitis. But before the closure of OAF, symptoms associated with inflammation in the sinus such as persisting pus discharge from OAF, malodor, nasal congestion and discharge, and postnasal drip should be eliminated medically with antibiotics, frequent antral irrigations, and decongestants. Patients should be carefully monitored and should be assessed often if the OAC or fistula has any acute sinusitis symptoms. Regardless of the chosen technique, two main points should be taken into account. First, sinus infection must be treated with adequate nasal drainage. This can be obtained by Caldwell-Luc procedure with nasal gastrostomy or endoscopic sinus surgery. Second is decreasing congestion by nasal decongestant and sterile saline water to obtain natural drainage and areolation from ostium. Avoid using long-term topical nasal decongestants that may cause rebound nasal congestion [16, 22].

5. Surgical management of OAFs

The preference of the technique to close an OAC depends on the size of the defect (which is sometimes difficult to estimate clinically), the health of the surrounding tissues, the health of the maxillary sinus, and the time of diagnosis. Also, postoperative prosthetic planning (e.g., dental-implant planning) should be taken into consideration [19, 23].

Success of the closure of an OAC, or an OAF, is closely related to the health of the involved maxillary sinus. If the drainage of the antrum via mucociliary transportation is impaired and osteomeatal complex is obstructed, a combined approach to the OAC may be necessary [23]. Even though an open approach to the maxillary sinus was used for a long time (Caldwell-Luc operation), functional endoscopic sinus surgery in combination with an intraoral closure technique is currently the treatment of choice in these patients [10, 21, 24].

The closure of the OAFs rarely requires a bony reconstruction except in patients with cleft repair or implant rehabilitation. When intraoral donor sites are insufficient, extraoral sites such as calvarial or anterior iliac crest may be used. Various authors previously described a variety of techniques for the closure of OACs. Agarwal [24] et al. have proposed the suturing of platelet-rich fibrin rolls to the communication site even though they did not mention their indication criteria for this technique. Noel et al. [17] used a pedicle nasoseptal flap in a patient who had previously undergone radiotherapy. The patient they described had an opening of 10 mm, which was closed successfully. The use of allogeneic materials or xenograft or alloplastic materials and the placement of a third molar tooth or a dental implant into the defect have all been proposed for the treatment of OACs. But all these methods are rarely used in the literature and are replaced with soft-tissue management techniques [16].

Several surgical techniques for OAF closure have been introduced in the literature. Buccal and palatal flaps are commonly used methods, while the other local flaps are mostly variations of the two techniques. Distant flaps such as the buccal pedicle fat pad, tongue, and temporal muscle flaps are also used techniques to close OAF. The size and localization of the defect, the presence of acute or chronic infection in the sinus, and the absence of sufficient vestibular depth or keratinized tissue surrounding the defect are all determinately important factors for the preference of surgical technique to close the defect. Additionally, during planning of the flap design, the surgeon should take into account whether it is immediate or delayed, whether there is thick and healthy tissue surrounding the defect, and whether the patient is healthy or medically compromised [16].

5.1. Buccal approach

5.1.1. Buccal advancement flaps

Buccal advancement flaps are among the most commonly used techniques for the OAC closure. This is due to the simplicity of the technique. Even though the literature states that OACs can heal spontaneously when the defect size is smaller than 1–2 mm, this may not be true in every small defect. [8, 11, 25, 26]. Some studies have even reported the spontaneous healing of OACs up to 5 mm size [8]. When there is infection in the communication site and the communication remains open for an extended period of time, this may lead to the formation of an OAF. Due to these facts, most surgeons may prefer buccal advancement flaps as the first treatment of choice even in small communications where closure may be possible by simple suturing [27].

Rehrman's flap and Môczár flap are the two most commonly used buccal advancement flaps. These two flaps may also have disadvantages when compared to simple suturing, because the reflection of a mucoperiosteal flap may result in swelling, and also requires the dentist to have proper training to perform this operation. Another disadvantage of the buccal advancement flap is the risk of losing the depth of the vestibular sulcus, even though the Môczár flap results in less vestibular sulcus flattening according to Vowern [8].

There are flapless closure methods which are simply the placement of resorbable materials into the socket such as oxidized cellulose [28]. These materials maintain a closure by stabilizing the blood clot in the socket. It must be kept in mind that there are currently no generally accepted guidelines to choose the method of closure. This is the reason why these flapless techniques are very commonly used by general practitioners due to their simplicity, which do not require extensive surgical skill. Even though some studies show these simple methods are as effective in obtaining closure as the buccal advancement flap, these studies are not always considered reproducible in terms of the method of analysis of the complications [27, 28]. It is generally not possible to know the exact size of the opening in the sinus floor without reflecting the flap. Therefore, dentists must be careful when deciding to use the flapless techniques and must keep in mind that the defect may be larger than they think it is. A plain radiograph (periapical film or orthopantomograph) can give an idea about the defect size. When an OAC occurs, success rate is very high when immediate closure is obtained. This rate drops significantly when the closure is performed secondarily [1, 29]. Infected tissues, apical cysts, and foreign bodies must be removed from the socket in case they may prevent healing [1, 11, 26].

To perform the buccal flap, two vertical diverging incisions are made at the mesial and distal ends of the socket. The incisions must extend beyond the defect and must lie on healthy bone. After elevation of the mucoperiosteal flap, the gingival edges of the socket are de-epithelialized by a sharp instrument. Then, the flap is positioned palatally and primary closure is obtained by multiple sutures. An apical periosteal release of the flap can sometimes be necessary. Following surgery, an antibiotic should be prescribed. Surgeons may sometimes prescribe postoperative nasal decongestants. When a fistula with sinus infection is present, the infection must be treated first. Some authors recommend daily irrigation of the perforated antrum by antibiotic solutions prior to surgery [30].

Falci et al. [30] have described a modification of this technique in a patient with OAF. They have sutured together the mucosal margins of the fistula prior to the reflection of the buccal flap. Then, the buccal flap was pulled over this sutured site and tucked under the palatal flap, which was elevated simultaneously with the buccal flap.

The main disadvantage of this simple and safe technique is the weak perfusion of the flap, which may lead to failure in the closure of large defects. Yalçın et al. [12] recommend this technique be used for smaller defects. As mentioned earlier, this technique may lead to a flattening of the vestibular sulcus, and in edentulous patients, a secondary vestibuloplasty may be required. In edentulous patients, a palatal flap technique can be preferred especially if the alveolar ridge is severely atrophied. In their study of 23 cases, Yaçın et al. have performed the buccal flap in 10 patients, and a loss of vestibular depth was observed only in 2 patients at the end of 6 months.

Buccal advancement flaps can be safely preferred in dentate patients with no alveolar resorption and a bony defect of less than 5 mm size in the sinus floor for the immediate closure of the OAC. Buccal flaps can be used in edentulous patient also if the fistula is on the buccal side of the alveolar crest [12]. Despite an initial successful closure, both the patient and the surgeon must be aware that there is always a risk of a recurring OAF formation [21]. Neuschl et al. [31] have reported a very rare complication, in which the duct of the parotid gland was iatrogenically sutured into the maxillary sinus during the closure of an OAC using a buccal flap.

5.1.1.1. Technique

After the fistula tract is excised, the trapezoidal buccal mucoperiosteal flap is reflected and the lateral wall of the maxilla exposed. Horizontal releasing incisions are made at the most apical part of the flap, which helps to move and extend the flap to the defect without tension. After flap release, it can be advanced upon the defect and sutured to palatal tissue (**Figure 1a–c**).

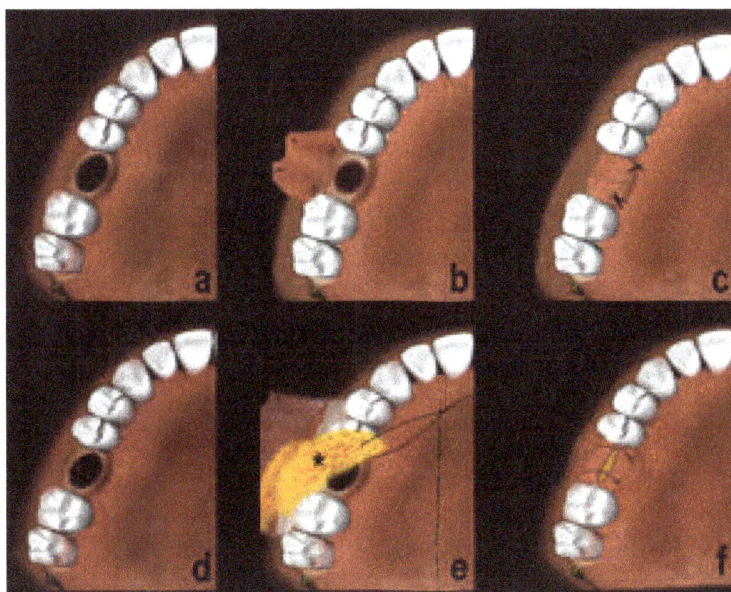

Figure 1. Illustration of buccal flaps: (a—c) Buccal advancement flap technique, (d—e) buccal fat-pad flap.

5.1.2. Buccal fat-pad flap

Another common buccal approach to OACs is the use of the buccal fat pad (BFP). The use of the BFP for the treatment of OAFs was first simply an alternative to the closure of small- and medium-sized defects; however, nowadays it is also used for large bony defects. The technique was first described by Egyedi in the late 1970s [32], and its use became more common following a study by Tideman et al. [33], which showed that the BFP epithelialized within 3–4 weeks. The technique is used not only in the treatment of OAFs but also in the reconstruction of medium-sized maxillary defects (as in tumor excisions) [34–36]. The buccal fat-pad flap has 10 ml of fat tissue. The fat pad is approachable through the oral cavity, and the buccal and temporal branches of the maxillary artery, facial artery, and superficial temporal artery perfuse it sufficiently, which make it a good choice as a material to close medium-sized defects of the maxilla [37].

The incision is similar to the buccal flap technique. In order to expose the BFP, the periosteum is incised behind the zygomatic buttress. The fat pad is manipulated by pressing extraorally below the zygomatic arc. Then, the fat pad is sutured to the palatal tissues, covering the fistula.

The success of the technique has been reported by many authors. Mohan et al. used the technique in 11 patients for various pathologies including pleomorphic adenoma excision, and observed partial loss of the graft only in one patient and hematoma in another patient [38]. Martin-Granizo et al. [39] have reported the successful application of the technique in their patients, even in those who have had partial necrosis of the flap. Nezafati et al. [40] performed a study comparing the buccal flap and buccal fat-pad flap techniques, and concluded that both were similarly successful. Infection of fat tissue is the main problem of this technique.

5.1.2.1. Technique

A circular incision with a 3-mm margin is made around the defect (**Figure 2**), the epithelial tract with any inflammatory tissue was completely excised, and two vertical incisions extended into the vestibule are made.

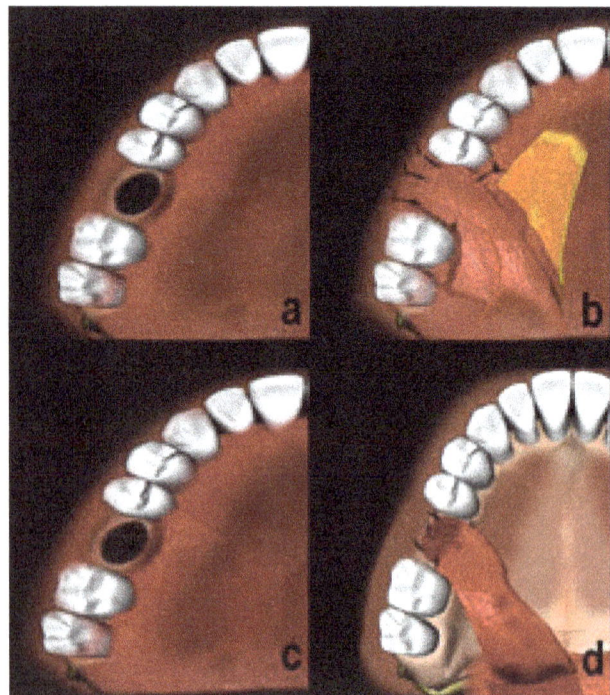

Figure 2. (a—c) Illustration of full-thickness rotational flap, (b—d) tongue flap technique for closure of large oroantral defects.

The trapezoidal buccal mucoperiosteal flap is reflected and the lateral wall of the maxilla is exposed. Buccal fat is exposed with a vertical incision through the periosteum posterior to the zygomatic buttress. Applying external pressure below the zygomatic arch helps herniation of the BFP. Following gentle extraction, the BFP is released with meticulous dissection via scissors. After gaining sufficient length, the flap is advanced to the oral defect from behind the molar teeth and was fixed on the fistula by absorbable polydioxanone sutures over the fat pad, which was gently advanced over the bong defect (**Figure 3**), and secured with sutures (**Figure 4**). Finally, the mucoperiosteal flap is replaced in its original position with sutures inserted between the BFP and the buccal flap. The fat is left exposed in the mouth without any coverage (**Figure 1d–f**).

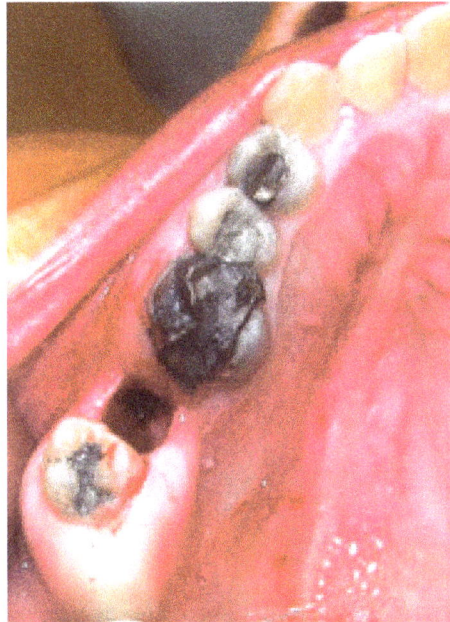

Figure 3. Excised fistula wall at the right maxillary molar region.

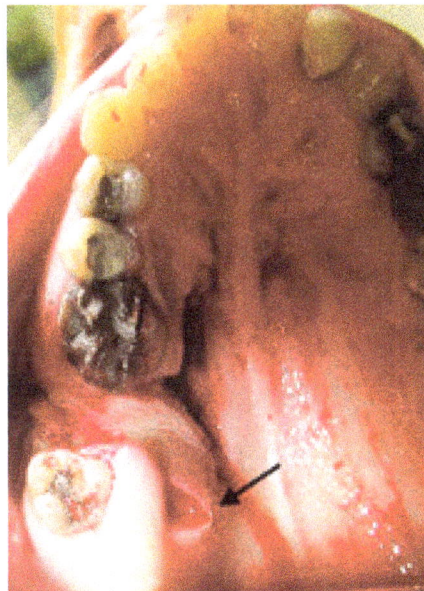

Figure 4. Dog-ear formation at full-thickness rotational flap at rotating point (marked with arrow).

5.1.3. Palatal flaps

The palatal flap has different forms that can be classified as straight-advancement, rotation-advancement, hinged, pedicle island, anteriorly based, submucosal connective tissue pedicle, and submucosal island flaps [1, 10].

5.1.4. Full-thickness palatal flap

Full-thickness rotational palatal flaps have the advantages of keratinized tissue, preservation of vestibular depth, and sufficient blood supply for better healing. However, the thick keratinized tissue limits rotation if the OAF is located at the maxillary tuberosity [1, 41]. With full-thickness palatal rotational flaps, at the pivot point, kinking or "dog-ear" formation can occur during flap rotation, which may compromise the vascular supply, predispose the patient to venous congestion, and impair the adaptation of the distal part of the flap. Kruger suggested that a V-shaped section be excised in the area of the greatest bend in the flap to prevent folding and wrinkling [3]. With full-thickness palatal rotational flaps, the technique exposes the bony structure of the hard palate and sometimes is required for re-epithelialization, causing severe complaints such as pain, burning, and edema of the hard palate.[13] There is also a risk of necrosis of the exposed bone at the donor site, especially in systemically compromised patients. Erdogan et al. [42] reported unexpected palatal bone necrosis in diabetics after the use of full-thickness palatal rotational flaps. Using a palatal stent is recommended after palatal rotational flap operations to reduce the edema and to stabilize the flap in its new position [43].

5.1.4.1. Technique

In the full-thickness mucoperiosteal palatal rotational flap technique, the flap design is arranged according to the greater palatine artery. About 1-cm length of additional flap is created to achieve tension-free closure of the fistula on the buccal bony base. Bone defect and

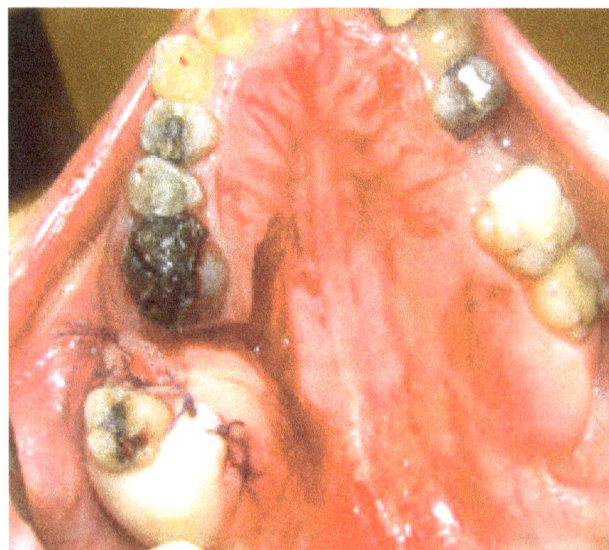

Figure 5. Dog ear was removed and adapted to defect and closed with full-thickness rotational flap.

angle of rotation are the key points in determining the width of the flap. Kinking formation at the rotation point of the flap should be evaluated; if dog-ear formation exists, it should be excised to obtain a better adaptation (**Figures 2 a–c** and **3–6**).

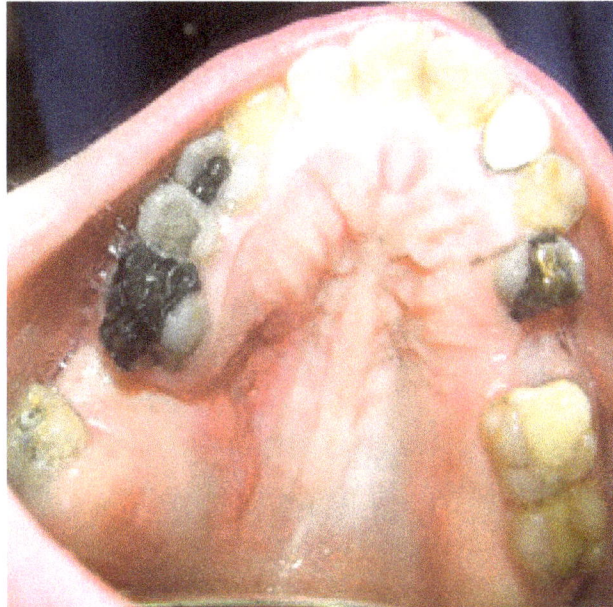

Figure 6. Healing of the fistula. After closing with FTPF (full-thickness palatal flap).

5.1.5. Modified submucosal connective tissue flap

Dergin et al. [44] reported a modified submucosal connective tissue flap for OAF repair. With a modified connective tissue flap, there is no folding or dog-ear formation because of its elasticity and it allows for better manipulation and adaptation in the closure of an OAF in the second and third molar region. In modified connective tissue flap techniques, all of the donor sites were closed with mucosal flaps that covered the underlying bone. In the modified connective tissue flap, no palatal acrylic plate is required postoperatively.

Ito and Hara [45] modified the pedicle palatal flap by developing a submucosal connective tissue pedicle flap, and reported that dividing the flap into an upper mucosal layer and underlying connective tissue layer overcomes the problem of bone exposure at the donor site. Healing at the donor site occurs within 1 month. The technique owes its success to the good blood supply and mobility without tension [46]. The only disadvantages of this technique are the difficulty of the dissection, possibility of injuring the blood supply, and the need for an experienced surgeon [45, 46].

The connective tissue-based pedicle palatal flap technique described by Dergin et al. [44] differs from the technique of Ito and Hara [45] in the design of the mucosal flaps and the preparation of the submucosal tunnel. Preparing a long, narrow mucosal flap carries a risk of necrosis and infection of the overlying mucosal flap at the donor site.

5.1.5.1. Technique

In the modified palatal connective tissue flap technique (**Figure 7a**), an H-type window-like incision was made in the palatal mucosa 4 mm from the gingival margins of the molar and premolar teeth, with the medial incision 2–3 mm from the midline. The fistula wall is excised circumferentially and the granulation tissue is curetted (**Figure 8**).

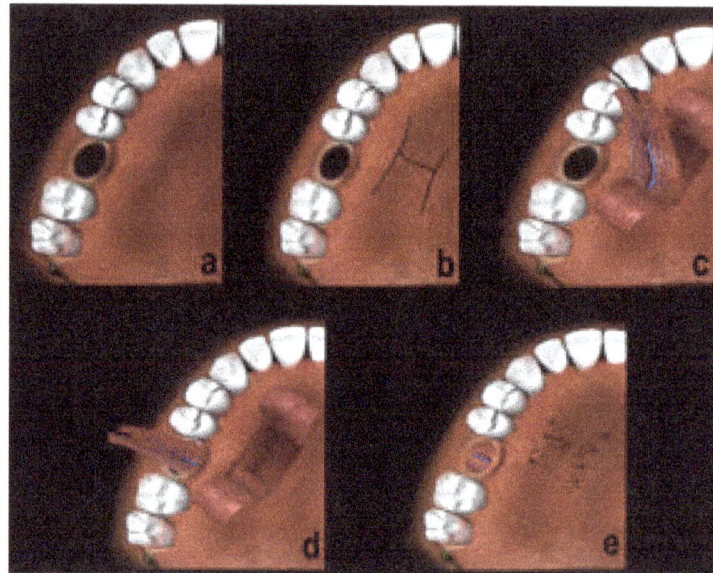

Figure 7. Illustration of the modified connective tissue technique a: excised fistulas wall, b: H incision, c: arterial palatal connective tissue window-like flaps and dissection of arterial connective flap, d: palatal tunnel maneuver, e: suturing.

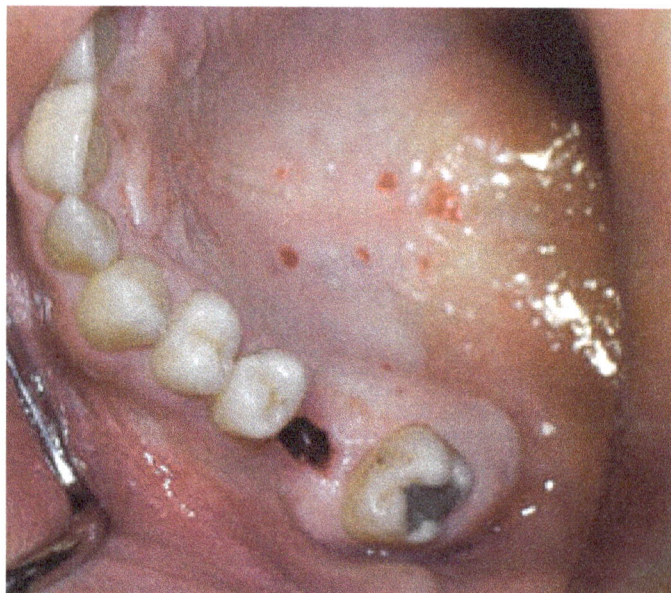

Figure 8. Oroantral fistula with excised fistula wall.

After excising the fistula, the mucosa of the two minor flaps of the H-type window-like incision (**Figures 7b** and **10**) was elevated and separated from the underlying connective tissue without jeopardizing the continuity of the mucosal flap (**Figure 9**).

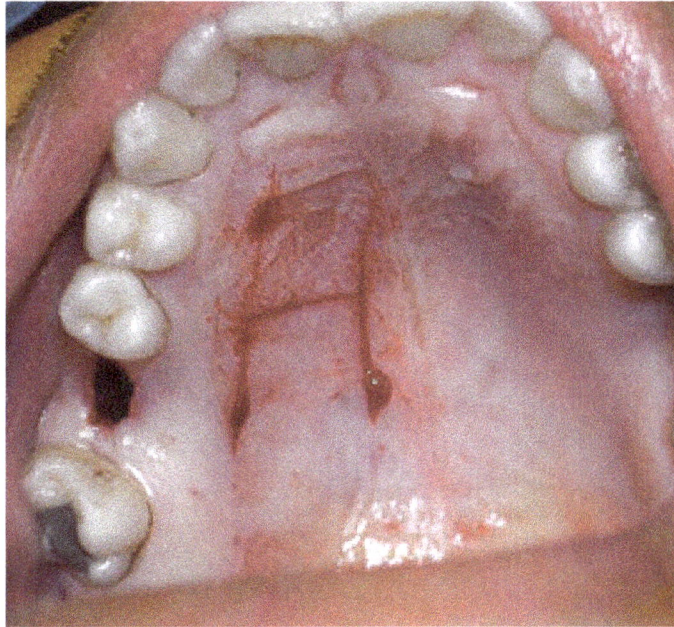

Figure 9. Intraoperative view of H-type incision.

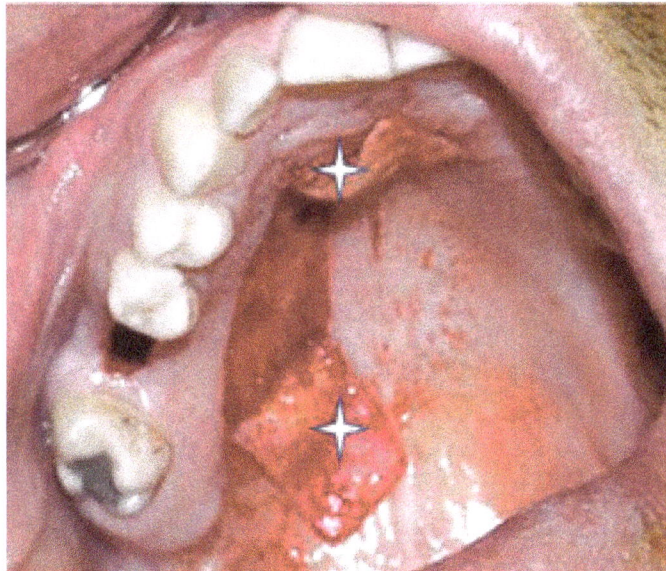

Figure 10. Elevated window-like mucosal H flap (marked with stars).

The underlying arterialized connective tissue was first dissected in the premolar-canine region, where the incisive and greater palatine arteries anastomose (**Figures 7c** and **11**).

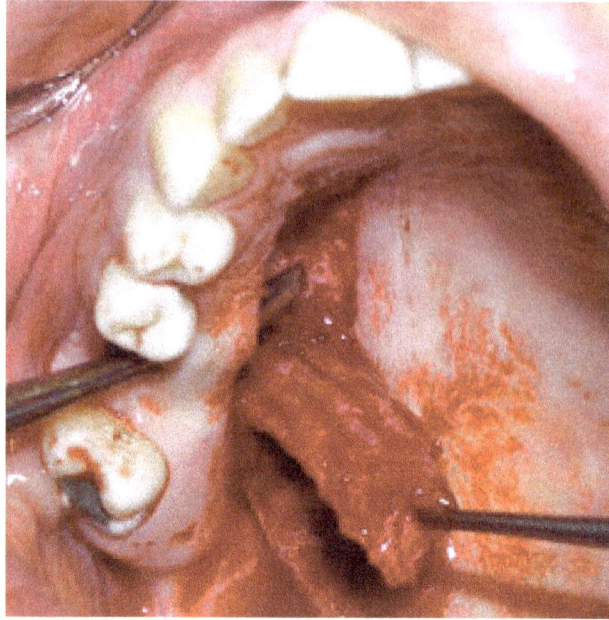

Figure 11. Intraoperative view of the elevated palatal connective tissue flap.

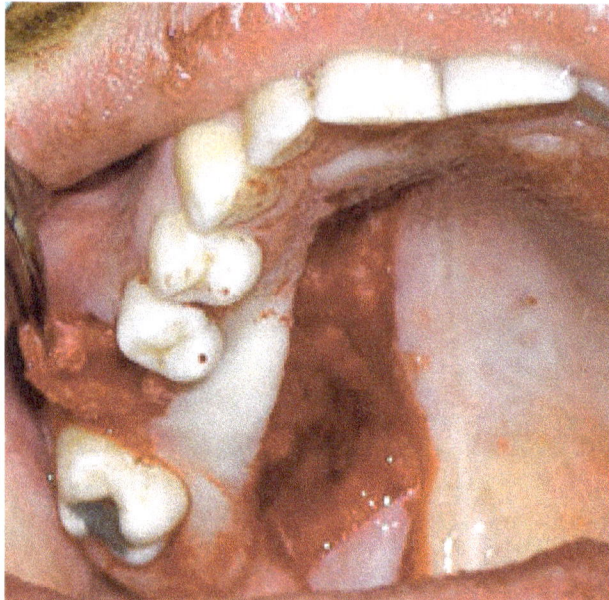

Figure 12. Orientation of the flap passing through the palatal tunnel to the underlying fistula during the operation.

The connective tissue was elevated with periosteum, as in palatal rotational flaps. The rotated flap was passed through a full-thickness tissue tunnel that was previously prepared on the palatal side of the OAF (**Figures 7d** and **12**).

The flap was inserted under the buccal mucosa and sutured with 4/0 polyglycan without any tension. The H-type minor flaps were sutured with 4/0 polyglycan and left for primary healing (**Figures 7e**, **13**, and **14**).

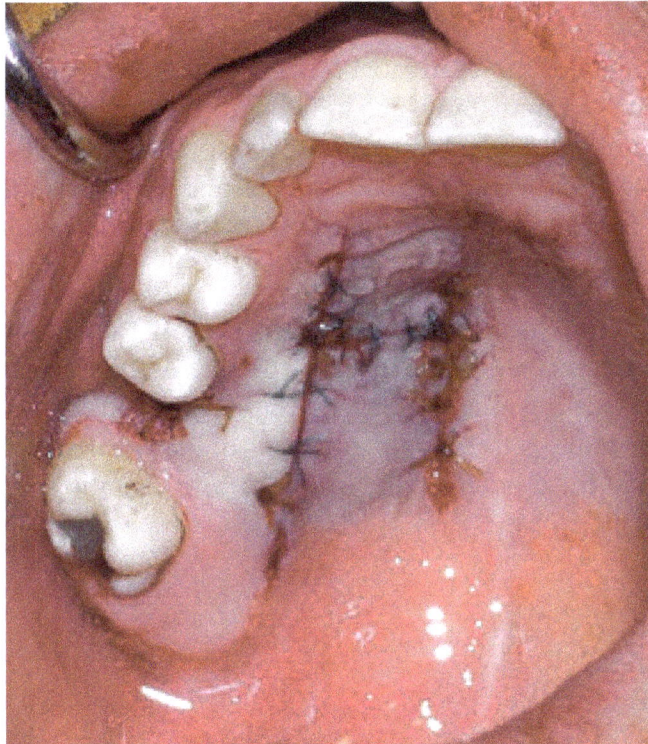

Figure 13. After the minor mucosal flaps were sutured, no area was left for secondary healing.

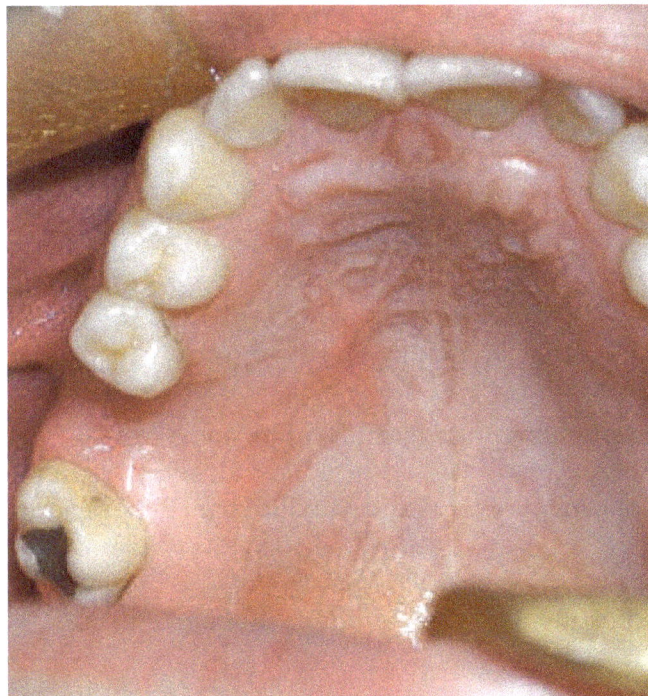

Figure 14. Healing of the fistula. After closing with MPCF (modified palatal connective tissue flap).

5.1.6. Distant flaps

Local flaps are the treatment of choice in most cases of OACs. However, sometimes these flaps may fail, and pedicle flaps from distant sites may be utilized in order to treat especially large defects. These flaps are usually selected from the anatomical sites in close proximity to the defect. Lateral tongue flap has been described as a method for the closure of OAF [47]. Lateral tongue flaps are used for the treatment of defects in the lateral palate and lateral alveolar process, and on the postoperative 14th day, the pedicle is severed [48] (**Figure 2c** and **d**).

The use of the temporalis flap has been described previously for intraoral reconstruction [49–51] and can be used for the reconstruction of large defects of the maxilla, especially following ablative tumor surgery. It is a well-vascularized flap with enough volume for the closure of large defects. The large bulk of this flap can also provide a soft-tissue bed if further bony reconstruction is planned for the defect site in the future. Distant flaps are preferred rarely, compared to local flaps [52].

6. Conclusion

OACs can be successfully treated if diagnosed at the time of occurrence or at an early stage. The size of the defect is an important factor in deciding which technique to use. Small openings can heal spontaneously, but the health of the sinus is an important factor which may lead to an incomplete healing and the formation of an OAF.

The clinician must make the correct diagnosis and decide the correct indication for treatment.

Local buccal and palatal flaps are the most proper for the closure of OACs resulting from dental procedures. However, large defects following tumor resection or trauma may require the use of more refined techniques for successful healing.

Author details

Guhan Dergin[1*], Yusuf Emes[2], Cagrı Delilbası[3] and Gokhan Gurler[3]

*Address all correspondence to: guhandergin@yahoo.com

1 Dentistry Faculty, Department of Oral and Maxillofacial Surgery, Marmara University, Istanbul, Turkey

2 Dentistry Faculty, Department of Oral and Maxillofacial Surgery, Istanbul University, Istanbul, Turkey

3 Dentistry Faculty, Department of Oral and Maxillofacial Surgery, Medipol University, Istanbul, Turkey

References

[1] Anavi Y, Gal G, Sifen R, Calderon S, Tikva Petah *et al*. Palatal rotation-advancement flap for delayed repair of oroantral fistula: a retrospective evaluation of 63 cases. Oral Surg Oral Med Oral Pathol Oral Radiol Endod. 2003 Nov;96(5):527–34.

[2] Lee JJ, Kok SH, Chang HH, Yang PJ, Hahn LJ. Repair of oroantral communications in the third molar region by random palatal flap. Int J Oral Maxillofac Surg. 2002 Dec; 31(6):677–80.

[3] Kruger GO, editor. Textbook of oral and maxillofacial surgery (6th ed). St Louis: CV Mosby; 1984: p. 291.

[4] Hanazawa Y, Itoh K, Mabashi T, Sato K. Closure of oroantral communications using a pedicled buccal fat pad graft. J Oral Maxillofac Surg. 1995 Jul;53(7):771–5.

[5] Skoglund LA, Pedersen SS, Holst E. Surgical management of 85 perforations to the maxillary sinus. Int J Oral Surg. 1983 Feb;12(1):1–5.

[6] Mustian WF. The floor of maxillary sinus and its dental, oral and nasal relations. J Am Dent Assoc. 1933;20:2175–87.

[7] Killey HC, Kay LW. An analysis of 250 cases of oroantral fistula treated by the buccal flap operation. Oral Surg. 1967 Dec;24(6):726–39.

[8] Von Wowern N. Closure of oroantral fistula with buccal flap. Rehrmann versus Moczair. Int J Oral Surg. 1982 Jun;11(2):156–65.

[9] Ehrl PA. Oroantral communication. Epicritical study of 175 patients, with special concern to secondary operative closure. Int J Oral Surg. 1980 Oct;9(5):351–8.

[10] Punwutikorn J, Waikakul A, V Pairuchvej V. Clinically significant oroantral communications-a study of incidence and site. Int J Oral Maxillofac Surg. 1994 Feb;23(1):19–21.

[11] Güven O. A clinical study on oroantral fistulae. J Craniomaxillofac Surg. 1998 Aug; 26(4):267–71.

[12] Yalçın S, Oncü B, Emes Y, Atalay B, Aktaş I. Surgical treatment of oroantral fistulas: a clinical study of 23 cases. J Oral Maxillofac Surg. 2011 Feb;69(2):333–9.

[13] Visscher SH, van Minnen B, Bos RR. Closure of oroantral communications: a review of the literature. J Oral Maxillofac Surg. 2010 Jun;68(6):1384–91.

[14] Nedir R, N. Nurdin N, El Hage M, Abi Najm S, Bischof M. Oroantral fistula: a complication of late implant failure. Clin Oral Implant Res. 2015; 26(Suppl. 12):408.

[15] Voss PJ, Vargas Soto G, Schmelzeisen R, Izumi K, Stricker A, Bittermann G, Poxleitner P. Sinusitis and oroantral fistula in patients with bisphosphonate-associated necrosis of the maxilla. Head Face Med. 2016 Jan; 6;12(1):3.

[16] Kuriyama T, Lewis MAO, Williams DW. Infections of the oral and maxillofacial region. In: Andersson L, Kahnberg K, Pogrel MA, editors. Oral and maxillofacial surgery. West Sussex: Blackwell; 2010: pp. 1197–1208.

[17] Noel J, Teo N, Divi V, Nayak JV. Use of pedicled nasoseptal flap for pathologic oroantral 23 fistula closure. J Oral Maxillofac Surg. 2016 Apr;74(4) 704.e1-6.

[18] Borgonovo AE, Berardinelli FV, Favale M, Maiorana C. Surgical options in oroantral fistula treatment. Open Dent J. 2012;6:94–8.

[19] Awang MN. Closure of oroantral fistula. Int J Oral Maxillofac Surg. 1988 Apr;17(2):110–5.

[20] El Hakim IE, El Fakharany AM. The use of the pedicled buccal fat pad (BFP) and palatal rotating flaps in closure of oroantral communication and palatal defects. J Laryngol Otol. 1999 Sep;113(9):834–8.

[21] Adams T, Taub D, Rosen M. Repair of oroantral communications by use of a combined surgical approach: functional endoscopic surgery and buccal advancement flap/buccal fat pad graft. J Oral Maxillofac Surg. 2015 Aug;73(8):1452–6

[22] Abuabara A, Cortez ALV, Passeri LA, et al. Evaluation of different treatments for oroantral/oronasal communications. Int J Oral Maxillofac Surg. 2006 Feb;35(2):155–8.

[23] Slack R, Bates G. Functional endoscopic sinus surgery. Am Fam Physician. 1998 Sep 1;58(3):707–18.

[24] Agarwal B, Pandey S, Roychoudhury A. New technique for closure of an oroantral fistula using platelet-rich fibrin . Br J Oral Maxillofac Surg. 2016 Feb;54(2):e31–2.

[25] Lazow SK. Surgical management of the oroantral fistula: flap procedures. Oper Tech Otolaryngol Head Neck Surg. 1999 Jun;10(2):148.

[26] Miloro M, Ghali GE, Larsen P, Waite P. Peterson's principles of oral and maxillofacial surgery, 3rd edition. St. Louis: CV Mosby; 1998: pp. 477–85.

[27] De Biasi M, Maglione M, Angerame D. The effectiveness of surgical management of oroantral communications: a systematic review of the literature. Eur J Oral Implantol. 2014 Winter;7(4):347–57.

[28] Gacic B, Todorovic L, Kokovic V, Danilovic V, Stojcev-Stajcic L, Drazic R, Markovic A. The closure of oroantral communications with resorbable PLGA-coated beta-TCP root analogs, hemostatic gauze, or buccal flaps: a prospective study. Oral Surg Oral Med Oral Pathol Oral Radiol Endod. 2009 Dec;108(6):844–50.

[29] Del Junco R, Rappaport I, Allison GR. Persistent oral antral fistulas. Arch Otolaryngol Head Neck Surg. 1988 Nov;114(11):1315–6.

[30] Falci SG, Dos Santos CR. Modification of the vestibular mucoperiosteal flap technique for closure of oroantral fistula. J Craniofac Surg. 2015 Oct;26(7):e659.

[31] Neuschl M, Kluba S, Krimmel M, Reinert S. Iatrogenic transposition of the parotid duct into the maxillary sinus after tooth extraction and closure of an oroantral fistula. A case report. J Craniomaxillofac Surg. 2010 Oct;38(7):538–40.

[32] Egyedi P. Utilization of the buccal fat pad for closure of oroantral communication. J Maxillofac Surg. 1977 Nov;5(4):241–4.

[33] Tideman H, Bosanquet A. Scott J use of the buccal fat pad as pedicled graft. J Oral Maxillofac Surg. 1986 Jun;44(6):435–40.

[34] Rapidis AD, Alexandridis CA, Eleftheriadis E, Angelopoulos AP. The use of the buccal fat pad for reconstruction of oral defects: review of the literature and report of 15 cases. Oral Maxillofac Surg. 2000 Feb;58(2):158–63.

[35] Hao SP. Reconstruction of oral defects with the pedicled buccal fat pad ap. Otolaryngo Head Neck Surg. 2000 Jun;122(6):863–7.

[36] Dean A, Alamillos F, Garcia-Lopez A, Sanchez J, Penalba M. The buccal fat pad in oral reconstruction. Head Neck. 2001 May;23(5):383–8.

[37] Loh FC1, Loh HS. Use of the buccal fat pad for correction of intraoral defects: report of cases. J Oral Maxillofac Surg. 1991 Apr;49(4):413–6.

[38] Mohan S, Kankariya H, Harjani B. The use of the buccal fat pad for reconstruction of oral defects: review of the literature and report of cases. J Maxillofac Oral Surg. 2012 Jun;11(2):128–31.

[39] Martín-Granizo R, Naval L, Costas A, Goizueta C, Rodriguez F, Monje F, Muñoz M, Diaz F. Use of buccal fat pad to repair intraoral defects: review of 30 cases. Br J Oral Maxillofac Surg. 1997 Apr;35(2):81–4.

[40] Nezafati S, Vafaii A, Ghojazadeh M. Comparison of pedicled buccal fat pad flap with buccal flap for closure of oro-antral communication. Int J Oral Maxillofac Surg. 2012 May;41(5):624–8.

[41] James RB. Surgical closure of large oroantral fistulas using a palatal island flap. J Oral Surg. 1980 Aug;38(8):591–5.

[42] Erdogan O, Esen E, Ustun Y. Bony palatal necrosis in a diabetic patient secondary to palatal rotational flap. J Diab Complications. 2005 Nov–Dec;196:364–7.

[43] Ward BB. The palatal flap. Oral Maxillofac Surg Clin N Am. 2003 Nov;15(4):467–73.

[44] Dergin G, Gurler G, Gursoy B. Modified connective tissue flap: a new approach to closure of an oroantral fistula. Br J Oral Maxillofac Surg. 2007 Apr;45(3):251–2.

[45] Ito T, Hara H. A new technique for closure of the oroantral fistula. J Oral Surg. 1980 Jul;38(7):509–12.

[46] Yamazaki Y, Yamaoka M, Hirayama M, et al. The submucosal island flap in the closure of oroantral fistula. Br J Oral Maxillofacial Surg. 1985 Aug;23(4):259–63.

[47] Sielgel EB, Bechtold W, Sherman PM, Stoopack JC. Pedicle tongue flap for closure of an oroantral defect after partial maxillectomy. J Oral Surg. 1977;35:746–9.

[48] Buchbinder D, St-Hilaire H. Tongue flaps in maxillofacial surgery. Oral Maxillofac Surg Clin North Am. 2003 Nov;15(4):475–86.

[49] Alonso del Hoyo J, Fernandez Sanroman J, Gil-Diez JL, Diaz Gonzalez FJ. The temporalis muscle flap: an evaluation and review of 38 cases. J Oral Maxillofac Surg. 1994;52:143–7.

[50] Demas PN, Sotereanos GC. Transmaxillary temporalis transfer for reconstruction of a large palatal defect: report of a case. J Oral Maxillofac Surg. 1989;47:197–202.

[51] Koranda FC, McMahon MF, Jernstrom VR. The temporalis muscle flap for intraoral reconstruction. Arch Otolaryngol Head Neck Surg. 1987;113:740–3.

[52] Campbell HH. Reconstruction of the left maxilla. Plast Reconstr Surg. 1948;3:66–72.

8

Advances in Management of Class II Malocclusions

Azita Tehranchi, Hossein Behnia,
Farnaz Younessian and Sahar Hadadpour

Abstract

Although mandibular advancement by bilateral sagittal split osteotomy seems to be a good mandibular treatment option to treat skeletal class II malocclusion, it is less stable than setback; relapse depends on a wide range of patient-centered and surgeon-centered factors relating to the skill and experience of the surgeon, proper seating of the condyles, the exact amount of mandibular advancement, the tension of the muscles and soft tissues, the mandibular plane angle, and the patient's age. In fact, patients with low and high mandibular plane angles have increased vertical and horizontal relapses, respectively. Nonsurgical management of class II malocclusion may be an option by which to effectively manage such cases. The present chapter discusses different treatment modalities for clinical management of class II malocclusion in growing and non-growing patients.

Keywords: class II malocclusion, diagnosis, treatment, management, advances

1. Introduction

Class II malocclusion is among the most common developmental anomalies with a prevalence ranging from 15 to 30% in most populations [1, 2]. This malocclusion is likely to produce significant negative esthetic, psychological, and social effects [3–6]. This dentofacial anomaly can be divided into two different categories based on the involved arch to maxillary excess or mandibular deficiency [7, 8]. The resulting anomaly may demonstrate various severities of class II malocclusion in different ages, which dictates the preferred approach to clinical management.

2. Etiology and pathogenesis of class II malocclusion

Like other types of malocclusions, the etiology of class II malocclusion has been linked to hereditary and environmental factors [9].

2.1. Class II division 1

Proclination of upper incisors and/or retroinclination of the lower incisors by a habit or the soft tissues can result in an increased overjet in any type of skeletal pattern [10]. In class II division 1, the lips of the parents are usually incompetent and they try to compensate it via circumoral muscular activity, rolling the lower lip behind the upper incisors, or moving the tongue forward between the incisors, or a combination of all these items [11]. Finger-sucking or other oral habits may also lead to the development of this malocclusion, mostly following imbalances of the buccinator muscles and tongue force, and narrowing the maxillary arch. In addition, habits usually procline the upper incisors and retrocline the lower incisors (**Figure 1**).

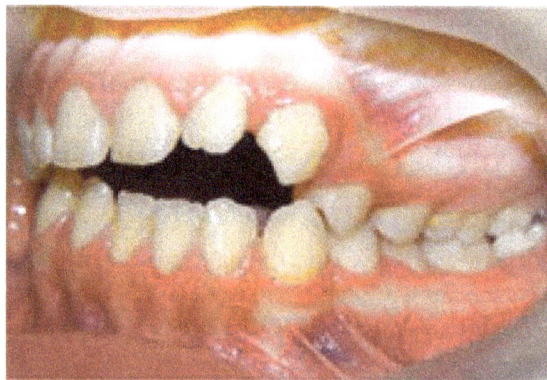

Figure 1. Prolonged thumb-sucking habit creating asymmetric open bite and class II malocclusion.

Dental features such as tooth size arch length discrepancies could be involved in developing class II malocclusion, which might be the reason for the labial movement of the upper incisors resulting in exacerbation of the overjet (**Figure 2**).

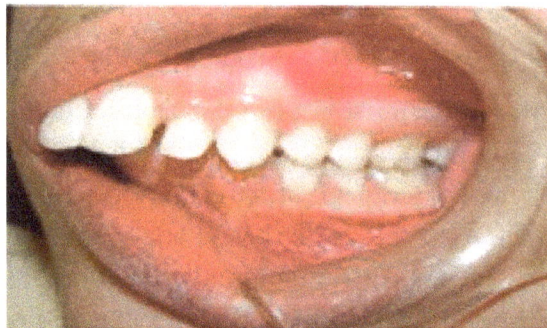

Figure 2. Class II div 1 malocclusion with class II molar and canine relationship and increased overjet and overbite.

2.2. Class II division 2

Vertical dimension of class II division 2 patients is usually decreased in comparison to other types, which may result in the absence of an occlusal stop on lower incisors and consequently an increase in the overbite [11]. Dental crowding also, in contrast to the div 1 category, is exacerbated by retroinclination of the upper incisors [11, 12]. Active muscular lips are responsible for upper and lower retroinclination in this type (**Figure 3**).

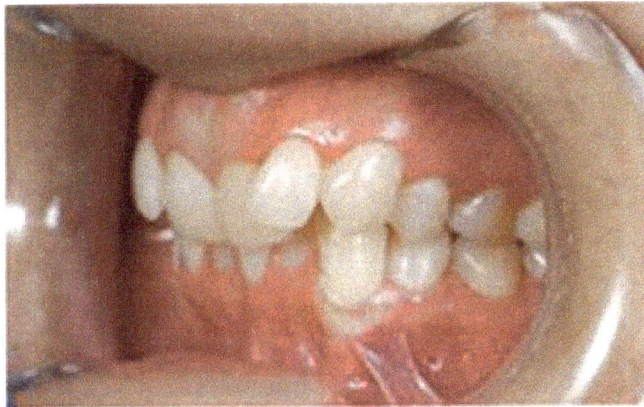

Figure 3. Retroclined upper central incisors, proclined laterals, and increased overbite in a class II div 2 case.

3. Diagnosis and clinical features of class II malocclusion

As in other types of malocclusions, class II malocclusion could be identified based on precise clinical evaluation (extra- and intra-oral features), diagnostic aids (history, photographic analysis, radiographic analysis, and cast analysis), and functional analysis (examination of postural rest position and maximum intercuspation, examination of the temporomandibular joint and orofacial dysfunction) of the patients [11–13]. The angle defined class II malocclusion as characterized by a distal relation of the lower to the upper permanent first molars to the extent of more than one-half the width of one cusp and the maxillary incisors being protrusive [14]. Class II division 1 patients demonstrate convex profile, dolichocephalic shape of the head, shallow/deep mentolabial sulcus, hyperactive mentalis, and upper lip. Class II division 2 patients present straight to convex profile, mesocephalic or dolichocephalic head shape, normal or hyperactive mentolabial sulcus, and normal or hyperactive upper lip [11, 12].

The presence of distal step molar relation, tooth size discrepancy, and/or excessive overjet may lead the clinicians to a false interpretation of skeletal class II malocclusion [9]. Skeletal class II malocclusion components may be classified by maxillomandibular relationship (mandibular retrognathism, midface protrusion or both), the cranial base length (increased length of the anterior cranial base: midface protrusion, while lengthening of the posterior cranial base: more retruded position of the temporomandibular articulation), vertical discrepancy (anterior upper face height often greater than normal), and steep occlusal plane (**Figure 4**) [9].

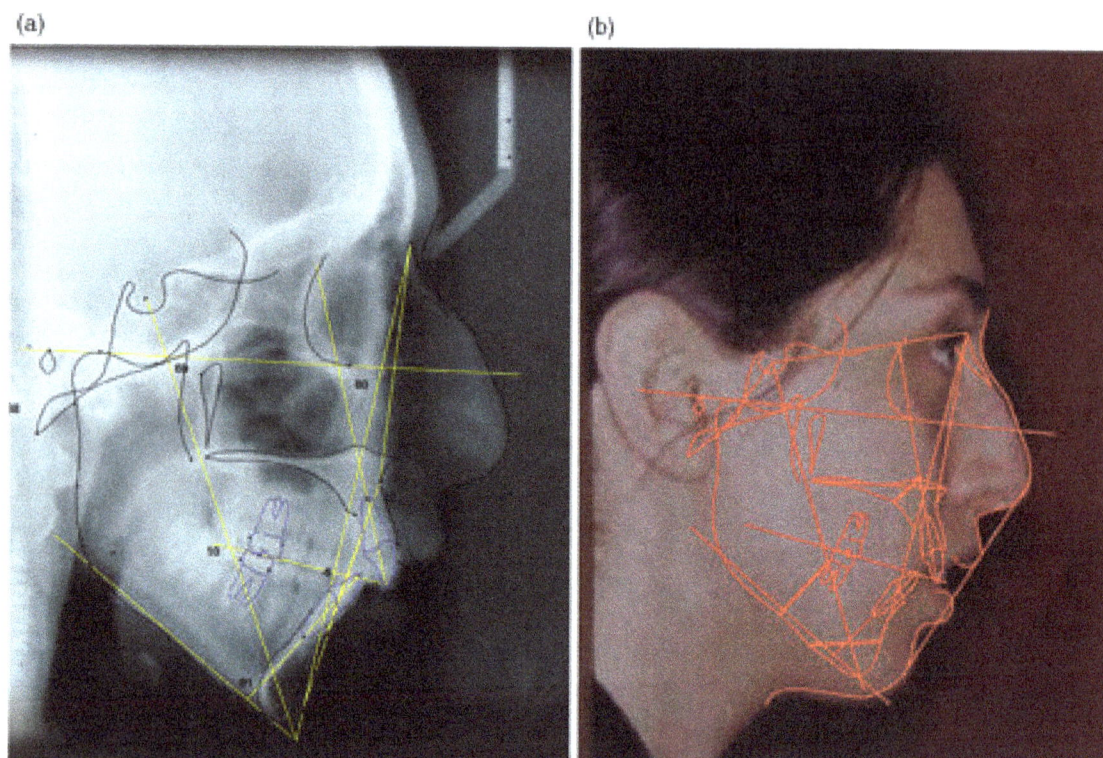

Figure 4. (a) Lateral cephalometric analysis of a patient with class II malocclusion and vertical growth pattern. (b) Superimposition of lateral cephalometric analysis on the soft-tissue profile of the patient (overlay tracing).

4. Treatment of class II malocclusion

Treatment strategies of class II malocclusion are categorized based on the growing and non-growing status of patients. Treatment timing of class II malocclusion has long been a topic of controversy for decades [15–17]. The literature is replete with research aimed at answering most clinical challenges of this type of malocclusion [18]. The existing evidence suggests that providing early orthodontic treatment for children with class II malocclusion and prominent upper front teeth is more effective in reducing the incidence of incisal trauma than providing one course of orthodontic treatment when the child is in early adolescence [19].

4.1. Early management in the mixed dentition

The best treatment modalities for class II malocclusion in growing patients include using functional appliances either removable (Activator, Bionator, Frankel, and Twin-block) or fixed appliances (MARA, cemented Twin-block, or Herbst appliance) that mostly enhance further mandibular growth via mandibular advancement and also headgear (Cervical, Highpull, and combination type), which provides extra oral force to restrict further maxillary growth [20–22] (**Figures 5** and **6**).

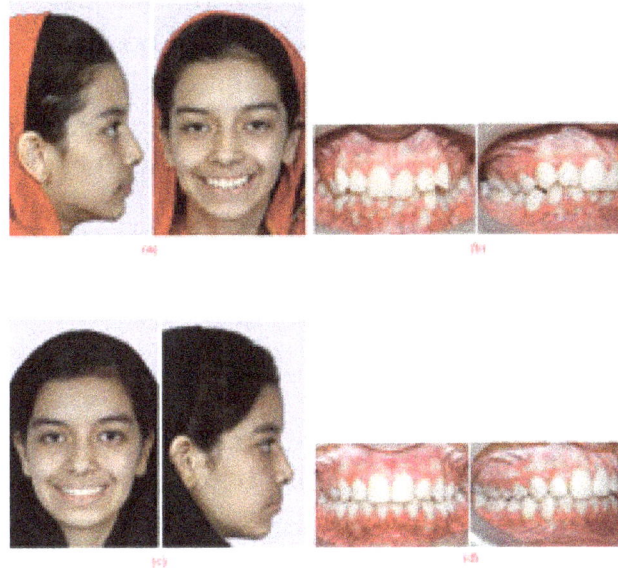

Figure 5. (a) Patient at age 11 years: frontal and profile photographs of the patient before treatment. (b) Intraoral photographs of the patient showing class II div 2 malocclusion. (c) Patient at age 13 years: photographs of the patient after treatment with cervical headgear and fixed orthodontic treatment. (d) Intraoral photographs of the patient after treatment.

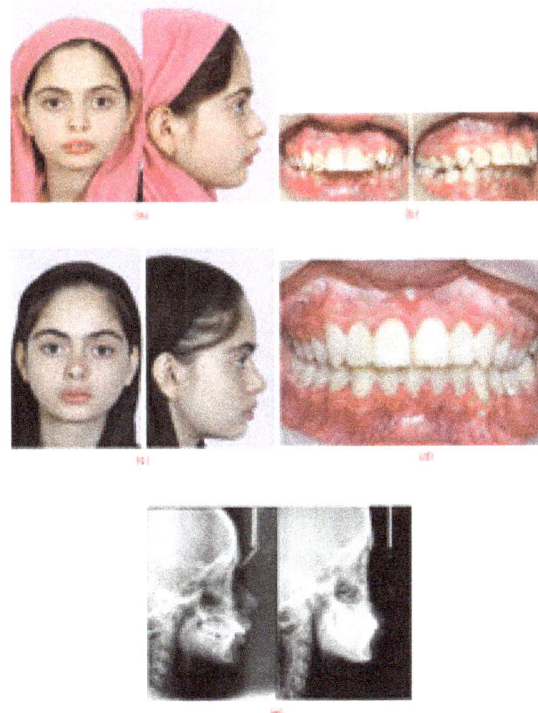

Figure 6. (a) Frontal and profile photographs of the patient at age 12 years prior to treatment. (b) Intraoral photographs of the patient showing class II div 1 malocclusion with increased overjet and overbite before treatment. (c) Photographs of the patient at age 14 years after an 8-month treatment with Twin-block, followed by fixed orthodontic treatment. (d) Intraoral photograph of the patient after treatment. (e) Pretreatment and posttreatment lateral cephalograms.

Both removable functional appliances and headgear therapy depend on the cooperation of the patients. However, in contrast to the theory, there would not be a clear cut between clinical indications of these two broad clinical interventions of class II malocclusions [23]. Among the different removable appliances, Twin-block is used more often [18], which can efficiently promote mandibular growth, restrict further forward growth of the maxilla, and improve skeletal relationships in growing skeletal class II individuals with mandibular retrusion [24, 25].

Figure 7 demonstrates a 14-year-old boy with class II malocclusion and bilateral buccal crossbite (Brodie syndrome). His mandible was totally locked and could not grow normally. Treatment began with a removable anterior bite plate, an open midpalatal screw in the acrylic portion for the upper arch in order to constrict the expanded ridge, and a Quad-helix appliance for the lower arch to expand the ridge. After 3 months, treatment was continued with a Twin-block appliance and an open screw in the maxilla. Fixed orthodontic treatment was performed for only 6 months.

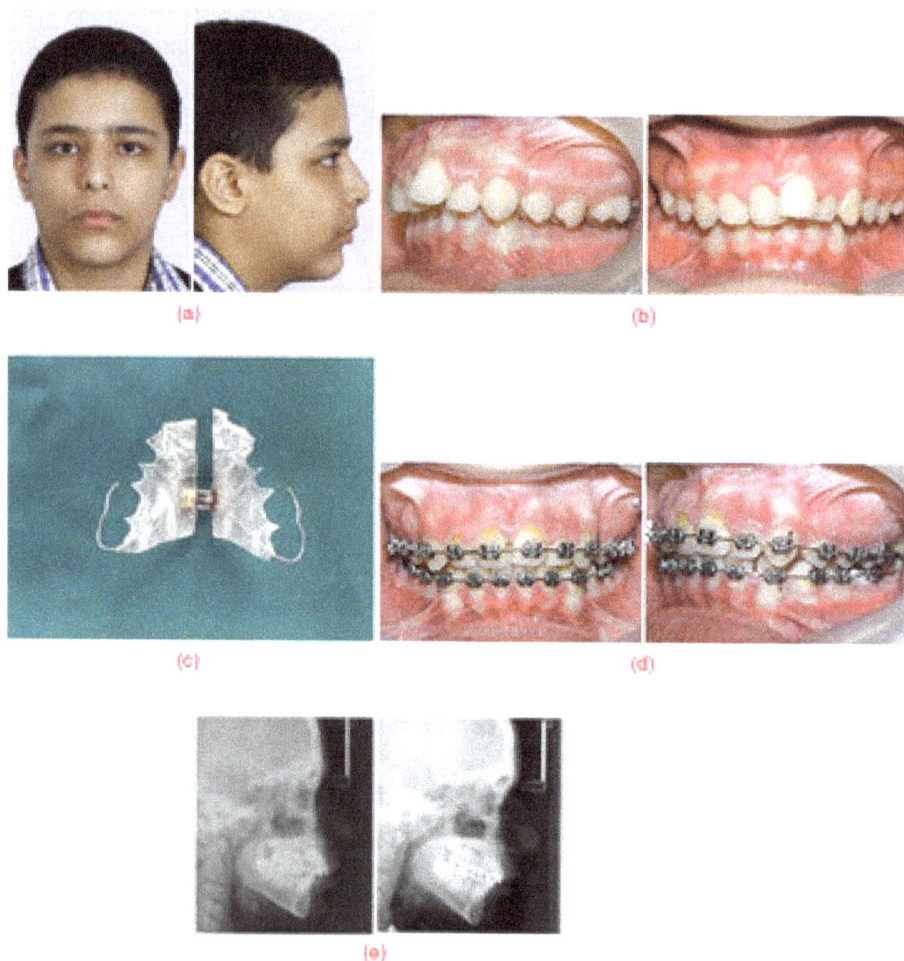

Figure 7. (a) Frontal and profile photographs of the patient before treatment. (b) Intraoral photograph before treatment. (c) Anterior bite plate and open screw in midpalatal portion. (d) Intraoral photograph of the patient 6 months after beginning the treatment. (e) Pretreatment and posttreatment lateral cephalograms.

Several systematic review studies have investigated the present literature on the effect of treatment with functional appliances in comparison with untreated controls and demonstrated that skeletal changes were statistically significant, but unlikely to be clinically significant [26]. The limited quality and heterogeneity of the present studies in this field restrict the power of pure clinical judgment. However, in two recent systematic review articles, removable functional appliances were effective in improving class II malocclusion in short term, although their effects are mainly dentoalveolar, rather than skeletal [27]. On the other hand, more long-term skeletal effects following removable functional appliances were seen in patients during their pubertal growth phase, compared to prepubertal phase [18, 25]. However, their soft-tissue changes were minimal from the clinical standpoint [28].

Fixed functional appliances were introduced first by Emil Herbst to overcome the cooperation obstacle of removable appliances [29]. The key differences between removable and fixed appliances are different working hours (intermittent vs. continuous), and also optimal treatment timing (before puberty growth vs. at or after puberty spurt) and direction of further growth [30]. To date, there are a limited number of studies evaluating clinical effectiveness and patient's experience and perceptions of these fixed functional appliances [23]. As it is stated in the literature, fixed functional treatment is effective when performed during the pubertal growth phase, and very little data are available on postpubertal patients [31]. Various types of fixed functional appliances (rigid, semirigid, and flexible) have been developed and used in clinical settings [13] (**Figure 8**). However, dental changes including mesial movement of lower molars and proclination of lower incisors were proven more significant than skeletal changes following their implication, compared to removable appliances [18, 32], which can negatively affect the long-term stability of the results. Many treatment modalities have been introduced to minimize the aforementioned side effects of these appliances including the application of increased-dimension arch wire, negative torque arch wire, and the use of lower incisor brackets with increased lingual crown torque [33, 34].

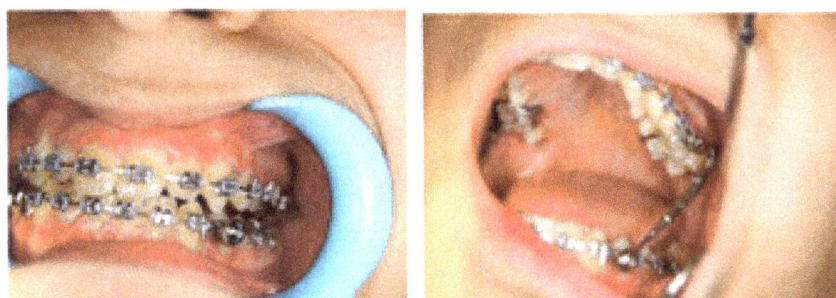

Figure 8. Fixed functional appliance.

Recently, clinicians tried to control the dentoalveolar side effects of fixed functional appliances by means of bone anchorage such as miniscrews and miniplates [35–37]. The results of the studies investigating the efficacy of skeletal anchorage were controversial and need further investigation [1, 38–40].

4.2. Late management of class II malocclusion

Currently, the number of adult patients seeking orthodontic treatment has gradually increased which focus mostly on camouflaging the malocclusion [41]. In contrast to growing patients, limited range of treatment modalities could be served for adult cases with class II skeletal and dental malocclusions. Depending on the severity of malocclusion, class II elastics, compensatory extraction (maxillary premolars and/or mandibular premolars) or even orthognathic surgical modalities may be used to alleviate the functional and esthetic problems associated with this type of malocclusion [42] (**Figures 9–11**).

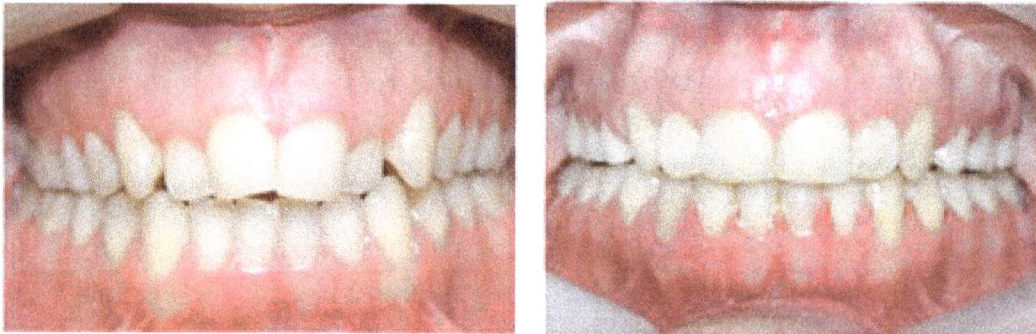

Figure 9. Pre- and posttreatment intraoral photographs of a patient using cervical headgear non-extraction treatment.

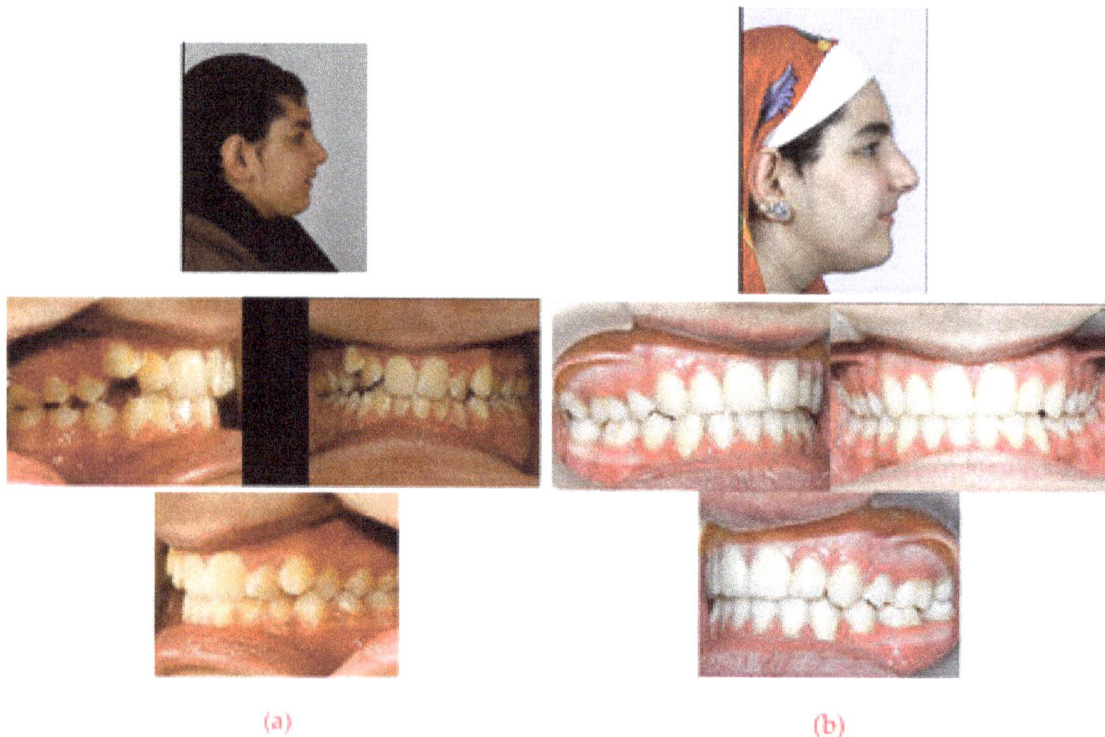

(a)　　　　　　　　　　　　　　　　　　　　(b)

Figure 10. (a) Profile and intraoral photographs of the patient at age 13 years. Treatment plan was to extract upper first premolars and lower second premolars. (b) Photographs of the patient after treatment at age 15 years.

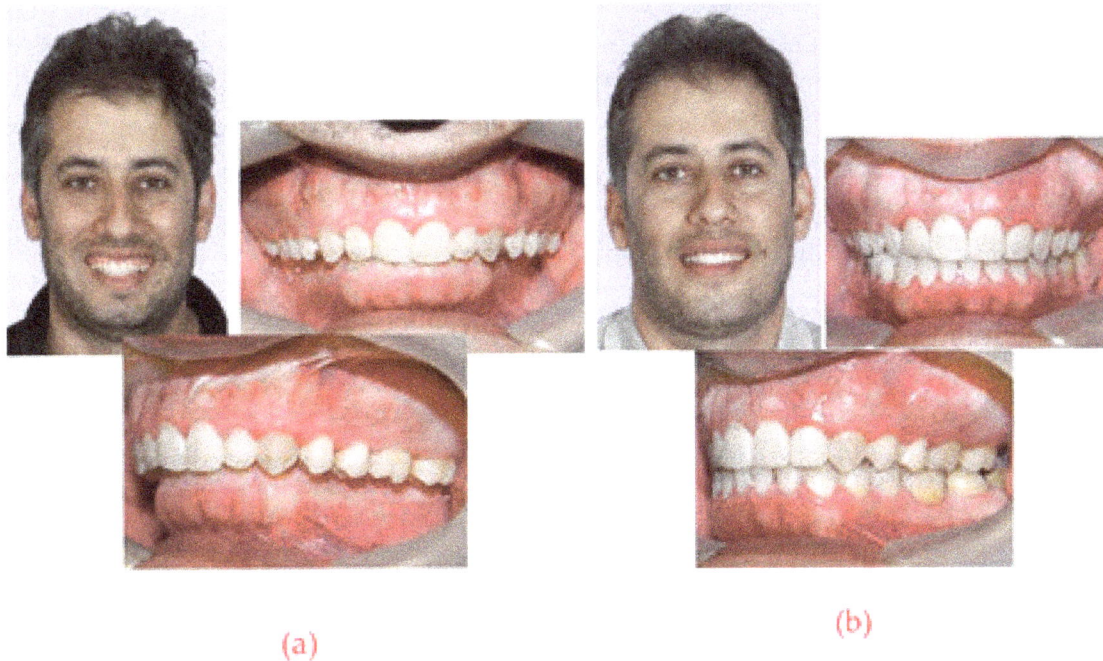

Figure 11. (a) Frontal and intraoral photographs of the patient with bilateral buccal crossbite. (b) Profile and intraoral photographs of the patient at the end of treatment.

The patient presented in **Figure 11** is another case of Brodie syndrome but at the age of 34 years. Fixed orthodontic treatment in combination with upper removable constriction plate and Quad-helix appliance in the lower arch was performed for 12 months, and then the patient underwent Lefort I (two-piece constriction and impaction) and mandibular advancement surgery. Postsurgical orthodontic treatment was continued for 5 months. Prevention of such complex orthognathic bimaxillary surgery could have easily been achieved in growing patients (**Figure 7**).

Class II elastics with non-extraction treatment plan is a typical interarch approach for managing mild class II malocclusion [43]. The effects of class II elastics include mesial movements of the mandibular molars, tipping of the mandibular incisors, distal movements and tipping of the maxillary incisors, extrusion of the mandibular molars and maxillary incisors, and consequently clockwise rotation of the mandibular plane [44]. As success of treatments based on interarch elastics depends heavily on patient compliance for their effectiveness, poor cooperation can lead to poor treatment outcomes and increased treatment time [45].

In many non-extraction cases, the pendulum appliance is the most effective and commonly used device for distalizing maxillary molars. Its significant clinical advantages include minimal dependence on patient compliance, allows for correction of minor transverse and vertical molar positions by incorporation of u-loop in adjustment springs (which further enhance additional space achievement), and laboratory-friendly fabrication. Palatal coverage concomitant to pendulum appliance mediated to reduce the moderate anchorage loss effect causing upper incisor proclination [46]. The expected distal movement of the first molars appears to be more significant if it could be used before the eruption of the upper second molars. To achieve proper distal movement of dentition after second molar eruption, clinicians may need to distalize the second molars first, followed by using a palatal arch bar (PAB) or Nance holding arch for retention. Then, the first molars are distalized. The extraction of erupted second molars can be done in case of great demand of distalizing first molars and the presence of erupting third molars, which may totally replace the second molar position [47] (**Figures 12** and **13**).

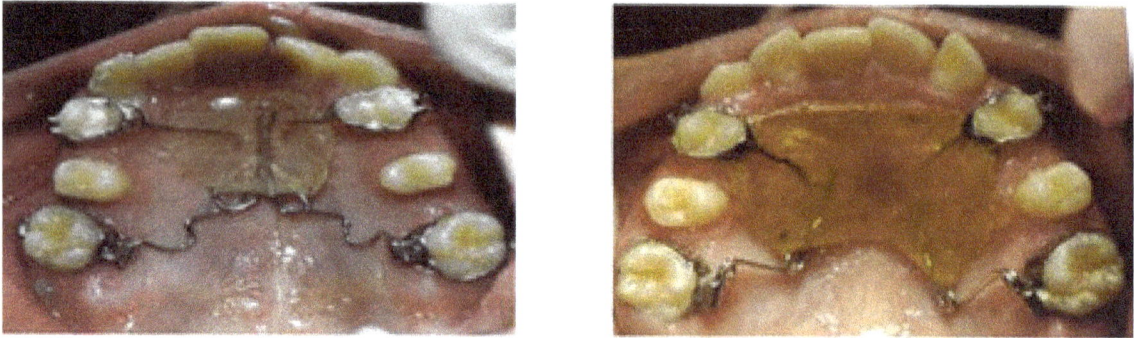

Figure 12. Distalizing maxillary molars by pendulum appliance, palatal coverage for anchorage control.

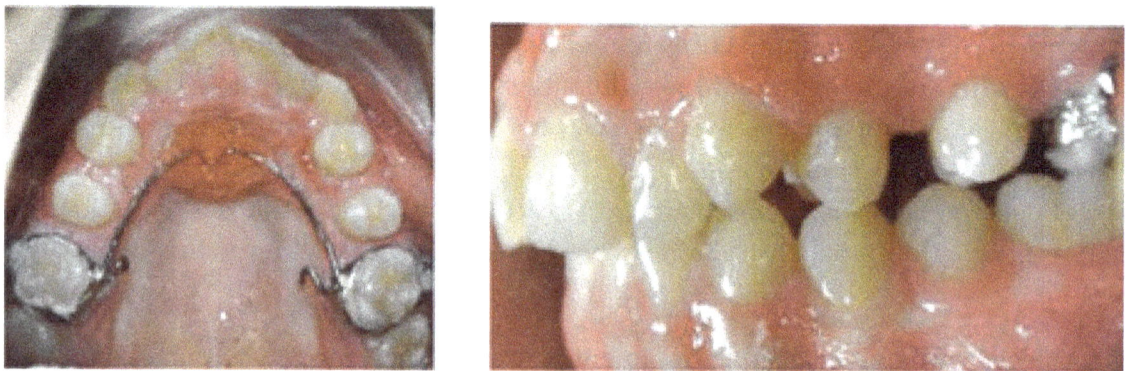

Figure 13. Nance holding arch for retention after achieving angle class I for the first permanent molars.

In a very recent study, both pendulum and distal screw seem to be equally effective in distalizing maxillary molars; however, greater distal molar tipping and premolar anchorage loss can be expected using the pendulum appliance [46].

Extractions of only upper premolars are indicated for some special patients. According to a current soft-tissue paradigm, clinicians must pay attention to several factors such as soft-tissue thickness, amount of pretreatment crowding or cephalometric discrepancy, when deciding their extraction regimens for adult patients [48, 49]. As it is stated in a very recent systematic review, when class II division 1 malocclusion is treated with maxillary and mandibular premolar extractions, the nasolabial angle increases and the lips are retracted. However, there is less retraction of the lower lip in the only upper premolar extraction protocol [50]. A delicate adjustment and trade-off between the amount of anterior retraction and the mesial movement of the posterior segment following extraction regimens in each vulnerable adult class II patient have to be considered to maintain the profile and the position of the upper lip at its most appropriate state. In order to reduce anchorage loss and space management obtained in extraction and non-extraction cases (distalizing appliances), temporary anchorage devices have been introduced in clinical orthodontic situations [51]. These devices serve considerable advantages including the ease of insertion and the removal in addition to the possibility of immediate loading [52, 53]. The only distinct factors predicting temporary anchorage device failures were soft-tissue inflammation surrounding a temporary anchorage device and early loading (within 3 weeks after insertion) [54].

In rare and very severe cases, distraction osteogenesis (DO) with or without further orthognathic surgery can be done to promote the situation [55, 56]. This procedure can be applied for very severe class II malocclusions following mandibular deficiencies with wide age range such as infants with Pierre Robbins syndrome, growing children with severe class II malocclusion (**Figures 14** and **15**), or even adult patients with the history of bilateral condylar ankylosis (**Figure 16**).

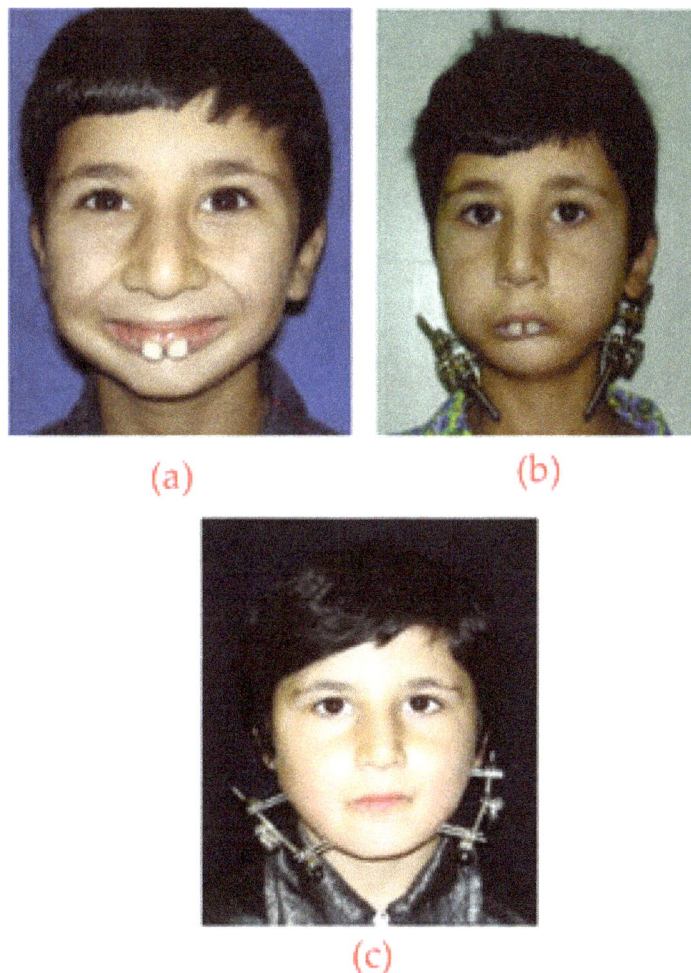

(a)   (b)

(c)

Figure 14. (a) Frontal photograph of the patient before distraction. (b) Bilateral extraoral distractors in place. (c) Post-distraction photograph after 30-mm activation.

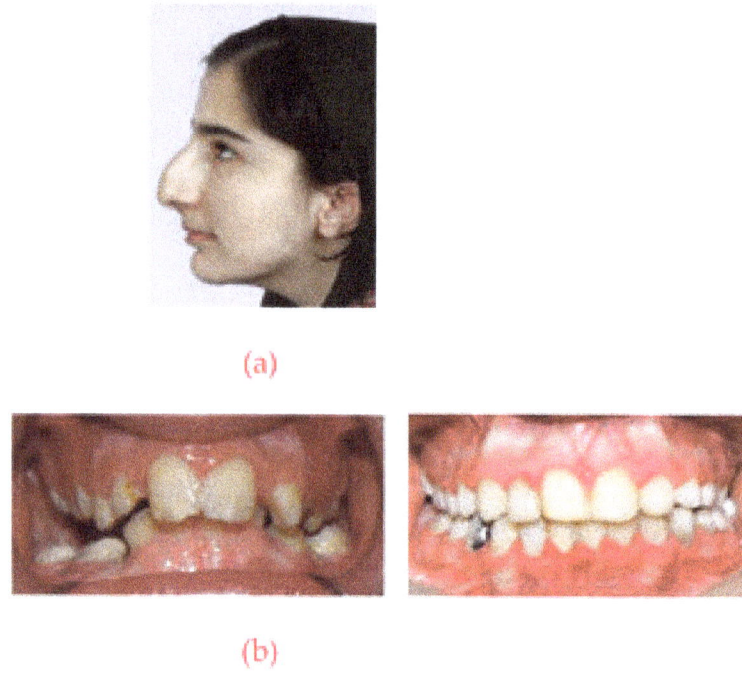

Figure 15. (a) Pre- and postdistraction photographs of patient's profile. (b) Intraoral photographs of the patient before and after bilateral DO.

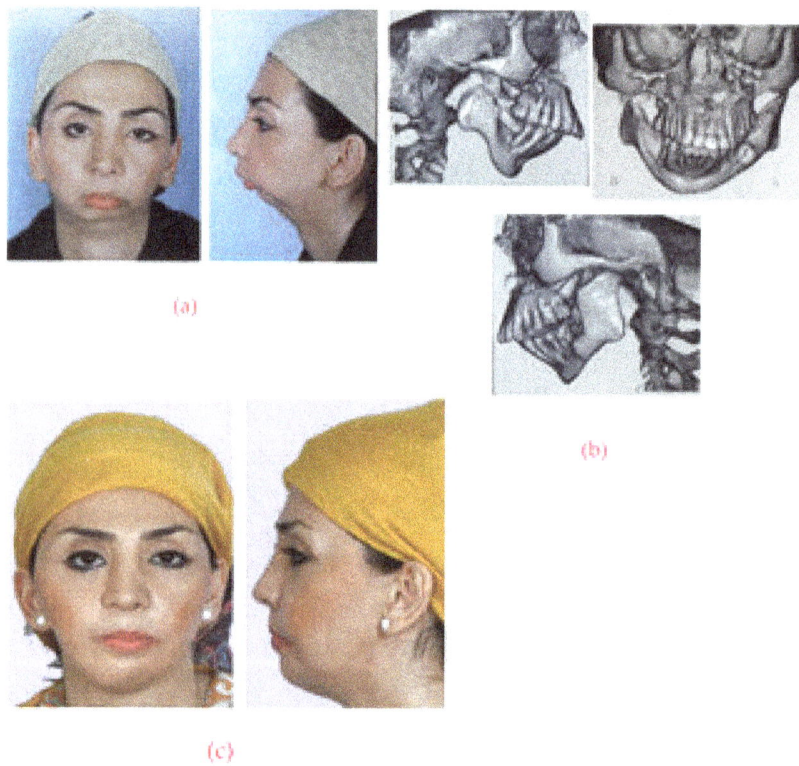

Figure 16. (a) A 29-year-old patient with bilateral condylar ankylosis. (b) CBCT scans of the patient. (c) At age 33 years after bilateral distraction osteogenesis, orthognathic surgery, and genioplasty.

In severe class II malocclusion cases, orthognathic surgery (mandibular advancement with or without maxillary impaction) can be done to enhance soft-tissue esthetic [57, 58]. The proper presurgical orthodontic tooth movements and alignment of arches are essential to maximize the amount of discrepancy correction during surgery [59]. Many class II patients present with proper mandible size, which is located downward and backward secondary to vertical maxillary excess. Superior impaction of the maxilla with proper center of rotation allows the mandible to rotate upwards and forwards, which enhance the facial height and increase chin prominence [59]. Although orthognathic surgery could be an efficient treatment modality in severe class II patients, both the cost of the surgery and the fear of undergoing surgery normally prevent patients from choosing this treatment option [60]. Furthermore, most of the studies on surgery-first approach are done on class III malocclusion cases, which significantly reduced treatment time with equal dentoalveolar short- and long-term results [61] (**Figures 17–20**).

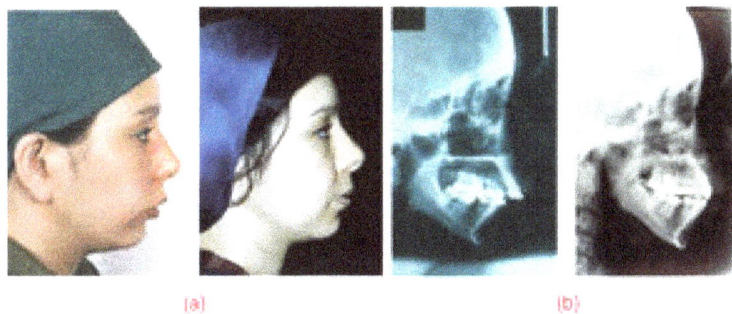

Figure 17. (a) Pre- and postsurgical (maxillary narrowing and mandibular advancement) photographs of the patient. (b) Pre- and postsurgical lateral cephalograms.

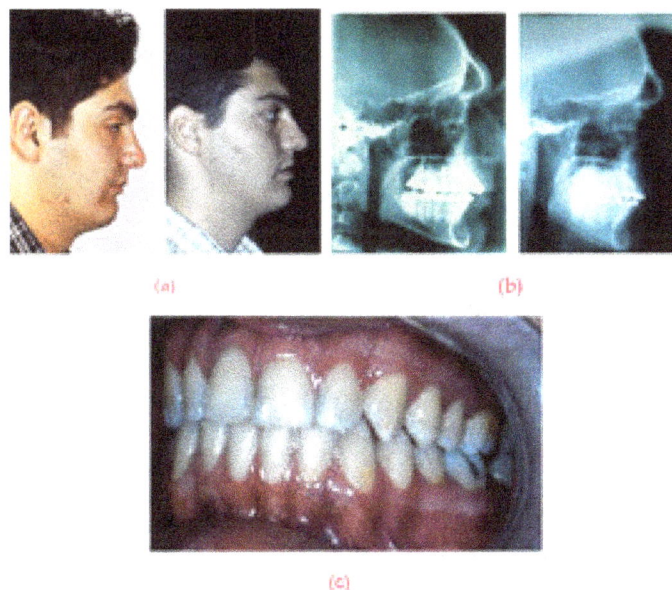

Figure 18. (a) Pre- and postsurgical (mandibular advancement) photographs of the patient. (b) Pre- and postsurgical lateral cephalograms. (c) Posttreatment occlusion.

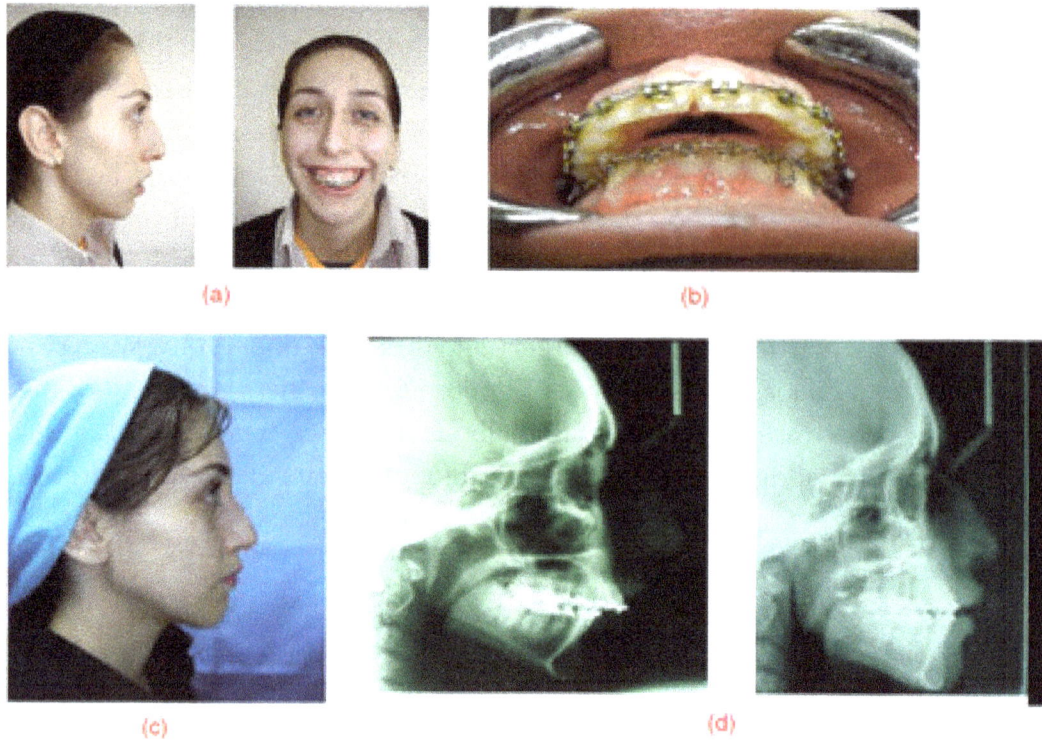

Figure 19. (a) Profile and frontal photographs of the patient before surgery. (b) Intraoral view of the patient prior to surgery. (c) Profile photograph of the patient after maxillary impaction and mandibular advancement surgery. (d) Lateral cephalograms of the patient before and after surgery.

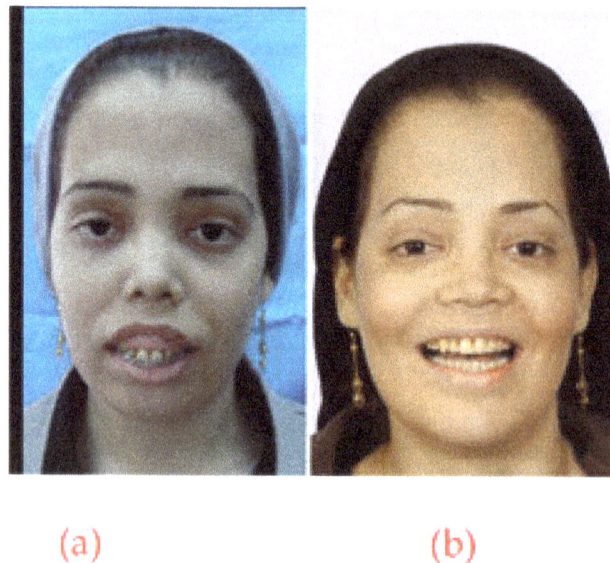

Figure 20. (a)Frontal photograph of an adult patient with major thalassemia, severe class II malocclusion 9-mm overjet, and 8-mm overbite before surgery. (b) Frontal photograph after 12-mm maxillary impaction and 8-mm setback plus genioplasty.

The clinical efficacy of orthognathic surgery on preexisting temporomandibular disorder (TMD) in class II patients is controversial [62, 63]. There are some reports of postsurgical condylar resorption in class II adult patients [64]. This could be the result of direct changes in the position of condyle, which may take place by inappropriate application of rigid fixation during surgery, worsening the TMD [65]. On the other hand, the improvement of clinical symptoms after orthognathic surgery can be explained by the better occlusal stability following surgery [66] (**Figure 21**).

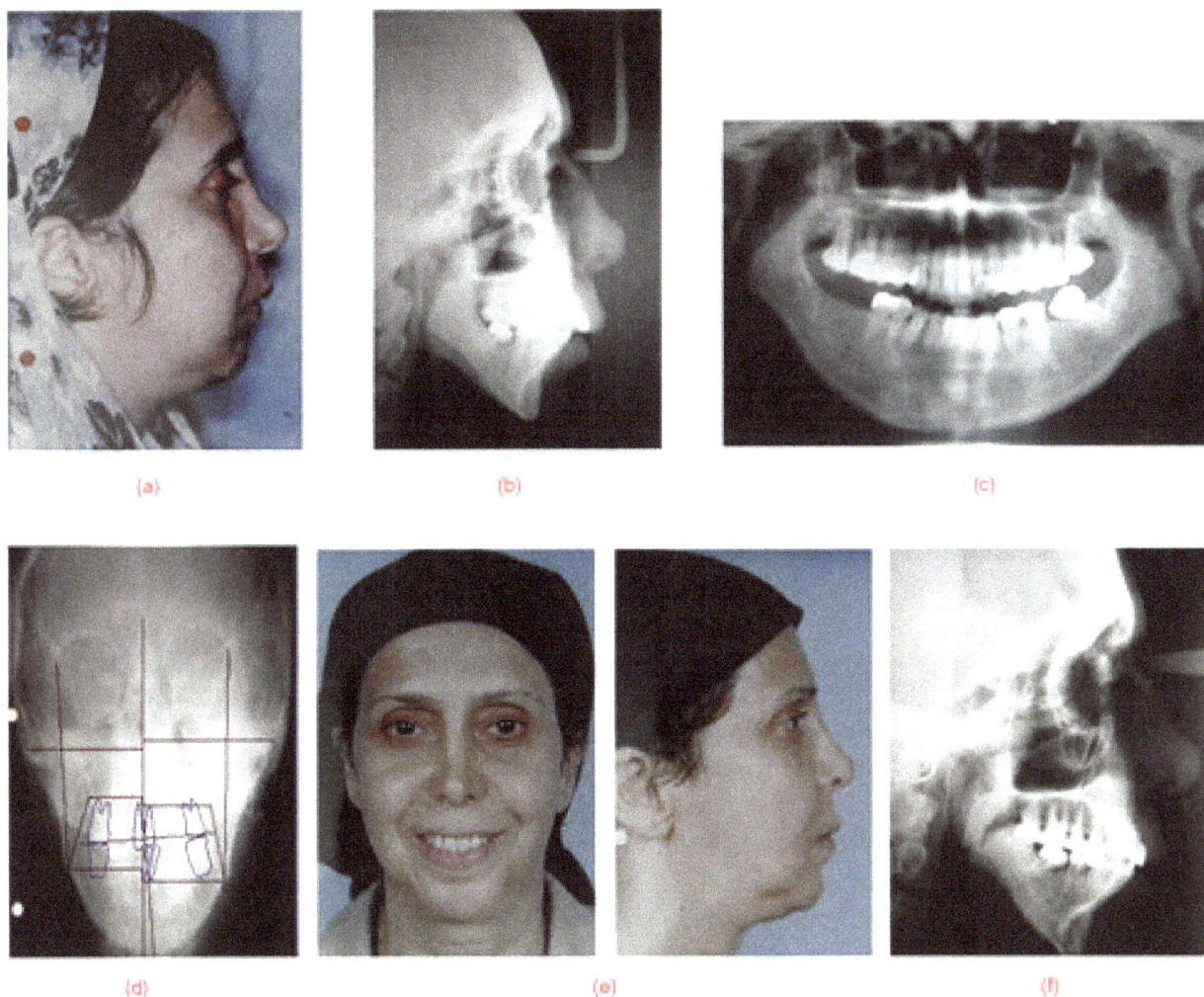

Figure 21. (a) Profile photograph of a patient with class II malocclusion and TMD. (b) Lateral cephalogram of the patient before treatment. (c) Panoramic view of the patient before treatment. (d) PA cephalogram showing cant of the maxilla and deviation of the mandible. (e) Frontal and profile photographs of the patient after mandibular advancement (nonrigid fixation). (f) Lateral cephalogram of the patient after surgery.

Mandibular DO has been introduced to correct severe skeletal discrepancies in class II adult patients [67]. This technique was first developed by Ilizarov for the long bones in the 1950s [68] and was ultimately applied for the facial skeleton [55, 69, 70]. At first, clinicians thought this method might end up in less neurosensory disturbances and a more stable result compared to the routine bilateral sagittal split osteotomies. However, these findings were not verified later by more controlled studies as they reported no considerable differences regarding neurosensory disturbances and short- or long-term skeletal stability [71] (**Figure 22**).

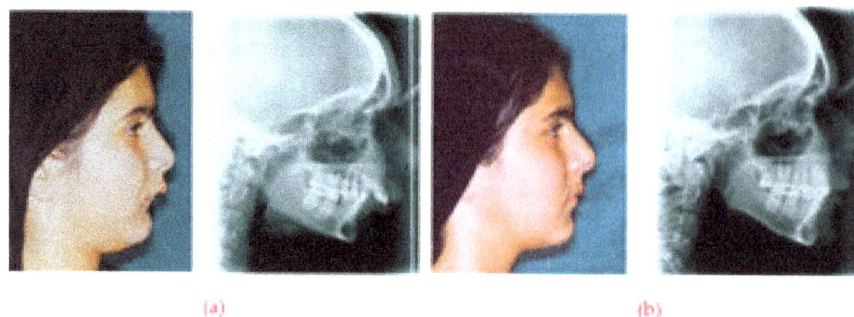

Figure 22. (a) Predistraction profile photograph and lateral cephalogram of an adult patient. (b) Postdistraction profile photograph and lateral cephalogram. (Bilateral intraoral distractors were used.)

5. Relapse

Despite the correction of a class II malocclusion, a considerable number of class II patients experience some level of unpredictable relapses in following years after treatment [28]. Reported relapse rates following these treatments range from 20 to 52% [72]. The only available evidence on stability of treatment regards the Herbst appliance [72]. Several factors including gender, muscular functions and pretreatment habits, different treatment modalities, and posttreatment occlusion have been considered as potential factors affecting stability of the result. However, a very recent systematic review concluded that currently, there is very limited evidence to support the influence of predictive factors on relapse or stability of treatment outcomes [73].

Although mandibular advancement by bilateral sagittal split osteotomy seems to be a good treatment option for skeletal class II, it is less stable than setback in the short and long terms [74]. Miniplates demonstrated better long-term results than bicortical screws of titanium, stainless steel, or bioresorbable material. However, their short-term relapse rate was approximately comparable in class II malocclusion patients. This observed relapse depends on a wide range of patient-centered and surgeon-centered characteristics involving the skill and experience of the surgeon in the proper seating of the condyles, the exact amount of mandibular advancement, the tension of muscles and soft tissue, the mandibular plane angle, and the patient's age. Patients with low and high mandibular plane angles have increased vertical and horizontal relapses, respectively [74].

6. Diagram

Class II Malocclusion Treatment

- Growing

  ○ Functional

- Removable
  - Activator
  - Bionator
  - Frankel
  - Twin-block
- Fixed
  - MARA
  - Cemented Twin-block
  - Herbst
  - Headgear (skeletal effect)
    - Cervical
    - High pull
    - Combination
- Non-growing
  - Camouflage
    - Non-extraction regimen with class II elastics
    - Distal movement of upper teeth ± second molar extraction
      - Pendulum
      - Headgear (dental effect)
      - Miniscrew-assisted distalizations
    - Extraction of maxillary premolars
  - Orthognathic surgery
    - Mandibular advancement
    - Bimax surgery
  - DO
- Relapse

Acknowledgements

The authors thank the staff of Orthodontic, Oral, and Maxillofacial Surgery departments for the general support of treatment procedures of the presented cases and specially wish to express their sincere gratitude to Prof. L Eslamian, Prof. M Nouri, and Prof. M Safavi.

Author details

Azita Tehranchi[1*], Hossein Behnia[2], Farnaz Younessian[3] and Sahar Hadadpour[4]

*Address all correspondence to: azitatehranchi@yahoo.com

1 Preventive Dentistry Research Center, Research Institute of Dental Sciences, Department of Orthodontics, School of Dentistry, Shahid Beheshti University of Medical Sciences, Tehran, Iran

2 Dental Research Center, Research Institute of Dental Sciences, Department of Oral and Maxillofacial Surgery, School of Dentistry, Shahid Beheshti University of Medical Sciences, Tehran, Iran

3 Dentofacial Deformities Research Center, Research Institute of Dental Sciences, School of Dentistry, Shahid Beheshti University of Medical Sciences, Tehran, Iran

4 Department of Orthodontics, School of Dentistry, Shahid Beheshti University of Medical Sciences, Tehran, Iran

References

[1] Elkordy SA, Aboelnaga AA, Salah Fayed MM, AboulFotouh MH, Abouelezz AM. Can the use of skeletal anchors in conjunction with fixed functional appliances promote skeletal changes? A systematic review and meta-analysis. European Journal of Orthodontics. 2015.

[2] Vasquez MJ, Baccetti T, Franchi L, McNamara JA, Jr. Dentofacial features of class II malocclusion associated with maxillary skeletal protrusion: a longitudinal study at the circumpubertal growth period. American Journal of Orthodontics and Dentofacial Orthopedics: Official Publication of the American Association of Orthodontists, Its Constituent Societies, and the American Board of Orthodontics. 2009;135(5):568.e1–7; discussion 9.

[3] Kiekens RM, Maltha JC, Hof MAt, Kuijpers-Jagtman AM. Objective measures as indicators for facial esthetics in white adolescents. The Angle Orthodontist. 2006;76(4): 551–6.

[4] Kalha AS. Early orthodontic treatment reduced incisal trauma in children with class II malocclusions. Evidence-based Dentistry. 2014;15(1):18–20.

[5] Seehra J, Fleming PS, Newton T, DiBiase AT. Bullying in orthodontic patients and its relationship to malocclusion,self-esteem and oral health-related quality of life. Journal of Orthodontics. 2011;38(4):247–56; quiz 94.

[6] Tehranchi A, Behnia H, Younessian F. Bipolar disorder: review of orthodontic and orthognathic surgical considerations. Journal of Craniofacial Surgery. 2015;26(4):1321–5.

[7] Feres MF, Raza H, Alhadlaq A, El-Bialy T. Rapid maxillary expansion effects in class II malocclusion: a systematic review. The Angle Orthodontist. 2015;85(6):1070–9.

[8] Perillo L, Padricelli G, Isola G, Femiano F, Chiodini P, Mataresei G. Class II malocclusion division 1: a new classification method by cephalometric analysis. European Journal of Paediatric Dentistry. 2012;13(3):192.

[9] Shaughnessy T, Shire L. Etiology of class II malocclusions. Pediatric Dentistry. 1988;10(4):336–8.

[10] Zaher AR, Kassem HE. Diagnostic considerations and conventional strategies for treatment of class II malocclusion. Skeletal Anchorage in Orthodontic Treatment of Class II Malocclusion: Contemporary Applications of Orthodontic Implants, Miniscrew Implants and Mini Plates. 2014:1.

[11] Moyers RE, Riolo ML, Guire KE, Wainright RL, Bookstein FL. Differential diagnosis of class II malocclusions: Part 1. Facial types associated with class II malocclusions. American Journal of Orthodontics. 1980;78(5):477–94.

[12] Baccetti T, Franchi L, McNamara JA, Tollaro I. Early dentofacial features of class II malocclusion: a longitudinal study from the deciduous through the mixed dentition. American Journal of Orthodontics and Dentofacial Orthopedics. 1997;111(5):502–9.

[13] Pfeiffer J, Grobéty D. The class II malocclusion: differential diagnosis and clinical application of activators, extraoral traction, and fixed appliances. American Journal of Orthodontics. 1975;68(5):499–544.

[14] Craig CE. The skeletal patterns characteristic of class I and class II, division I malocclusions in Norma Lateralis 1. The Angle Orthodontist. 1951;21(1):44–56.

[15] Wheeler TT, McGorray SP, Dolce C, King GJ. The timing of class II treatment. American Journal of Orthodontics and Dentofacial Orthopedics: Official Publication of the American Association of Orthodontists, Its Constituent Societies, and the American Board of Orthodontics. 2006;129(4 Suppl):S66–70.

[16] Dolce C, McGorray SP, Brazeau L, King GJ, Wheeler TT. Timing of class II treatment: skeletal changes comparing 1-phase and 2-phase treatment. American Journal of Orthodontics and Dentofacial Orthopedics: Official Publication of the American Association of Orthodontists, Its Constituent Societies, and the American Board of Orthodontics. 2007;132(4):481–9.

[17] Burden D, Johnston C, Kennedy D, Harradine N, Stevenson M. A cephalometric study of class II malocclusions treated with mandibular surgery. American Journal of Orthodontics and Dentofacial Orthopedics: Official Publication of the American Association of Orthodontists, Its Constituent Societies, and the American Board of Orthodontics. 2007;131(1):7.e1–8.

[18] Giuntini V, Vangelisti A, Masucci C, Defraia E, McNamara JA, Jr., Franchi L. Treatment effects produced by the twin-block appliance vs the forsus fatigue resistant device in growing class II patients. The Angle Orthodontist. 2015;85(5):784–9.

[19] Thiruvenkatachari B, Harrison JE, Worthington HV, O'Brien KD. Orthodontic treatment for prominent upper front teeth (class II malocclusion) in children. The Cochrane Database of Systematic Reviews. 2013;11:Cd003452.

[20] Firouz M, Zernik J, Nanda R. Dental and orthopedic effects of high-pull headgear in treatment of class II, division 1 malocclusion. American Journal of Orthodontics and Dentofacial Orthopedics. 1992;102(3):197–205.

[21] Hubbard GW, Nanda RS, Currier GF. A cephalometric evaluation of nonextraction cervical headgear treatment in class II malocclusions. The Angle Orthodontist. 1994;64(5):359–70.

[22] Behnia H, Motamedi MHK, Tehranchi A. Use of activator appliances in pediatric patients treated with costochondral grafts for temporomandibular joint ankylosis: analysis of 13 cases. Journal of Oral and Maxillofacial Surgery. 1997;55(12):1408–14.

[23] Pacha MM, Fleming PS, Johal A. A comparison of the efficacy of fixed versus removable functional appliances in children with class II malocclusion: a systematic review. European Journal of Orthodontics. 2015.

[24] Gong Y, Yu Q, Li PL, Wang HH, Wei B, Shen G. Efficacy evaluation of fixed Twin-block appliance and tooth extraction in skeletal class II malocclusion. Shanghai Journal of Stomatology. 2014;23(5):597–600.

[25] Perinetti G, Primozic J, Franchi L, Contardo L. Treatment effects of removable functional appliances in pre-pubertal and pubertal class II patients: a systematic review and meta-analysis of controlled studies. PloS One. 2015;10(10):e0141198.

[26] Marsico E, Gatto E, Burrascano M, Matarese G, Cordasco G. Effectiveness of orthodontic treatment with functional appliances on mandibular growth in the short term. American Journal of Orthodontics and Dentofacial Orthopedics: Official Publication of

the American Association of Orthodontists, Its Constituent Societies, and the American Board of Orthodontics. 2011;139(1):24–36.

[27] Koretsi V, Zymperdikas VF, Papageorgiou SN, Papadopoulos MA. Treatment effects of removable functional appliances in patients with class II malocclusion: a systematic review and meta-analysis. European Journal of Orthodontics. 2015;37(4):418–34.

[28] Flores-Mir C, Major PW. A systematic review of cephalometric facial soft tissue changes with the activator and bionator appliances in class II division 1 subjects. European Journal of Orthodontics. 2006;28(6):586–93.

[29] Rondeau B. Herbst appliance fixed-functional appliance class II skeletal malocclusion. Journal of General Orthodontics. 2001;12(3):7–17.

[30] Shen G, Hagg U, Darendeliler M. Skeletal effects of bite jumping therapy on the mandible – removable vs. fixed functional appliances. Orthodontics and Craniofacial Research. 2005;8(1):2–10.

[31] Perinetti G, Primozic J, Furlani G, Franchi L, Contardo L. Treatment effects of fixed functional appliances alone or in combination with multibracket appliances: a systematic review and meta-analysis. The Angle Orthodontist. 2015;85(3):480–92.

[32] Zymperdikas VF, Koretsi V, Papageorgiou SN, Papadopoulos MA. Treatment effects of fixed functional appliances in patients with class II malocclusion: a systematic review and meta-analysis. European Journal of Orthodontics. 2015.

[33] Dowsing P, Murray A, Sandler J. Emergencies in orthodontics. Part 2: management of removable appliances, functional appliances and other adjuncts to orthodontic treatment. Dental Update. 2015;42(3):221–4, 7–8.

[34] Gonner U, Ozkan V, Jahn E, Toll DE. Effect of the MARA appliance on the position of the lower anteriors in children, adolescents and adults with class II malocclusion. Journal of Orofacial Orthopedics: Fortschritte der Kieferorthopadie : Organ/official journal Deutsche Gesellschaft fur Kieferorthopadie. 2007;68(5):397–412.

[35] Markic G, Katsaros C, Pandis N, Eliades T. Temporary anchorage device usage: a survey among Swiss orthodontists. Progress in Orthodontics. 2014;15(1):29.

[36] Jing Y, Han X, Guo Y, Li J, Bai D. Nonsurgical correction of a class III malocclusion in an adult by miniscrew-assisted mandibular dentition distalization. American Journal of Orthodontics and Dentofacial Orthopedics. 2013;143(6):877–87.

[37] Leung MT-C, Lee TC-K, Rabie ABM, Wong RW-K. Use of miniscrews and miniplates in orthodontics. Journal of Oral and Maxillofacial Surgery. 2008;66(7):1461–6.

[38] Cozzani M, Fontana M, Maino G, Maino G, Palpacelli L, Caprioglio A. Comparison between direct vs indirect anchorage in two miniscrew-supported distalizing devices. The Angle Orthodontist. 2015.

[39] Munoz A, Maino G, Lemler J, Kornbluth D. Skeletal anchorage for class II correction in a growing patient. Journal of Clinical Orthodontics. 2009;43(5):325–31.

[40] Pattabiraman V, Kumari S, Sood R. Mini-implant-supported sliding jig. Orthodontics: The Art and Practice of Dentofacial Enhancement. 2011;12(4):396–9.

[41] Alvirde AE, Acevedo JA, GonzálezII RMA. Treatment of a class II division 1 malocclusion in an adult patient. A case report. Revista Mexicana de Ortodoncia. 2015;3(1): 39–46.

[42] Cleall JF, Begole EA. Diagnosis and treatment of class II division 2 malocclusion. The Angle Orthodontist. 1982;52(1):38–60.

[43] Jones G, Buschang PH, Kim KB, Oliver DR. Class II non-extraction patients treated with the forsus fatigue resistant device versus intermaxillary elastics. The Angle Orthodontist. 2008;78(2):332–8.

[44] Pancherz H, Malmgren O, Hägg U, Ömblus J, Hansen K. Class II correction in Herbst and Bass therapy. The European Journal of Orthodontics. 1989;11(1):17–30.

[45] Skidmore KJ, Brook KJ, Thomson WM, Harding WJ. Factors influencing treatment time in orthodontic patients. American Journal of Orthodontics and Dentofacial Orthopedics. 2006;129(2):230–8.

[46] Caprioglio A, Cafagna A, Fontana M, Cozzani M. Comparative evaluation of molar distalization therapy using pendulum and distal screw appliances. The Korean Journal of Orthodontics. 2015;45(4):171–9.

[47] Hilgers J. The pendulum appliance for class II non-compliance therapy. Journal of Clinical Orthodontics. 1992;26(11):706–14.

[48] Kachiwala VA, Kalha AS, Machado G. Soft tissue changes associated with first premolar extractions in adult females. Australian Orthodontic Journal. 2009;25(1):24–9.

[49] Erdinc AE, Nanda RS, Dandajena TC. Profile changes of patients treated with and without premolar extractions. American Journal of Orthodontics and Dentofacial Orthopedics: Official Publication of the American Association of Orthodontists, Its Constituent Societies, and the American Board of Orthodontics. 2007;132(3):324–31.

[50] Janson G, Mendes LM, Junqueira CHZ, Garib DG. Soft-tissue changes in class II malocclusion patients treated with extractions: a systematic review. The European Journal of Orthodontics. 2015:cjv083.

[51] Păun A, Stanciu R, Pătraşcu I. Skeletal anchorage in orthodontic treatment of a class II malocclusion. Romanian Journal of Oral Rehabilitation. 2015;7(1).

[52] King KS, Lam EW, Faulkner MG, Heo G, Major PW. Vertical bone volume in the paramedian palate of adolescents: a computed tomography study. American Journal of Orthodontics and Dentofacial Orthopedics: Official Publication of the American

Association of Orthodontists, Its Constituent Societies, and the American Board of Orthodontics. 2007;132(6):783–8.

[53] Tehranchi A, Behnia H, Younessian F, Ghochani MS. Rapid, conservative, multidisciplinary miniscrew-assisted approach for treatment of mandibular fractures following plane crash. Dental Research Journal. 2013;10(5):678.

[54] Chen YJ, Chang HH, Lin HY, Lai EHH, Hung HC, Yao CCJ. Stability of miniplates and miniscrews used for orthodontic anchorage: experience with 492 temporary anchorage devices. Clinical Oral Implants Research. 2008;19(11):1188–96.

[55] Behnia H, Tehranchi A, Morad G. Distraction osteogenesis. 2013.

[56] Tehranchi A, Behnia H, Soheilifar S. Evaluation of skeletal, dental, soft tissue and airway cephalometric changes in severe class II malocclusions treated by bilateral mandibular distraction osteogenesis. Iranian Journal of Orthodontics. 2012;7(3).

[57] Proffit WR, Phillips C, Tulloch JF, Medland PH. Surgical versus orthodontic correction of skeletal class II malocclusion in adolescents: effects and indications. The International Journal of Adult Orthodontics and Orthognathic Surgery. 1992;7(4):209–20.

[58] Tehranchi A, Behnia H, Ghochani M, Younessian F. Oro-facial characteristics and the surgical correction of patients affected by beta-thalassaemia: a review of the literature and report of a case. Australian Orthodontic Journal. 2015;31(1):98–106.

[59] Balachander R, Karthik K, Katta A, Rajasigamani K. Surgical correction of class II skeletal malocclusion in an adult patient. Journal of Orofacial Sciences. 2014;6(1):58.

[60] Shetty A, Patil A, Ganeshkar S. Comparison of skeletal, dental and soft tissue changes in young adults with class II malocclusion, treated either by camouflage, fixed functional appliance or orthognathic surgery—a prospective study on Indian subjects. Open Journal of Stomatology. 2012;2(04):373.

[61] Huang CS, Hsu S, Chen Y-R. Systematic review of the surgery-first approach in orthognathic surgery. Biomedical Journal. 2014;37(4):184.

[62] Magnusson T, Ahlborg G, Svartz K. Function of the masticatory system in 20 patients with mandibular hypo- or hyperplasia after correction by a sagittal split osteotomy. International Journal of Oral Maxillofacial Surgery. 1990;19(5):289–93.

[63] Sanders B, Kaminishi R, Buoncristiani R, Davis C. Arthroscopic surgery for treatment of temporomandibular joint hypomobility after mandibular sagittal osteotomy. Oral Surgery, Oral Medicine, and Oral Pathology. 1990;69(5):539–41.

[64] Catherine Z, Breton P, Bouletreau P. Condylar resorption after orthognathic surgery: a systematic review. Revue de stomatologie, de chirurgie maxillo-faciale et de chirurgie orale. 2015.

[65] Behnia H, Tehranchi A, Younessian F. Comprehensive management of temporomandibular joint ankylosis—state of the art. 2015.

[66] Jang J-H, Choi S-K, Park S-H, Kim J-W, Kim S-J, Kim M-R. Clinical evaluation of temporomandibular joint disorder after orthognathic surgery in skeletal class II malocclusion patients. Journal of the Korean Association of Oral and Maxillofacial Surgeons. 2012;38(3):139–44.

[67] Azumi Y, Sugawara J, Takahashi I, Mitani H, Nagasaka H, Kawamura H. Positional and morphologic changes of the mandibular condyle after mandibular distraction osteogenesis in skeletal class II patients. World Journal of Orthodontics. 2003;5(1):32–9.

[68] Ilizarov GA. The principles of the Ilizarov method. Bulletin of the Hospital for Joint Diseases Orthopaedic Institute. 1987;48(1):1–11.

[69] Tehranchi A, Behnia H. Treatment of mandibular asymmetry by distraction osteogenesis and orthodontics: a report of four cases. The Angle Orthodontist. 2000;70(2):165–74.

[70] Tehranchi A, Behnia H. Facial symmetry after distraction osteogenesis and orthodontic therapy. American Journal of Orthodontics and Dentofacial Orthopedics. 2001;120(2): 149–53.

[71] Vos M, Baas E, de Lange J, Bierenbroodspot F. Stability of mandibular advancement procedures: Bilateral sagittal split osteotomy versus distraction osteogenesis. International Journal of Oral and Maxillofacial Surgery. 2009;38(1):7–12.

[72] Bock NC, von Bremen J, Ruf S. Stability of class II fixed functional appliance therapy —a systematic review and meta-analysis. The European Journal of Orthodontics. 2015:cjv009.

[73] Wins SM, Antonarakis GS, Kiliaridis S. Predictive factors of sagittal stability after treatment of class II malocclusions: a systematic review. The Angle Orthodontist. 2015.

[74] Joss CU, Vassalli IM. Stability after bilateral sagittal split osteotomy advancement surgery with rigid internal fixation: a systematic review. Journal of Oral and Maxillofacial Surgery. 2009;67(2):301–13.

9

State-of-the-Art Immediate Implant Therapy

Peter R. Hunt and Laura M. Ceccacci

Abstract

Implantology is the newest major branch of dentistry and one that is rapidly becoming more and more important. A subject that was ridiculed 40 years ago is now transforming dentistry. Implantology gives hope for the end-stage edentulous patient unable to wear dentures. It enables those facing loss of a tooth to avoid bridgework or removable partial dentures. It is often simpler, faster, and far more effective over the long term to replace a failing tooth with an implant with a restoration than to do a root canal, post-core, and crown. This chapter discusses immediate implant therapy, which greatly reduces surgical interventions and shortens total treatment time, while preserving the alveolar structures which are rapidly lost when a tooth is extracted.

Keywords: immediate implant therapy, socket regeneration with implants, single-stage implant surgery, immediate placement, immediate loading

1. Introduction

Traditionally, implants have been placed into healed ridges where the teeth had been removed from a previous procedure. For an edentulous patient there was no other option, but to remove the teeth quickly before placing implants, which became a standard. The traditional protocol was then to reflect a soft tissue flap, to prepare a channel in the bone, to place the implant with a cover screw, and then to cover the soft tissue flap back over the region for a period of three to six months. At that time, another soft tissue flap was raised and a connection made to bring the implant transgingivally so that it could be brought into function. This meant the patient was subject to three surgical interventions: the extraction, the implant placement, and the second-stage exposure. With healing cycles in place, therapy from extraction to second-stage exposure and final restoration could take a year or more to complete.

Although this protocol can ensure a stable and functioning implant, it has some unfortunate sequelae. Most obvious are the time, expense, and discomfort for the patient associated with the three surgical procedures. Only recently have we started to appreciate that there is another, more significant issue with this three-stage protocol. This is the significant loss of alveolar bone and the periodontal soft-tissue complex in the region of the extraction. This can be extremely difficult to correct with augmentation procedures. Aesthetic and functional deformities remain. Immediate implant therapy can reduce the number of surgical procedures and expedite therapy, while at the same time minimizing the loss of alveolar and gingival structures, thus reducing aesthetic and functional deformities.

2. Post-extraction course

2.1. Ridge collapse

When a tooth is removed, the hard and soft tissue complex surrounding the tooth undergoes a series of changes. The soft tissues immediately collapse down, having lost the support from the tooth (**Figure 1**).

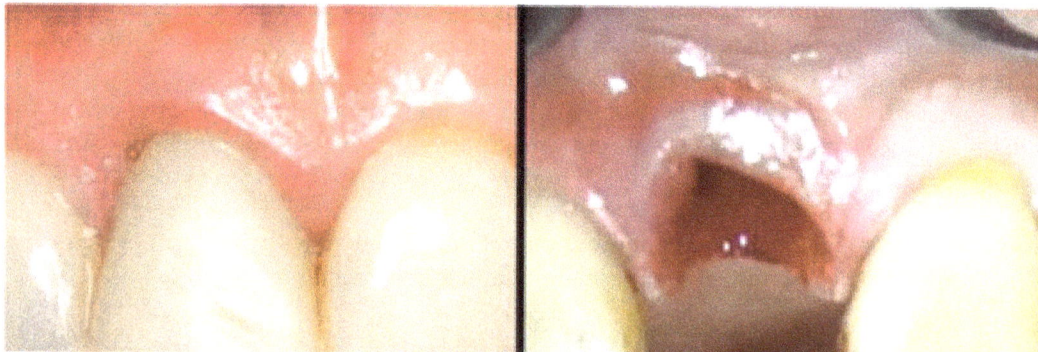

Figure 1. As soon as the right central incisor is removed, the soft-tissue complex starts to collapse.

Bleeding into the socket rapidly turns to a blood clot. Very quickly epithelium starts to migrate over the top of the blood clot. By this time blood vessels have invaded the blood clot and stem cells are proliferating, differentiating, and maturing. The region becomes progressively organized so that connective tissue and then bone start forming (**Figure 2**).

In time, there are major changes in the soft tissue covering the ridge. After the ridge epithelializes over, the new "Ridge" gingiva blends with the remnants of the original marginal attached gingiva. This lasts for a relatively short time because the region of attached gingiva starts to shrink, sometimes so much that only a very narrow band of attached gingiva remains on the alveolar crest (**Figure 3**).

As time passes, the bone in the crestal region shrinks, more so on the labial than on the lingual. The ridge height diminishes and the overall bone volume decreases. The tough cortical bone thins and the medullary bone starts to atrophy as there is less function with the teeth missing.

The more time that passes, then the more bone loss that is likely to occur [1–3]. All these factors suggest that it would be better to do everything possible to stop the shrinkage process starting when the tooth is removed. Immediate interceptive therapy is required.

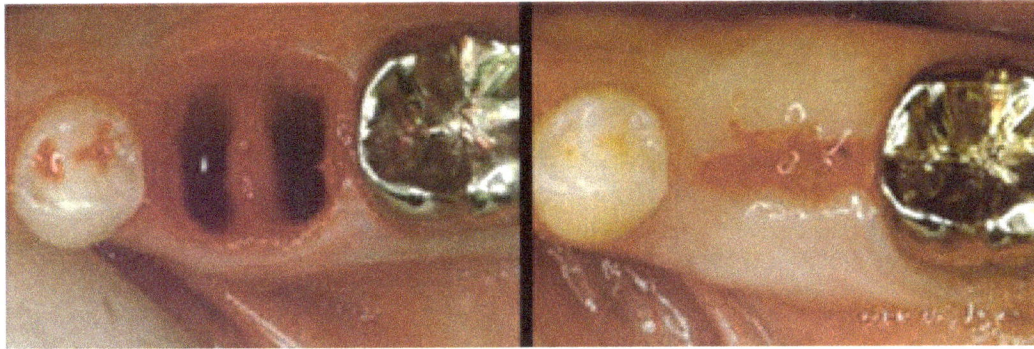

Figure 2. Left: The first molar has just been removed. Right: One month later.

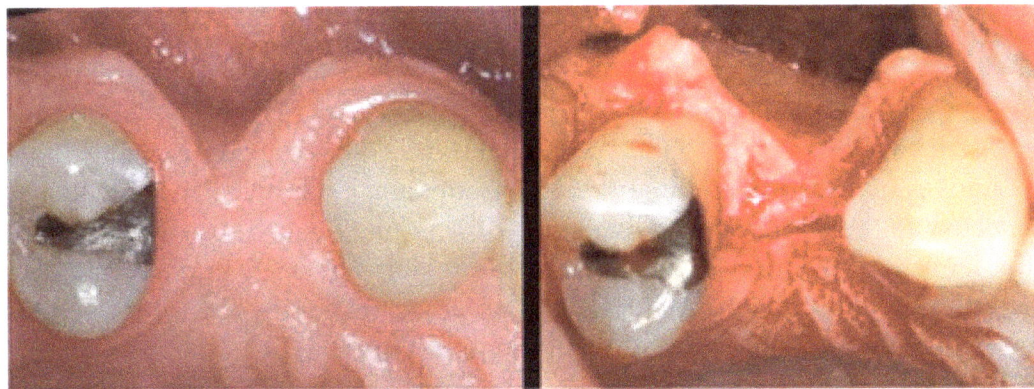

Figure 3. In this case, following the loss of the premolar, both the attached gingiva and the alveolar bone shrunk down extensively.

3. Requirements for immediate implant placement

3.1. Successful removal of the tooth

Immediate placement is precluded upon careful removal of teeth. The prime aim is to leave a socket with intact bone walls with sufficient residual bone to stabilize an implant. Unfortunately, this is one of the major uncertainties in the whole protocol, because some teeth can be extremely resistant to removal, others can fracture readily. If not careful, the bone housing for the tooth can easily be lost in the tooth removal process. For these reasons, it is quite standard to split multi-rooted teeth into their individual roots. Each root can then be removed individually. Removing labial bone to get at decayed or fractured off at the gum level teeth is generally quite harmful as this reduces the height of the residual socket. Instead, periotomes are better used for loosening and elevating the roots. Ultrasonic periotome tips are particularly useful to expedite root removal (**Figure 4**).

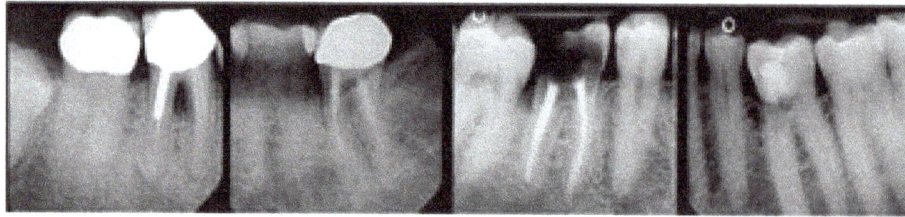

Figure 4. Teeth difficult to remove. Left: Large post in distal root with bulbous root end. Left Center: Long, thin deep roots. Right Center: Deep decay, poor tooth structure, large root canal fillings. Right: External resorption, very deep roots, proximity to neighboring tooth.

3.2. Removal of infection and granulation tissues in the region

Once the tooth has been removed from the socket, it is critical to remove three tissues from the socket: Remnants of the gingival complex, deeper granulomas, and periapical lesions.

3.2.1. Remnants of the gingival complex

Where the teeth have been periodontally involved it may take some time to work around the socket to remove any soft tissue remnants with curettes and excavators. In some sockets, there may be infected epithelial remnants which pass down quite deep. These need to be removed so that they are not taken down deeper into the region when an implant is placed. Both infections and epithelial down-growths are both associated with loss of osseointegration; removing them allows for successful implant therapy (**Figure 5**) [4].

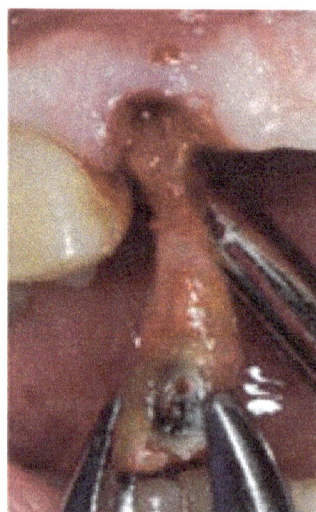

Figure 5. When this tooth was being removed, a considerable amount of epithelial remnants and connective tissue granulations came out with it. Granulations can often be more extensive than expected. They take time and considerable effort to remove.

3.2.2. Deeper granulomas

More difficult to remove are deeper granulomas residing between roots. These can be of periodontal or endodontic origin. It is necessary to work around and under the granuloma with spoon excavators. Once they have been separated then they can be lifted up and out of the socket. Ultrasonic debridement and/or de-granulation with rough-cut burs can speed the process (**Figure 6**).

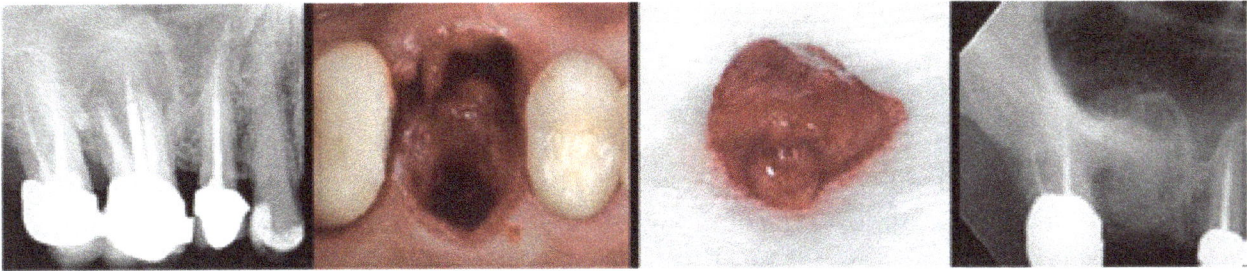

Figure 6. This molar has obvious trifurcation involvements and periapical infection. With the tooth removed, the granulations are apparent, considerably more than expected. When cleaned out, a large sinus perforation to the distal was apparent. There was no ability to stabilize an implant, so the procedure was changed to a "Socket Regeneration" procedure.

3.2.3. Periapical endodontic lesions

The most difficult region to remove residual infection from is the apical region. Sometimes an apical granuloma will come out with the root and this is always good to see. There are other times where it may be necessary to open up the apical region beneath the root space or to access the lesion from a lateral approach. No matter what, it is critical to do this de-granulation for an implant placed in the region to be successful (**Figure 7**).

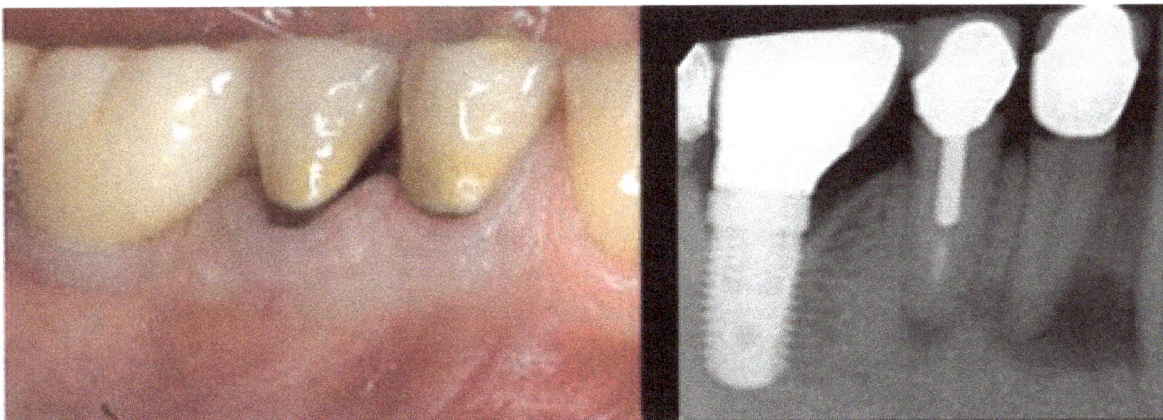

Figure 7. Both these premolars have apical infections and may break off at the gum level because of marginal decay. A procedure is needed to remove the teeth, debride the region and place implants. See **Figures 35** and **36** for treatment.

4. Ability to position and stabilize an implant in the remaining bone volume

Once the tooth has been removed and the region de-granulated, attention must turn to positioning and stabilizing an implant correctly. There are two different and sometimes incompatible considerations.

4.1. Implant positioning

These days it is the abutment which produces the desired emergence form as it exits the soft tissue collar. An implant platform is round but the form of a tooth as it emerges from the gingiva is highly variable. So the abutment that starts out round at the implant platform needs some vertical height, thickness of gingiva or "running room" to change to the desired form as it exits the gingiva. This implies two things: first, positioning the implant platform is critical, as it needs to serve as the base for the abutment; second, the angle of the implant, the diameter of the implant, and the length of the implant are less critical (**Figure 8**).

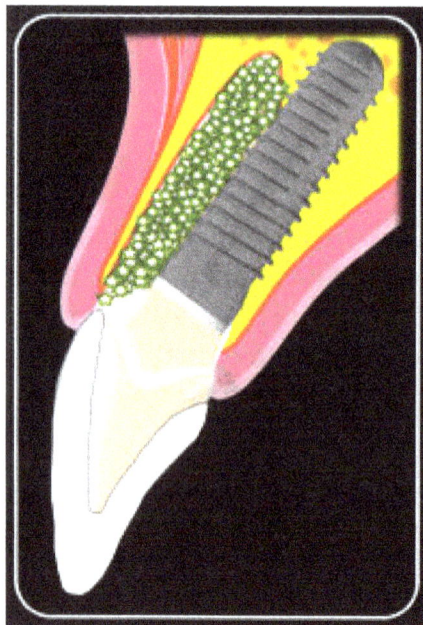

Figure 8. Modern implant environment principles.

Implant: oriented into palatal bone wall to gain stability.

Platform Placement: deeper to allow room for Emergence Profile Development

Augmentation: to fill out the residual socket, preserve labial bone wall, and prevent resorption

Abutment: to develop the desired "Tooth Form" and to support hard and soft tissue contours

Positioning an implant into a healed bony ridge is in many respects simpler than placing one into an extraction socket for several reasons.

4.1.1. The original socket may divert drills and take them off course

This is most common in multi-rooted sockets where the central core of bone can be very hard and it can be very difficult to establish a starting point for a pilot drill. The drill tends to be diverted down and into one of the root spaces (**Figure 9**).

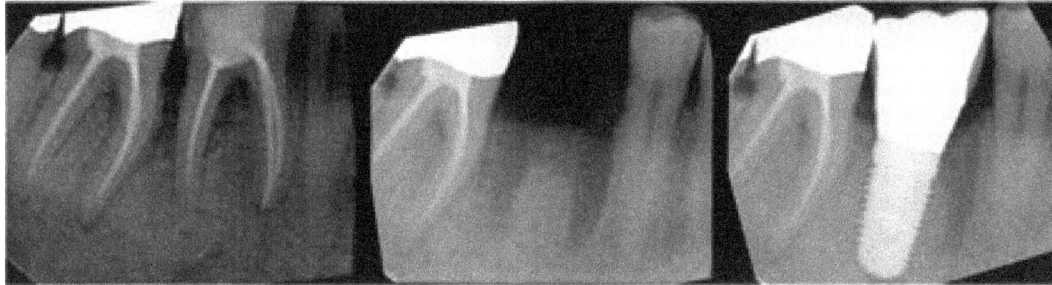

Figure 9. This vertically fractured molar was removed. Instead of the channel being established centrally in the furca region, it was diverted down the distal root space. A custom abutment was needed to manage the situation.

4.1.2. The original socket is not where implant support is available

A common example of this is in the maxillary anterior region where it is not a good idea to place an implant down the socket as this will mean that the implant gets placed too labial. This jeopardizes the thin labial bone wall of the socket. It is better to intentionally angle the implant into the palatal wall of the socket to gain the desired stability and position (**Figure 10**).

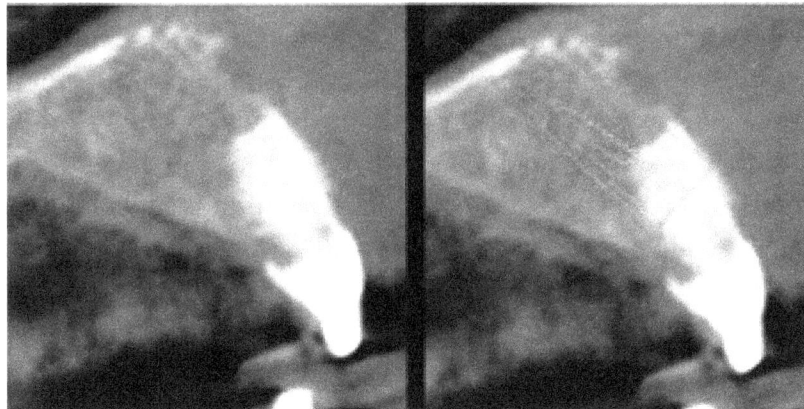

Figure 10. This central incisor needs replacing. The labial bone wall is very thin. The implant needs to be set into the palatal bone wall. The proposed position is outlined.

4.1.3. The original position of the tooth may not be the best position for an implant

The tooth may have an original malocclusion or have drifted, rotated, or changed position as part of a mesial drifting or bite collapse process. This can mean that it would be better to have the implant in a slightly different position (**Figure 11**).

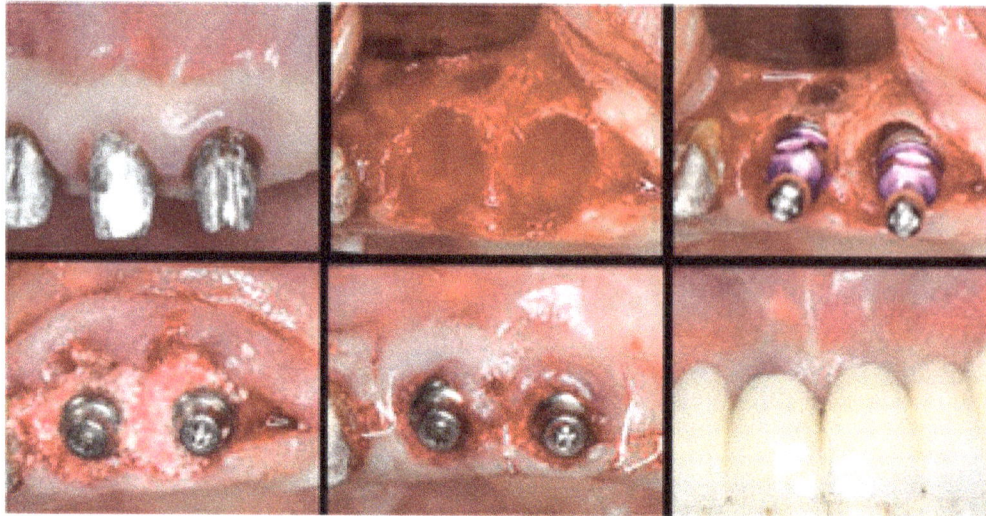

Figure 11. This case shows failing incisor teeth. These were extracted and immediately replaced with Camlog® implants and gingivaformers. Notice how the implants were moved laterally in the sockets to improve the midline of the final case.

4.2. Stabilizing regions

The ability to gain stability for a dental implant in extraction sockets very much depends on the form of the socket. The bone walls in a socket are generally quite firm and stable, so a small amount of bone can provide adequate stability for an implant. Of course, if immediate loading is required at the same time then a much higher level of stability is required [5, 6].

The region providing stabilization for an implant within a recent extraction socket can be quite limited and requires careful planning. Most times the socket will be larger than the implant. Often the only place where the implant engages the bone is in the apical region where the bone walls converge. However, one must be careful because all too often the socket is compromised in one way or another. For example, many sockets have little or no labial bone and this means that the implant needs to be positioned more centrally within the available bone complex. In socket management, it is always necessary to appreciate how the socket is liable to heal, both with or without an implant.

Sometimes, particularly in the molar regions, there is no obvious place for stabilizing an implant in the former socket. If bone is available beyond the residual socket, it may be possible to use as little as 2–3 mm to stabilize the implant. In the mandible, it is necessary to carefully check the location of the mandibular nerve as this may prevent this "Going beyond the socket" procedure. All that is needed is to make sure that the implant is stable. Obviously, it will not be possible to immediately load the implant with this limited amount of stabilization (**Figure 12**).

In the maxilla, it may be necessary to perform an intentional sinus lift to gain stability for the implant. The bone of the sinus floor, though it may be thin, is generally very stable. All that is necessary is to penetrate the floor in a safe way, such as with an ultrasonic device. The hole is then expanded with a hand-held osteotome. The final diameter of the channel should be matched to the apical diameter of the tapered implant that will be placed.

The sinus floor membrane is lifted with the osteotome. Bone graft is then placed and taken up into the sinus with the osteotome. A tapered, screw-threaded implant is placed into the channel. As it is screwed to place, the implant will gain increasing stability as the wider part of the implant gains traction. The sinus-lifted portion will also provide enhanced long-term stability (**Figure 13**).

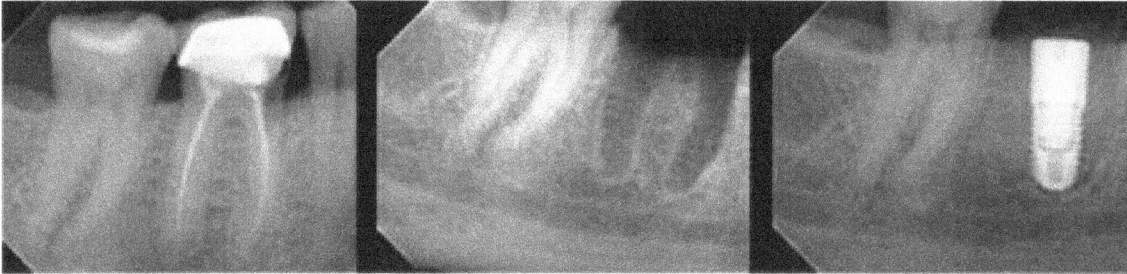

Figure 12. It would not have been sensible to take the channel deeper to gain stability because of the proximity of the nerve. Instead, the Pilot Drill was angled down the mesial root space, and then the channel was uprighted and expanded with progressively larger drills. The final implant placement was nicely centered and the implant was stable.

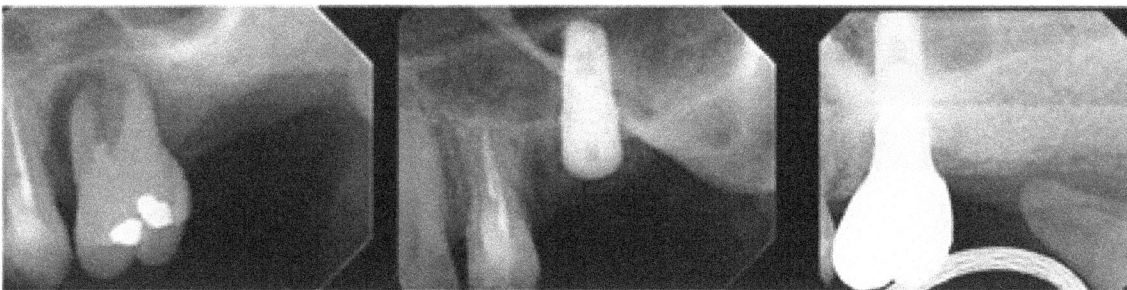

Figure 13. There was nothing much holding this molar in place. It was removed, the region debrided, and an intentional sinus lift performed to gain additional bone volume to stabilize an implant, so gaining additional support. Both the sinus region and the residual socket were grafted. Both regions healed to provide adequate support for the implant and restoration.

5. Provision of an osseous coagulum surrounding the implant

If an implant is adequately stabilized in a fresh socket, then much of the implant surface is liable to be exposed to the oral environment, allowing it to become contaminated; the result is that the implant will fail to osseointegrate. Instead of just leaving a blood clot around the implant, most operators feel more comfortable with filling the voids between the implant and the bony walls of the socket with a bone graft; this not only helps with implant osseointegration but also helps in preventing ridge collapse [7]. The term "Osseous Coagulum" implies supplying all the components which surround and protect the implant following placement.

These help stabilize the blood clot and allow a secure environment for it to develop stem cells, to re-organize, develop osteoblasts, and develop native bone ready to osseointegrate to the implant.

Certain types of bone graft, the slow-resorption materials, have been shown to resist or slow down the ridge resorption process which starts as soon as a tooth is removed [7–9]. At the same time, they encourage new bone to develop. The two aspects are synergistic. They help each other, so the term "osseous coagulum" implies a region which will in time become bone.

New bone formation occurs most predictably within the four walls of a socket. This is why everything possible is done to preserve the four walls of a socket during tooth removal and why the implant platform is placed down below the bone crest. If one bone wall is missing, then a membrane is always placed to provide the environment for its regeneration (**Figure 14**).

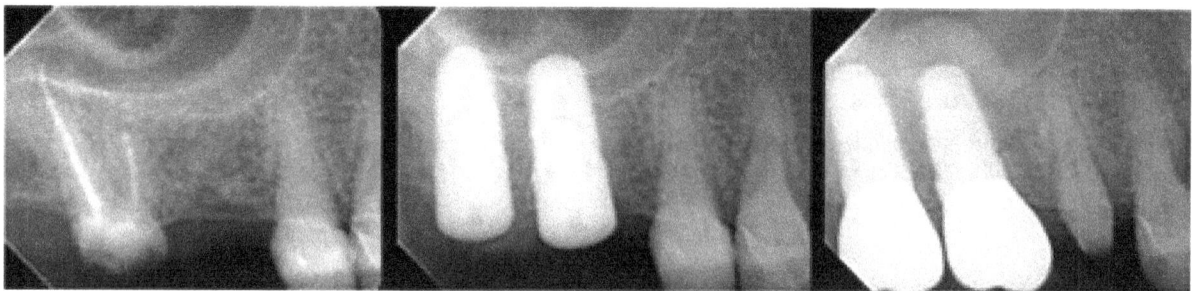

Figure 14. In this case an Osseous Coagulum Zone was needed in the region of the extracted roots of the second molar and also in the sinus lift region for the first molar implant. This was all managed in one surgical procedure when the second molar was extracted.

6. Wound closure

Closing the wound is the last part of the procedure. The aim is to protect the implant within the osseous coagulum, contain the graft materials, prevent early contamination and infection, stabilize the blood clot, and prevent bleeding. It is not just a matter of flap closure. One also has to consider the devices used to cover the implant including cover screws, extended height healing caps, and abutments of one form or another. Each of these components has a specific indication.

6.1. Component options

6.1.1. Cover screw

Cover screws are flat, low-profile devices often supplied with the implant. These are mostly used in traditional therapy where primary closure of the flaps over the region containing the new implant is desired (**Figure 15**).

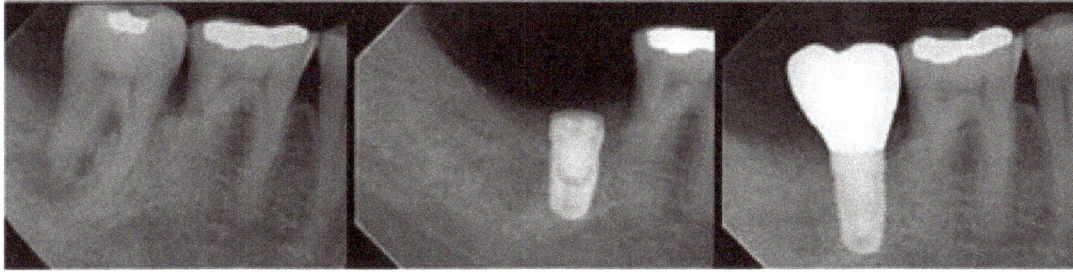

Figure 15. This case had a large periodontal defect with complete involvement of the distal root. The tooth was extracted, the region debrided and an implant with a cover screw placed at the same time. The deficient region in the distal root region was augmented with Bio-Oss Collagen® (Geistlich). There was primary closure over the implant. The region recovered and was restored with a custom abutment and final crown.

6.1.2. Gingivaformer

Gingivaformers come in various heights and configurations. Traditionally they have been placed at second-stage implant exposure surgery to form a trans-gingival passage into the mouth. These days they are often placed at the time of implant placement, with flaps being brought up around the outside of the gingivaformer (**Figure 16**).

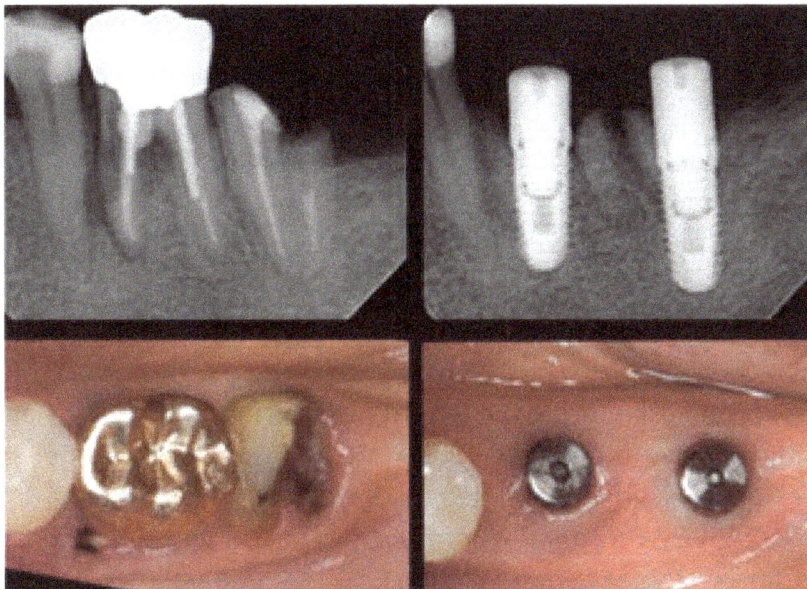

Figure 16. Left: Two failing molars. They were removed and immediately replaced with implants and hard- and soft-tissue augmentation. Right: Three months later, healing is evident. The case is now ready for restoration.

6.1.3. Abutment

Abutments provide an emergence and form which is more tooth-shaped. They also carry a restorative post, so these devices are used for immediate implant placement where immediate loading and a provisional restoration are required. Custom zirconia sleeves secured to a Ti-CAD base devices are generally more useful than off-the-shelf components because they allow for custom form, good gingival reaction, and tooth-like color. Zirconia has better gingival adhesion than Titanium or PEEK plastic components. We use them for both temporary and final restorations (**Figure 17**).

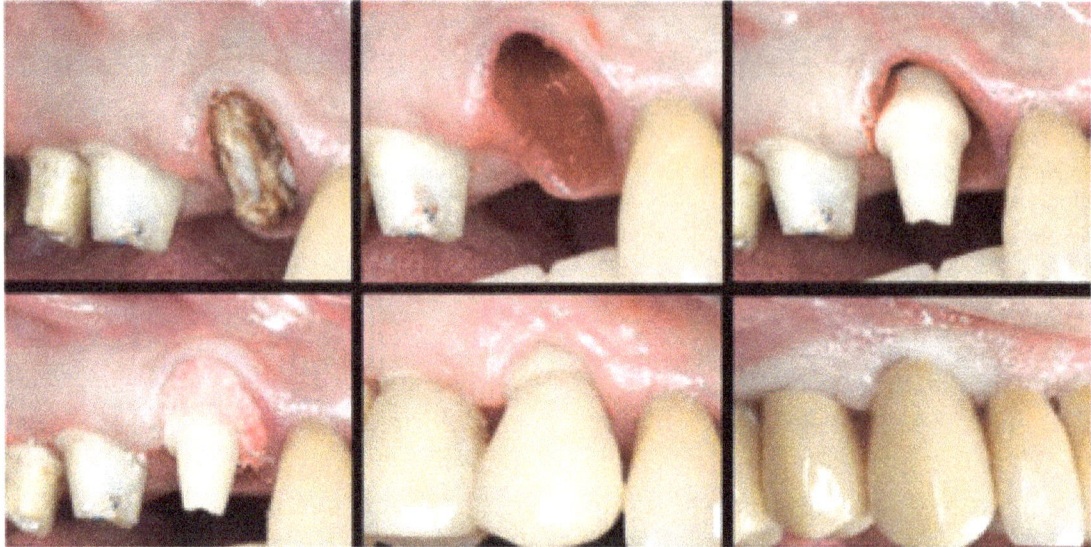

Figure 17. In this case, when the tooth was extracted, an implant was placed which supported a provisional abutment. Graft material was placed around the abutment to fill the channel defects. Despite the exposed graft material which was stabilized by cyanoacrylate (not shown), the wound healed-over fast and at one month appears very normal. Notice how the gingival margin healed well up on the abutment. The final implant-supported restoration improved the form and appearance of the original tooth.

6.2. Soft tissue closure

6.2.1. Primary closure

Traditionally, implant placement has been done by raising soft tissue flaps in the region adjacent to the implant site to allow access to prepare the bone channel and to place the implant(s). At the end of the procedure, the soft tissue flaps were closed back over the wound with what is called Primary Closure. With immediate placement of implants into extraction sockets, getting primary closure is more complex. To accomplish this, it is necessary to raise flaps and advance them to cover over the socket. The bigger the socket the more difficult it is to close over. If bone and soft tissue augmentation has been done, then more bulk has been added to the region, and this can increase the problems of getting closure. Finally, swelling and hematoma formation can make obtaining and maintaining primary closure still more difficult. The traditional solution to this problem is to make the flaps more mobile by raising them further and by severing the periosteum under the free mucosal part of the flap. However, this has the effect of moving attached gingiva from the sides of the socket to the top of the socket. There's no real problem with that in the short term, but in the long term it's essential to have attached gingiva attached to the alveolar bone outside and around an implant. It means an additional surgical procedure is needed not only to place a trans-gingival component, but also to raise the attached gingiva in the region and to displace it out and around the gingiva-former.

However, unless large-scale augmentation is being used, or the patient has a predisposition to implant failure, then primary closure is not required. Partial closure is quite adequate in most situations.

6.2.2. Partial closure

"Partial closure" is where the flaps are brought up around a gingivaformer or abutment placed in the implant, instead of a cover screw. This has several advantages. The surgical procedure is less invasive and it makes for a "single-stage" procedure. This is where there is no need for a secondary implant exposure procedure. It means that the overall treatment time is reduced by several months. The soft tissue complex is also more mature and stable than would be normal in a traditional two-stage procedure. It is easy to provide augmentation under the flaps, with bone graft and thickness increasing membranes, thus increasing the gingival thickness and providing a "safety zone" to protect the rough surface of the implant from becoming contaminated at an early stage. Finally, it means that attached gingiva surrounds the gingivaformer or abutment and this provides better protection for the implant and a more "Natural" appearance as the implant restorative component emerges through the gingiva. We tend to add a collagen-based bone graft at the base of the gingivaformer to fill any channel defects that may be present between the implant and the inner walls of an extraction socket. This is heaped up to increase gingival thickness. This provides a "safety zone" to protect the rough surface of the implant from becoming contaminated and infected at the outset (**Figure 18**).

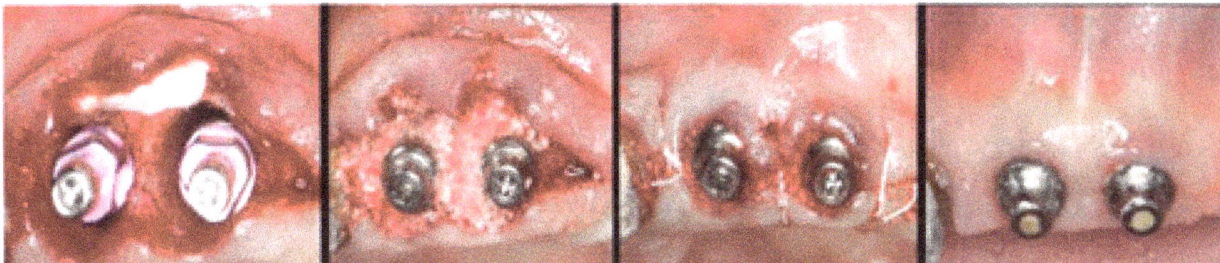

Figure 18. These front teeth were failing, so they were removed. Camlog® implants and gingivaformers were placed. The region was augmented with Mucograft® and Bio-Oss Collagen® (Geistlich) and the flaps were approximated. Healing proceeded nicely and a good final outcome was obtained.

6.2.3. Membrane closure

It is useful to think of ways which avoid extensive soft tissue mobilization and primary closure, one which leaves the attached gingiva where it is, or increases and thickens it. The trend is to use membranes of one form or another to cover the socket, the implant, the gingivaformer, and the bone graft within the osseous coagulum and the whole area.

Essentially, this is taking up the well-established principles of "socket regeneration" [7–9]. This is where extraction sockets are filled with bone graft of one form or another, and then covered over with various membranes. These range from Teflon-based plastic membrane, to collagen membranes to artificial membranes derived from polylactic acid or biodegradable co-polymers. Most of these seem to work quite satisfactorily, although as healing occurs, some shrinkage of the complex can be anticipated. The key is to get "wall-to-wall" regeneration within the socket. The membrane has several functions. First, it stabilizes the blood clot and bone graft mixture which enables it to consolidate, start healing, and become organized. With some membranes such as collagen membranes, the membrane material becomes partly or completely incorporated into the blood clot. The region soon becomes epithelialized. In others, such as the Teflon membranes, epithelialization starts to occur underneath the membrane. The individual processes do not matter too much as all the membranes serve to protect the healing wound and to reduce the potential for trauma, contamination, and infection. By about three weeks, the region is able to manage on its own because it is covered by epithelium with connective tissue immediately underneath. In short, it is not essential for complete primary closure of soft tissue flaps over a socket regeneration site. Instead, it is possible to achieve wound closure, implant osseointegration, bone regeneration, and good soft tissue healing by using artificial membrane; all the more reason to use these proven socket regeneration techniques to provide protection in a healing socket which contains a newly placed implant. Another benefit is with the implant there will be less shrinkage of the complex. A 4.0 mm height gingivaformer is generally placed into the implant instead of a cover screw and this helps "tent up" and stabilize the region. Bone graft generally fills up to and slightly over the top of the gingivaformer, and then the membrane covers the whole region.

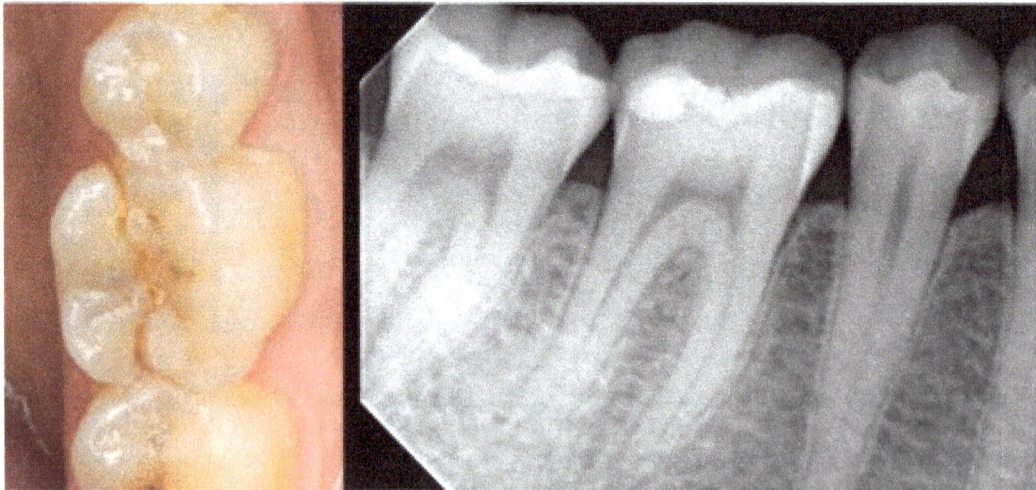

Figure 19. This mandibular first molar is vertically fractured and the crack extended sub-osseously.

As healing progresses there is some shrinkage. The top of the gingivaformer generally becomes exposed and at the appropriate time, it can easily be removed for impression taking. Emergence profile development and placement of a final abutment and restoration are then routine (**Figures 19–21**).

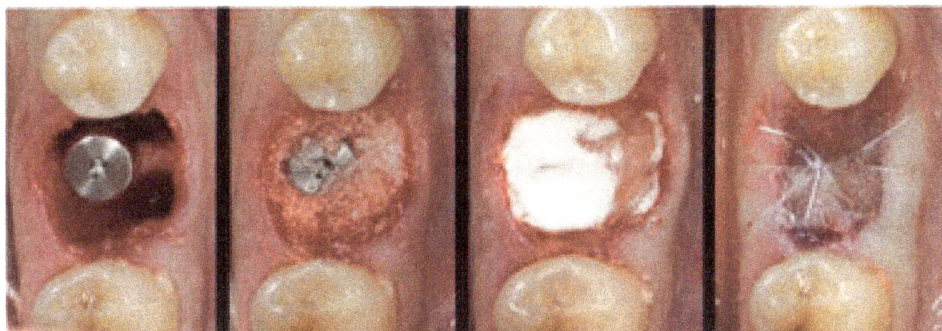

Figure 20. The tooth was removed and a Camlog® implant and gingivaformer placed. Bio-Oss Collagen® was placed down and around the implant. A Mucograft® membrane was placed over and the region sutured and sealed with Tissue Glue.

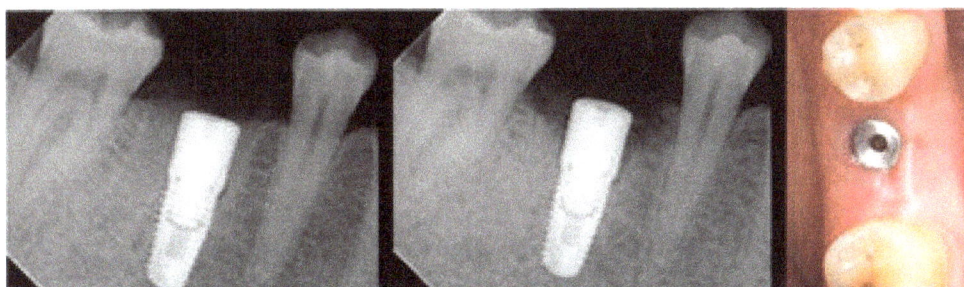

Figure 21. The radiograph on the left was taken immediately following the procedure. The one alongside was taken 3 months later as was the photograph. The case is now ready for a final restoration.

7. Regional considerations

7.1. Maxillary anteriors

Maxillary anterior teeth immediate replacement is very demanding. It can be very difficult to provide a final result where it is hard to know if a crown is implant-supported or tooth-supported. All too often, the give-away is that the implant-supported unit has recession of the interproximal papillae and labial gingival margin. This can be very difficult to reverse surgically. The obvious way to approach these situations is to be prepared for an immediate implant replacement and to make sure that the original hard and soft tissues in the region are maintained.

It's critical not to place the implant directly down the extraction socket as this will lead to the implant being set far too labial, leading to greater recession of the labial bone and soft tissue complex [9–14]. What is needed instead is to reinforce and regenerate the labial plate of bone. This is done by generating an osseous coagulum by placing a slow-resorbing bone graft between the labial bone and the implant. This allows adequate time for native bone to grow into the region. Instead of stabilizing the implant into the bone at the apex of the socket, the implant needs to be stabilized into the palatal bone wall. This requires an abutment which can be angled towards the palatal which means the screw access channel will come out labially. To manage, this requires a separate abutment with an angle change and a separate crown. To facilitate the desired abutment form and angle change, it is necessary to set the implant platform quite deep within the bone complex. The case shown below illustrates all of these considerations (**Figures 22–28**).

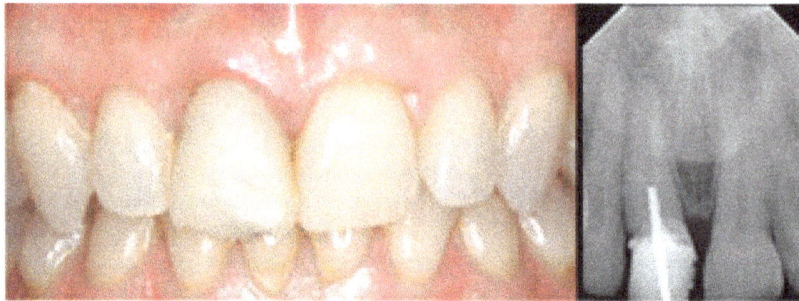

Figure 22. The patient had the misfortune to have a crown on a maxillary central incisor fracture off while she was under anesthesia for a minor surgical procedure.

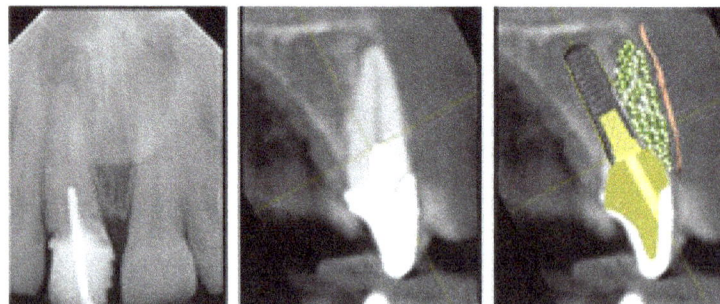

Figure 23. The cross-sectional CBCT cut showed that the tooth had little or no labial bone plate, but that there was a good volume of stable bone in the palatal wall of the socket. The principle of the procedure then is to anchor an implant into this palatal wall. The empty bone socket then needed to be filled with a bone graft and the outer wall of the socket needed to be protected with a membrane.

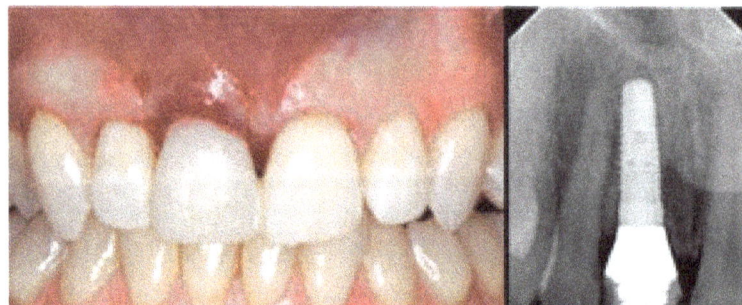

Figure 24. Here was the situation immediately following the procedure. An implant has been placed, all the augmentation materials are present and a temporary abutment with a provisional crown has been secured. It is screw-retained.

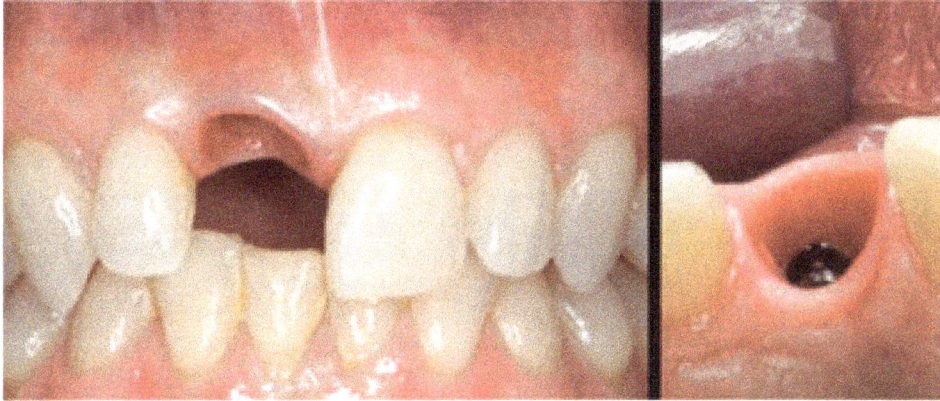

Figure 25. Four months later when the temporary abutment and crown are removed, the region looks very healthy. Notice the well-keratinized sulcus and freedom from inflammation.

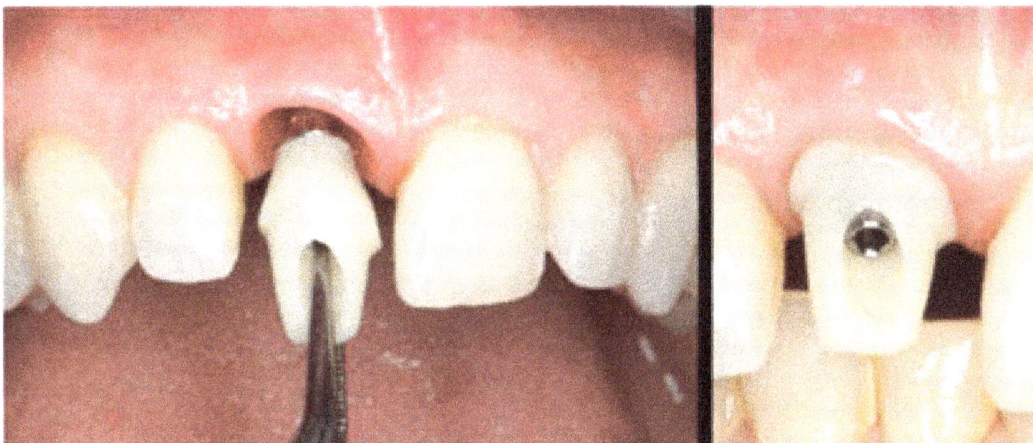

Figure 26. Now the final abutment is placed. This is a custom Zirconia sleeve secured onto a Titanium Base CAD-CAM component.

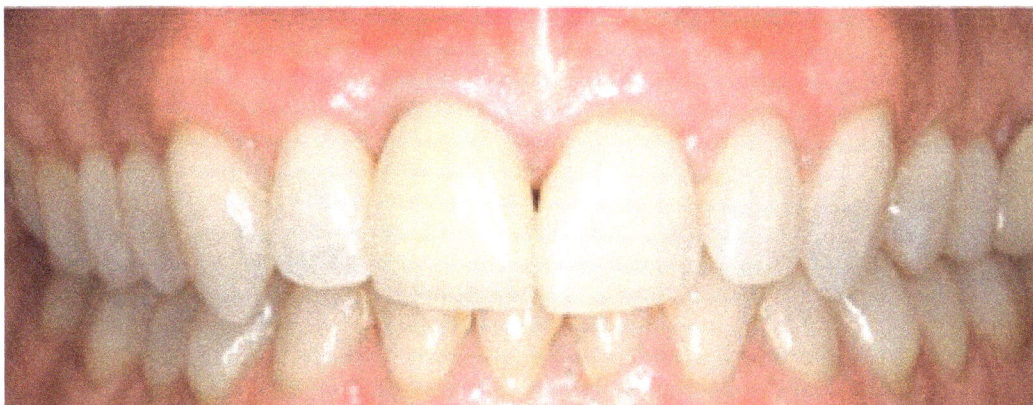

Figure 27. The final result.

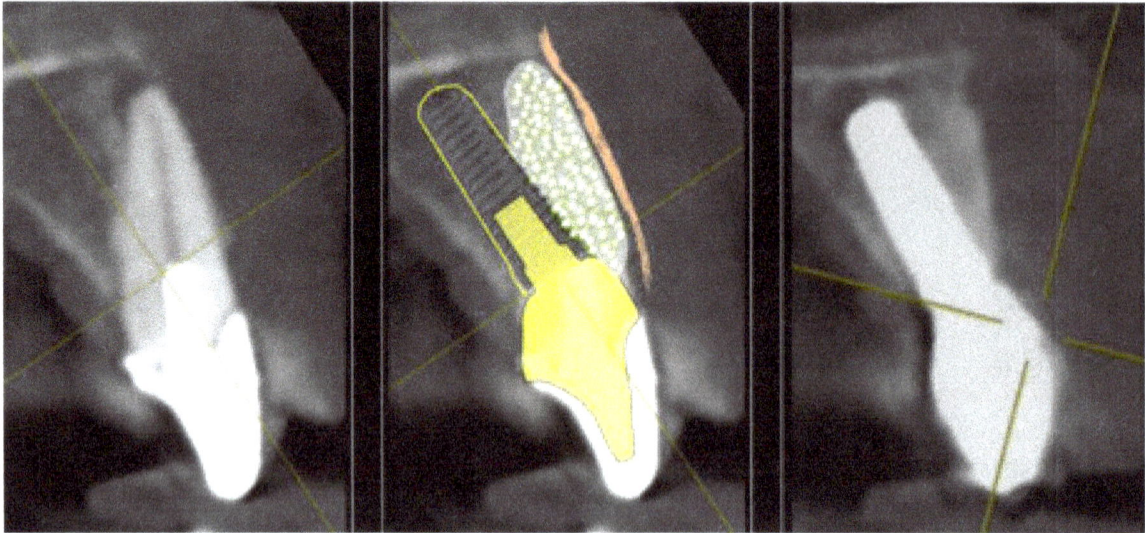

Figure 28. On the right is a cross-sectional CBCT slice taken 6 months following treatment showing that the labial region is stable and has filled in nicely.

7.2. Mandibular anteriors

The guidelines for mandibular anterior replacements are completely different from those of the maxillary anteriors. The situation can be much more variable and requires very careful analysis. The essential thing to appreciate is that one has to be very careful to make sure there is adequate bone volume within which to place an implant. The case which follows is a good illustration of some of the problems that can occur (**Figures 29–32**).

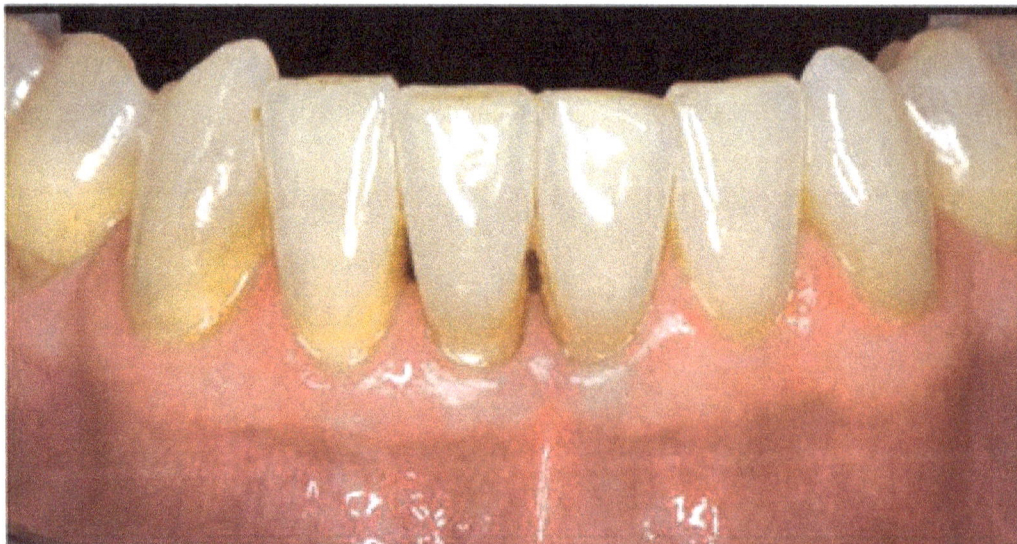

Figure 29. These lower anterior teeth seem almost perfect. On a routine examination the general dentist noticed there was a radiographic defect in the root canal chamber of the right central incisor. He referred the case to an endodontist for evaluation who diagnosed an external resorption of the tooth. He declined to treat the case and recommended an implant consult.

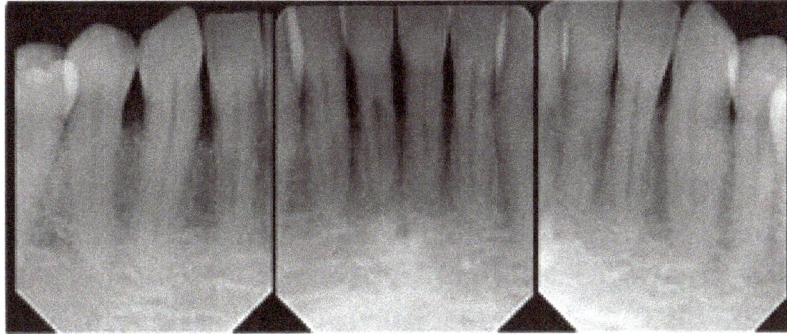

Figure 30. The patient came to see us. We took a CBCT and in the cross-sections it was obvious that the two central incisors had minimal supporting bone on the lingual and very little on the labial aspect.

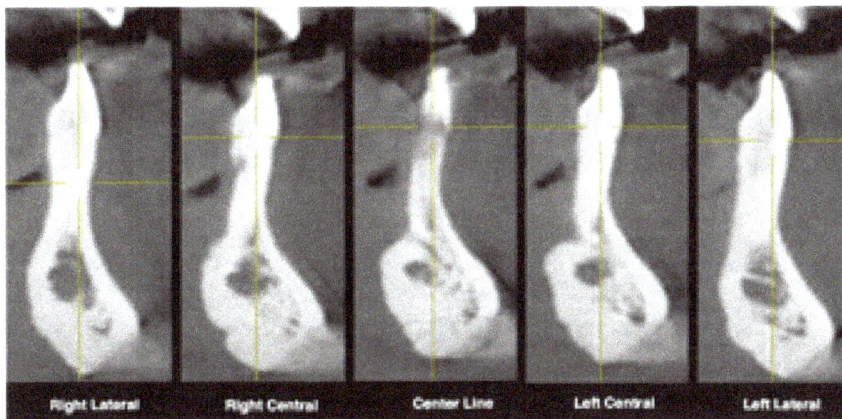

Figure 31. In addition in the midline, there was a very strange invagination of the bone structure. In short, this was not a suitable place for an implant.

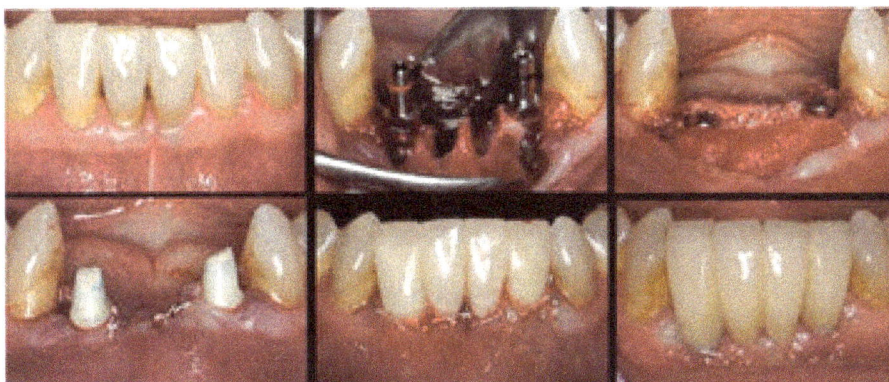

Figure 32. Two implants were placed in the lateral incisor regions, with extensive regional augmentation. An immediate provisional restoration was placed at the same time. After healing, for 6 months a final restoration was able to be constructed by the referring dentist, Dr. Peter Flaherty, Devon, PA.

One last point, the mandibular anterior region is the only region of the mouth where the bone width can decrease from the crest to the apical region. Although there may appear to be ample bone at the crest it can be relatively easy to perforate out of the bone during the channel preparation and implant insertion. Usually the perforation is out to the labial.

7.3. Maxillary premolars

Maxillary premolars can be quite difficult to replace with implants. There can be two, sometimes even three roots of a premolar, particularly the first premolar, so the tooth can be difficult to remove in the first place. The labial roots are generally set very close to the outer plate of bone, so in this respect they are similar to the maxillary anterior teeth. It can be tempting to want to choose a palatal root space to place the implant into, but this may be set too palatally. It is better to prepare the initial channel down between the labial and the palatal roots. An ultrasonic tip can establish the ideal starting point for a pilot drill which allows the channel to be finalized using drills. Premolar roots are much wider palatal-to-buccal than they are mesial-to-distal, so it may not be possible to get great initial stability. What stability can be achieved is obtained in the apical one third of the channel. It can be tempting to use a larger diameter implant to get greater stability but this should be resisted because it can leave minimal interproximal space.

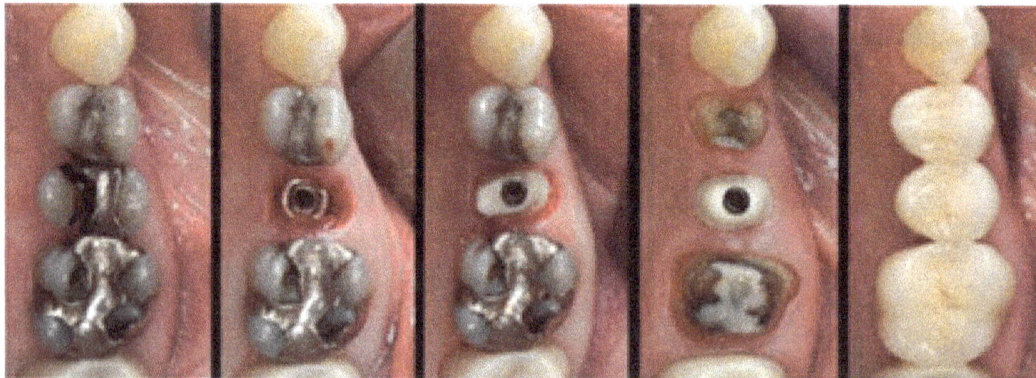

Figure 33. This case started with the sub-osseous fracture of the palatal cusp of a maxillary second premolar. The tooth was not restorable. It was extracted and immediately replaced with an implant to which a temporary Zirconia Sleeve abutment was then attached.

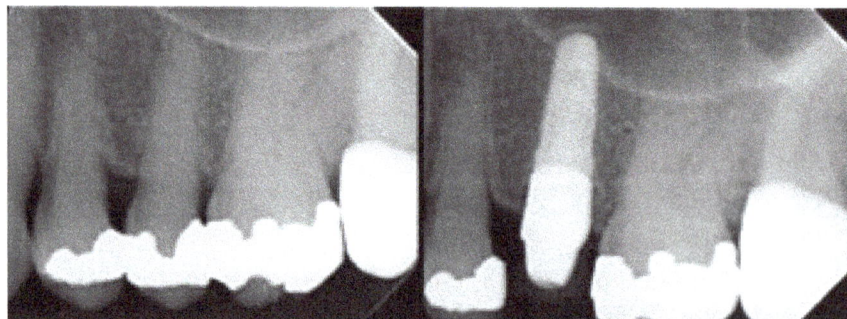

Figure 34. As is often the case with premolars, there was not enough initial stability of the implant to load it immediately. By taking the implant a little higher, into the sinus region, additional stability was gained.

One relatively common problem is for the implant to penetrate out of the bone apically. The reason for this is that the operator fails to appreciate that the bone housing tapers in medially as the alveolus progresses apically. This can be avoided if the drill path parallels that of the outer plate of bone. It is also necessary to sink the implant platform deeper than usual so that the abutment placed on the platform can flare out buccally and lingually to develop an elliptical, pre-molar form (**Figures 33–35**).

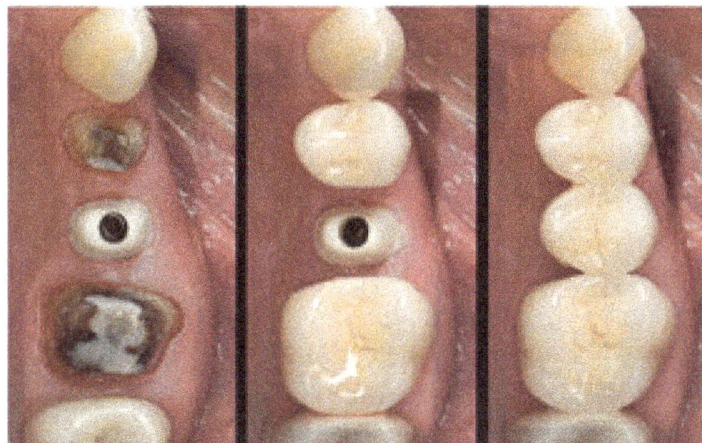

Figure 35. The deep position of the implant platform made it easy to develop the optimal emergence form for the abutment and for the final crown.

7.4. Mandibular premolars

The anatomy of the mandibular premolar region can be challenging. The labio-lingual bone dimension can be narrow even when it contains teeth. When the teeth are removed, the ridge shrinks more. The labial bone can be particularly thin and rapidly disappears after an extraction. The mandibular nerve can be very close which makes it impossible to gain extra stability for an implant by preparing the implant channel deeper (**Figures 36** and **37**).

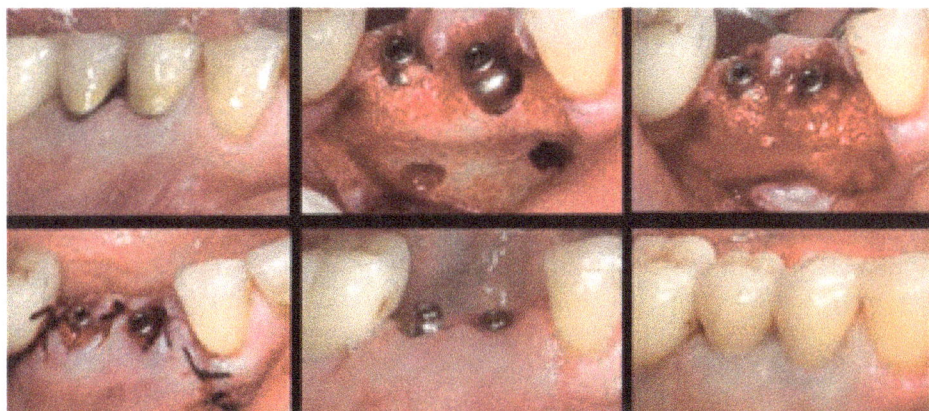

Figure 36. These two premolars were painful and had apical lesions. A labial flap allowed access to remove the teeth, to debride the region and to place implants and gingivaformers.

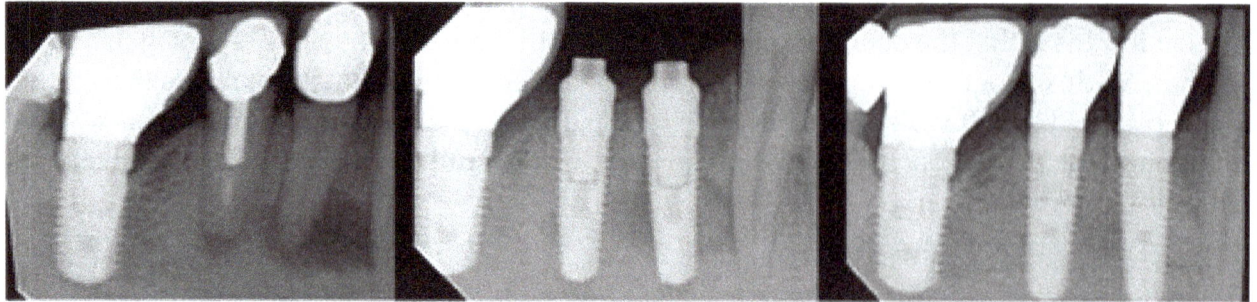

Figure 37. The radiographic series shows good healing. The molar implant was one with a 1.4 mm machined collar placed five years earlier.

7.5. Maxillary molars

The critical factor to appreciate with maxillary molars is that they have relatively little bone supporting them in the first place. What bone there is usually closely follows the form of the roots with the covering of bone around each root being quite thin. This bone covering can easily be taken away by recession, occlusal trauma, and furcation involvements. What is left can be inadequate to support an implant. It is critical to retain what bone there is in the region. An adequate volume of bone to support an implant is found in less than 5% of cases in our experience. This is why when replacing a maxillary molar with an implant it is necessary to consider providing a sinus lift. Once these principles are appreciated, then immediate molar replacement is both predictable and successful (**Figures 38–40**) [15].

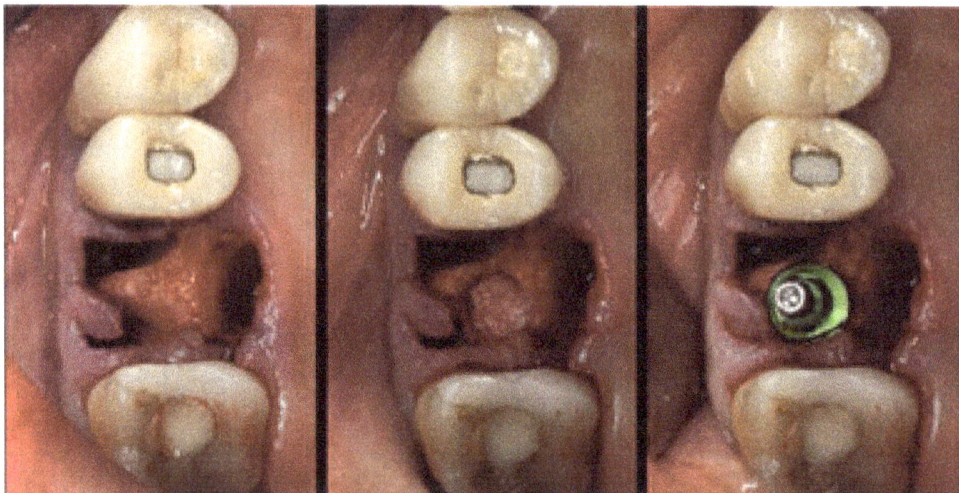

Figure 38. The first molar was failing and was removed. The labial and lingual walls were almost non-existent and the socket was expected to collapse. The central core bone in the trifurcation region was adequate to prepare a trephine channel, to raise the sinus floor, to augment the sinus region with bone graft and to place an implant.

Where the trifurcation region of bone is unable to stabilize an implant, such as when there is a large furcation involvement, it will be necessary to obtain apical stabilization by an intentional sinus lift procedure.

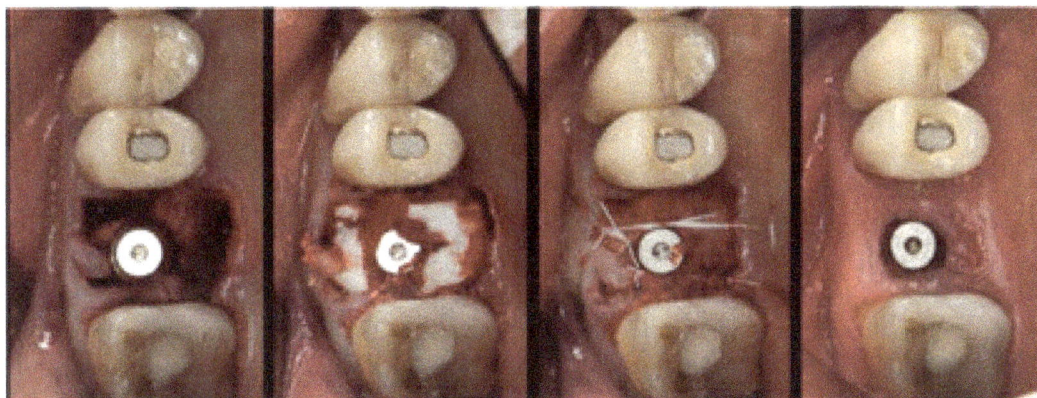

Figure 39. The former root spaces are then filled with bone graft, covered with a membrane and sutured. There was no advancement of the marginal gingival flaps.

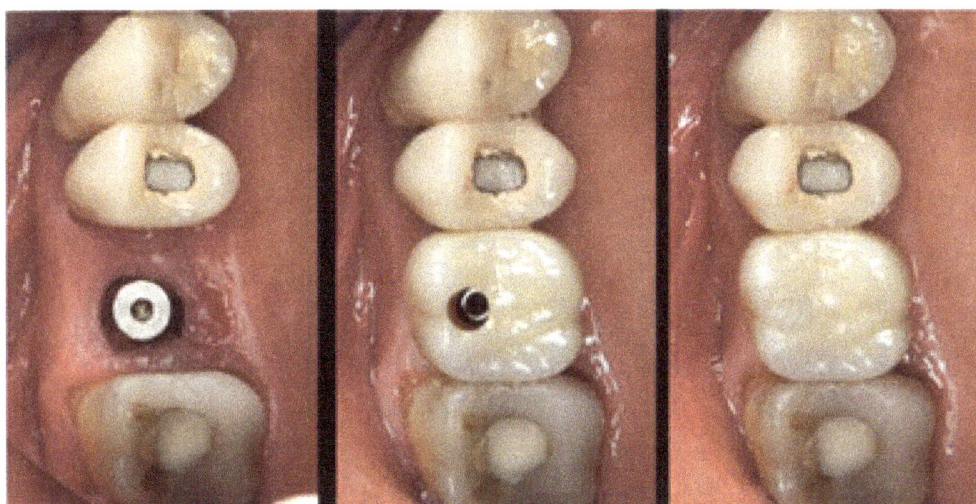

Figure 40. The region healed well and a restoration was placed.

Here is an example of such a case (**Figures 41–44**).

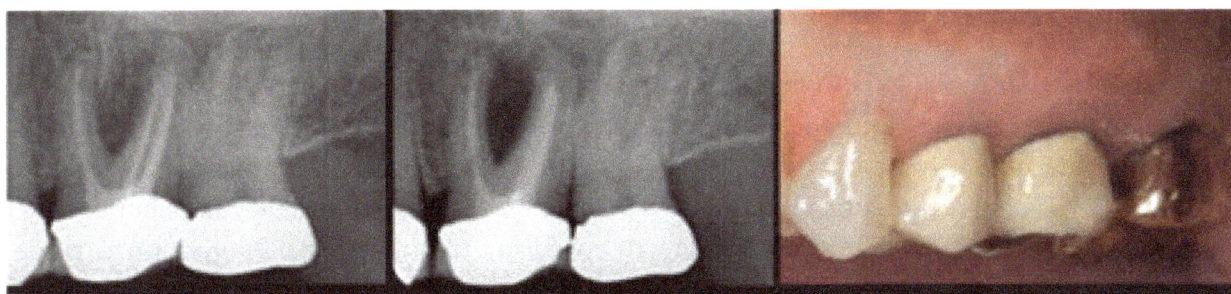

Figure 41. Left: On initial presentation the patient was advised to have the molar replaced by an implant. Center: Five months later, with no therapy, the furcation defect had increased greatly. Right: An abscess is now pointing out labially.

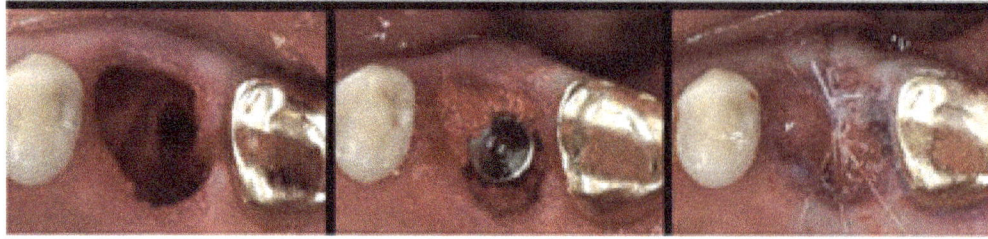

Figure 42. The tooth was sectioned and removed. A sinus floor perforation was obvious, so this was used as the starting point for the stabilization of the implant, even though it was a little distal. After a small sinus lift with bone graft, the implant was placed, surrounded by more bone graft, sutured and covered by a membrane.

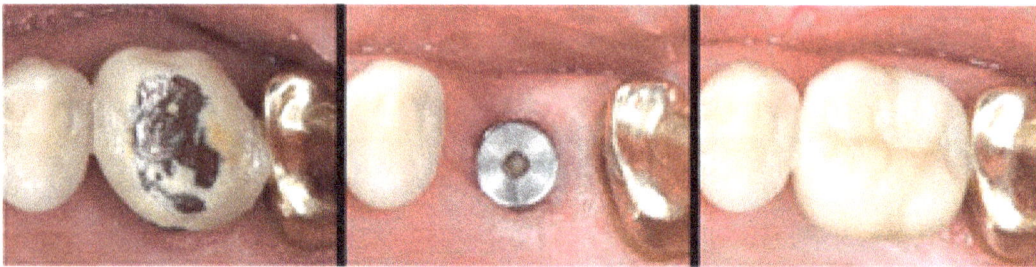

Figure 43. Here is the original, after healing and with the final restoration.

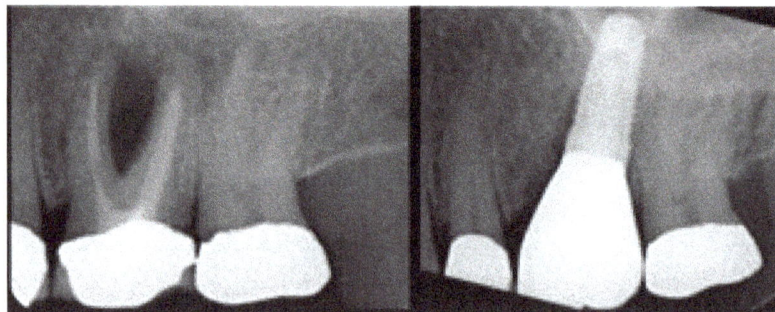

Figure 44. Before and after radiographs.

7.6. Mandibular molars

When mandibular molars are extracted, there tends to be a fairly rapid collapse of the labial plate with loss of ridge height and recession of the ridge to the lingual. Part of the reason for this is that the buccal roots of mandibular incisors often have very little bone coverage. In addition, traditional extractions with forceps can be fairly destructive on the labial bone plate. In short, it can be very difficult to rebuild a collapsed mandibular ridge. Prevention of ridge loss is better, simpler, easier, and faster. In the extraction procedure, everything possible should be done to preserve the labial and lingual plates.

Removing the roots can be difficult and time-consuming. Once this is done and granulation tissues have been removed, there should be a four-wall defect. Establishing the right position for and stability of the implant can be difficult. Sometimes this is possible in a former root socket. It may be possible to use the inter-radicular septum. Often it is necessary to make the channel for the implant a little deeper than the socket of the tooth. However, it is critical to ensure that there is clearance above the mandibular nerve. If this is not available, then it will be necessary to perform a socket regeneration procedure. The case which follows is typical of a situation which could be managed immediately (**Figures 45–47**).

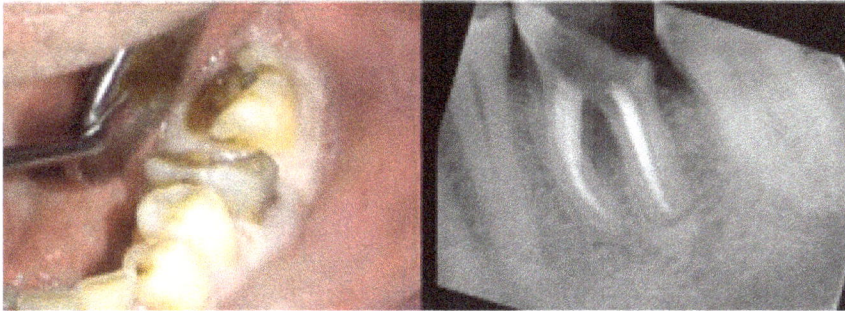

Figure 45. This mandibular molar had never been restored after the root canal therapy. Now the tooth is hopeless and there is considerable bone destruction in the region.

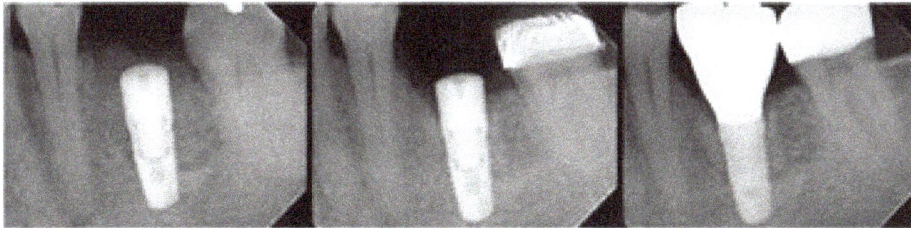

Figure 46. The tooth was removed, the region debrided, stabilization for the implant was generated apically, an osseous coagulum was developed with a bone graft and a membrane covered over the region while it healed. The final restoration was placed five months following the procedure.

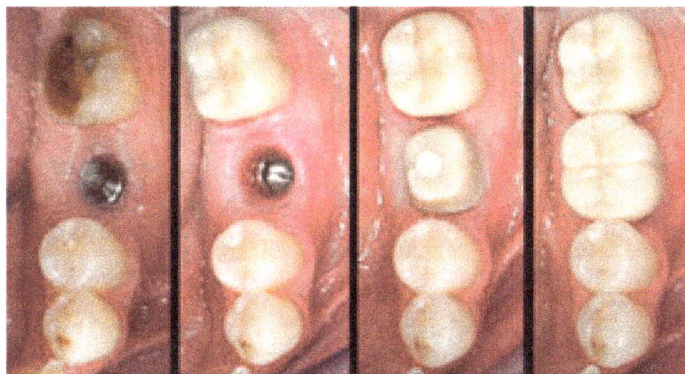

Figure 47. As is typical the gingivaformer is exposed by the time the case is ready to be restored. A custom zirconia emergence attached to a Camlog® Titanium Base CAD-CAM component is placed. This allows the final crown to appear very natural.

8. Larger scale immediate replacements

The success of immediate single tooth replacement has led us to take on larger scale cases with multiple missing teeth. These are always difficult situations because the hard and soft tissue defects that can arise from the loss of multiple adjacent teeth are more extensive and much more difficult to repair. The principles applied are much the same as for the individual tooth situation. The teeth are removed carefully with care being taken to preserve whatever bone is in the region. The region is thoroughly debrided, implant channels prepared, implants placed with adequate stability, an osseous coagulum with membrane coverage provided, and closure. The one real difference in these cases is that flap access to the region is required. The case shown below would generally not be treated using an immediate protocol. Traditional therapy would have been very complex because the teeth would have been removed, the ridge would shrink away almost completely, and re-building the region would have been exceedingly difficult, multi-staged, and lengthy. The patient, a graduate student in his late twenties, was about to leave the region and requested an accelerated protocol (**Figures 48–52**).

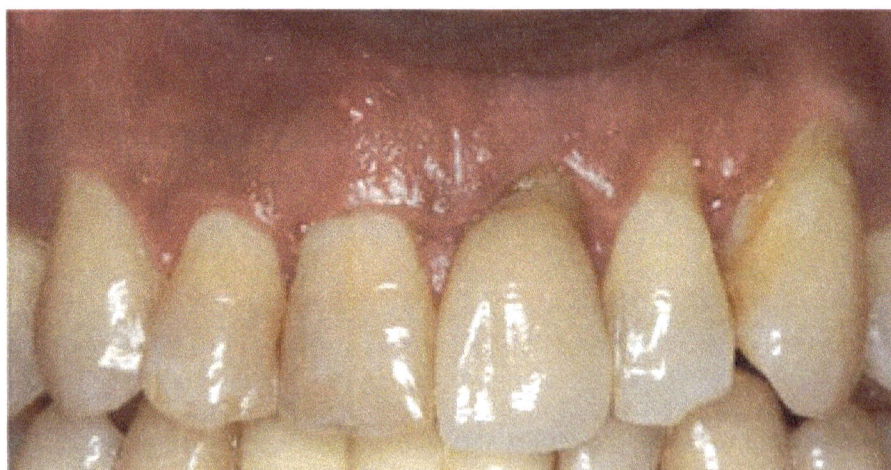

Figure 48. Clinical view of the dentition.

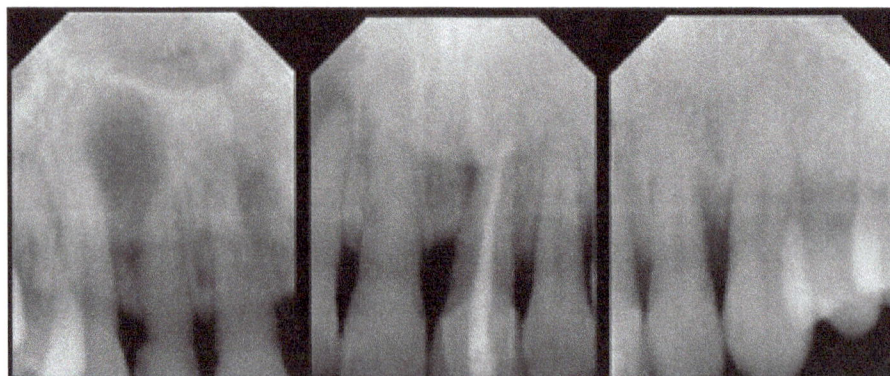

Figure 49. Periapical radiographs of the region.

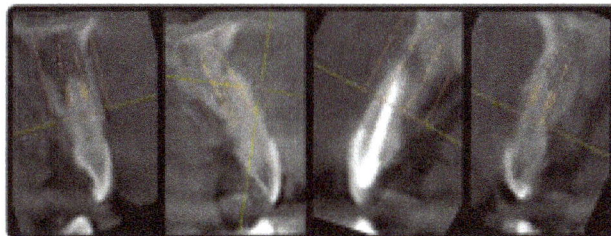

Figure 50. CBCT slices through the teeth show a variety of advanced lesions including almost complete loss of facial bone on three teeth.

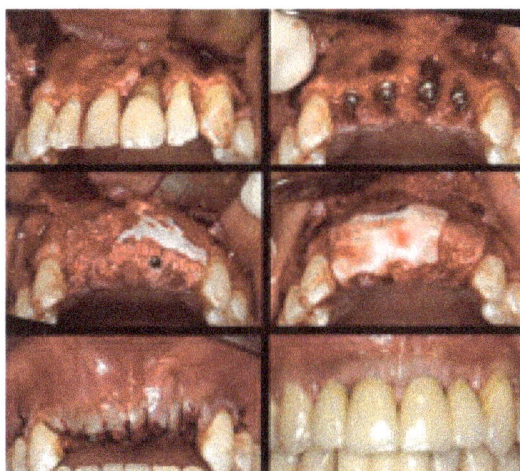

Figure 51. The region was open flapped for debridement. Camlog® implants were placed in all four sockets. An osseous coagulum was developed using BioOss Collagen particulate bone graft and covered with Bio-Gide® and Mucograft® collagen membranes (Geistlich). The region was closed without primary closure. Five months later the case was restored with individual abutments and restorations.

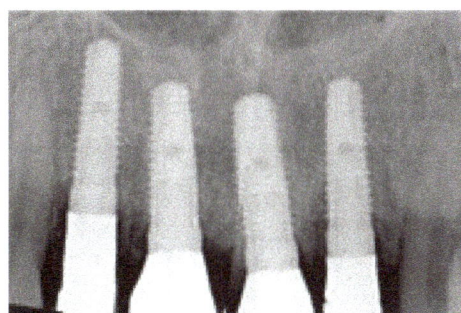

Figure 52. Post-therapy radiographs show that the region is continuing to recover.

Traditional therapy for this case would have been extremely complex, time consuming, and difficult. While this result cannot be considered ideal, it was relatively simple, fast, and effective. The basic principles of debridement, positioning, and stabilization of implants, developing an osseous coagulum and wound closure described above were used throughout therapy. All things being considered, the result in this case is very encouraging.

8.1. Failing individual teeth with aesthetic concerns

The case shown below also has many problems. They can all be handled individually, but what is really needed is to blend them all into a treatment plan that works towards a harmonious end result. It is a real challenge to make implant-supported restorations look natural alongside restorations supported on natural teeth but that was what was needed in this case (**Figures 53–56**).

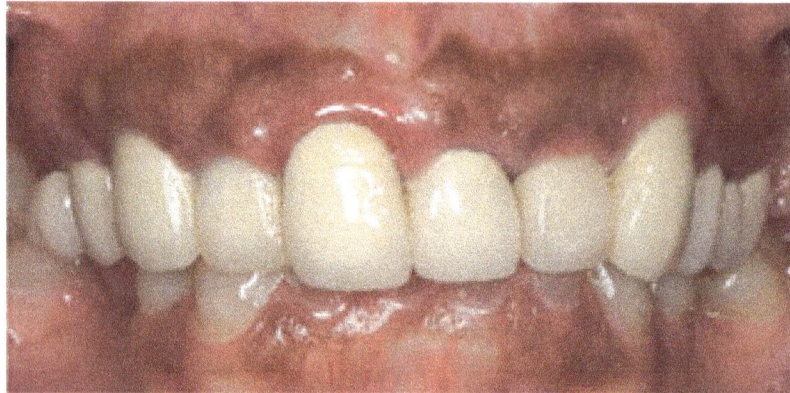

Figure 53. The patient was concerned about the puffy gums and the poor appearance of the teeth.

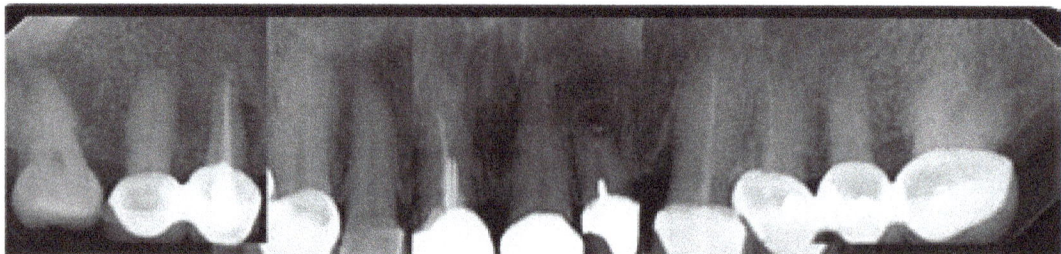

Figure 54. The radiographs show some failing teeth but the bone support is basically good.

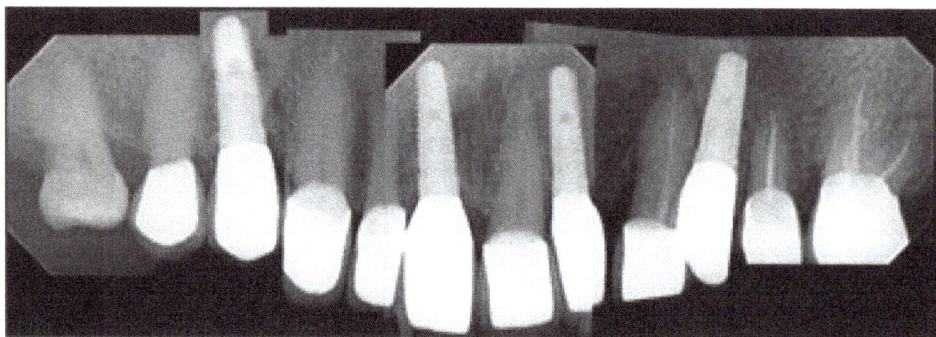

Figure 55. Four implants have replaced the failing teeth using an immediate replacement protocol. In the process the gingival lines have been re-aligned and the gingival health of the implants and natural teeth is now good. The aesthetics have been greatly improved.

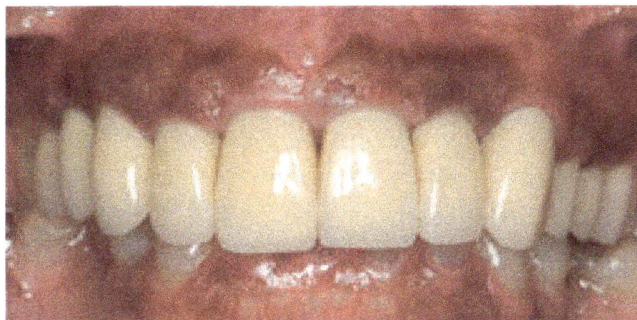

Figure 56. Therapy is completed, the appearance is now very natural.

9. Complications

Complications can occur with any procedure, but in immediate replacement these tend to be infrequent and relatively insignificant. The critical requirement is for careful monitoring of healing during the post-surgical process. If problems arise they should be managed as rapidly as possible.

9.1. Early loss of implant stability

This is an infrequent but very serious complication, usually occurring on immediately loaded implants with restorations. Loss of implant stability requires immediate action.

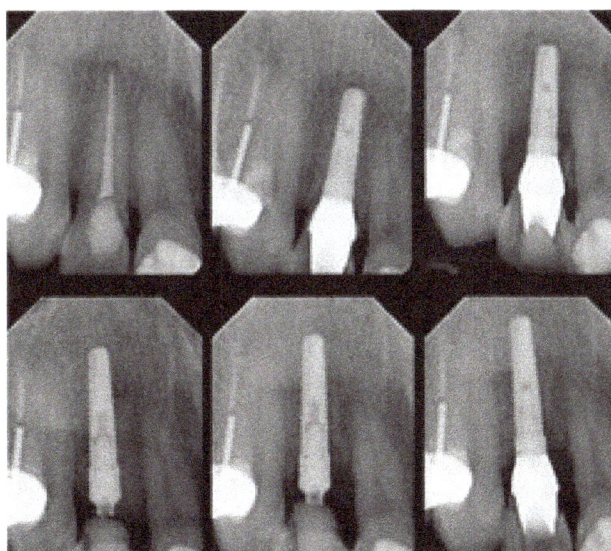

Figure 57. This lateral incisor was fractured at the gum level. It was removed and immediately replaced with an immediate load implant and provisional. Four weeks later he reported it was mobile. The referring dentist bonded it to the adjacent teeth. He was referred back to us 10 days later when it was more obvious that the region was quite compromised.

There are three options. First is to remove the abutment and to replace it with a gingivaformer. For this to work there must be no signs of inflammation or infection in the region, just slight mobility. The second alternative is to remove the implant, clean the region, and to replace it with another fresh, un-contaminated implant. Preferably this will gain additional stability with a larger size or length. However, it should be converted to a gingivaformer procedure to be sure of getting rid of the potential for breakdown. The third alternative is to remove the implant, to clean out the region, and do socket regeneration in the region. The case shown below was managed with the second option protocol (**Figure 57**).

The implant was removed and the region thoroughly cleaned out. A longer implant was then placed, with a gingivaformer positioned; the region was then augmented extensively with more bone graft before the region was closed. Three months later the healing was satisfactory, though there was some medial papillary recession.

9.2. Connection abscess (abutment screw loosening)

These occur because of loosening of the abutment retaining screw. Usually an abscess is a rather late occurrence. At an earlier stage there is inflammation of the marginal gingiva. If this is allowed to continue for too long, then the abscess may penetrate through the gingiva as seen in the case below. The way to check this is to rock the crown and to see if there is any mobility. The axis of the rotation will be at the connection. It is important to differentiate this from mobility of the implant which is where the axis of rotation would be more apical.

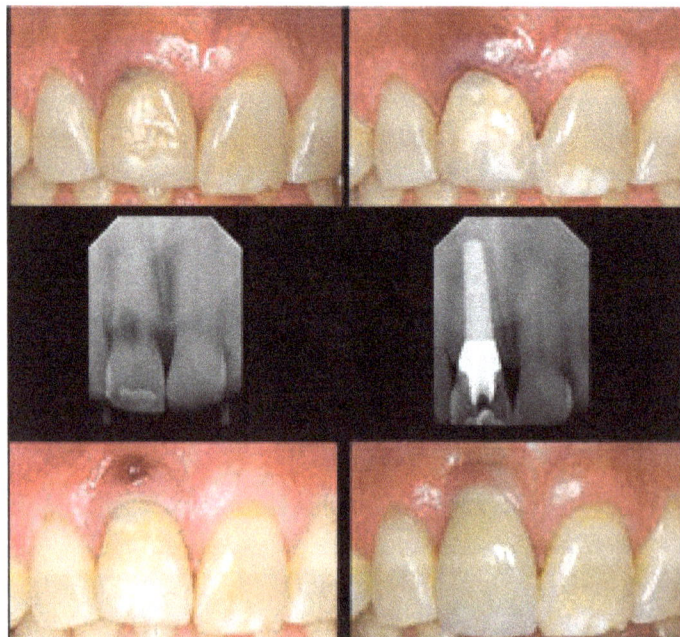

Figure 58. Top left: Situation with internal tooth resorption. Top Right: Following immediate replacement. Center left: Original radiograph. Center right: With implant and provisional. Bottom left: Four months later with connection abscess due to mobility of connection. Bottom right: Final case with healed situation but with increased marginal recession.

This sometimes occurs because at the time of implant placement, there is a hesitance about over-tightening the abutment retaining screw, as this may cause the implant to rotate. If this rotation does occur, it can be interpreted as the wrong choice of post-surgical restoration in that the implant was really not stable enough to immediately load.

There can be one other cause for this problem. It occurs when bone graft used for the augmentation gets trapped between the abutment and the implant platform when the abutment is placed. A radiograph should always be taken at the end of the procedure to check that this has not occurred. Although the connection may be tight at the outset, as the graft softens, the joint will loosen (**Figure 58**).

9.3. Marginal gingival recession

This is a rather complex subject. Stability of the marginal gingival complex depends on many factors which can be grouped into three main considerations: structure, replacement structure, and pathology.

Structure: We start working with the pre-existing condition. A normal gingival complex is supported over marginal bone; if that bone is lost for one reason or another then the gingival margin can more easily recede. Gingiva is usually differentiated into attached gingiva and free marginal gingiva. Everybody appreciates that attached gingiva should be attached to the tooth, but there is not so much appreciation for it also being attached to the marginal bone complex. Many of our surgical procedures raise up and move this marginal attached gingiva, sometimes to places where there is no bone for it to re-attach to, for example when a flap is mobilized to cover over a socket. When replacing a tooth with an implant, it is critical that it be surrounded by attached gingiva, which is attached to the bone and then comes up over the gingivaformer or abutment.

Replacement Structure: Some teeth when replaced by an implant will have considerable amounts of native bone remaining in the region. Although this will be affected by the change-over, in most cases the hope is that it remains, regenerates, and starts to support the implant. However, in some of our most critical situations, such as in the maxillary anterior region, the implant is set back palatally and at an angle to get stability in the palatal bone. The void between the implant and the labial wall of the socket has to be augmented with a bone graft. We usually over-augment to make sure that this consolidates without receding. Similarly, the gingival complex is usually augmented with a gingival allograft or more traditionally a connective tissue graft. Another factor to take into account is the material and form of the temporary abutment as this is often used to bulk out and support the augmented regions. These should be of materials which are bio-compatible with the soft and hard tissues in the region. We use custom formed Zirconia sleeves secured on a titanium base to accomplish this in our cases.

Pathology: Inflammation and infection can affect marginal soft and hard tissues. They can induce a wide-range of responses ranging from swelling to hyperplasia, from fibrosis to tissue breakdown, and for attached tissues to become detached (**Figure 59**).

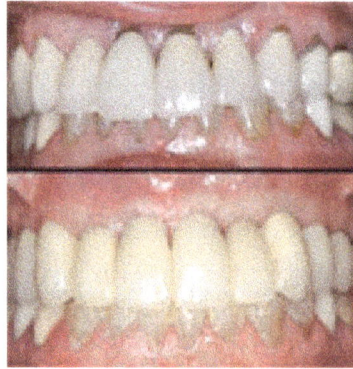

Figure 59. This patient had marginal recession and recurrent decay around the maxillary anterior teeth. Neither the patient nor the referring dentist was comfortable with another round of conventional restorative therapy. The teeth were all replaced with implants. Notice the change in gingival form and structure. Restorative dentistry by Dr. Chris Furlan, Havertown, PA, USA.

9.4. Peri-implantitis

Peri-implantitis is an inflammatory reaction in the tissues surrounding an implant, both gingiva and bone. One has to be careful to differentiate it from marginal gingivitis or inflammation of the gingival tissues about an implant. If there are changes in the marginal bone below the rough surface of the implant, then one should assume that osseointegration in that region has broken down and that the rough surface on the implant has become contaminated. If this is the case then it is doubtful if it can be "re-treated" or made so that re-osseointegration can develop. It may be possible to get short-term benefits, but it is often better to replace the implant (**Figure 60**).

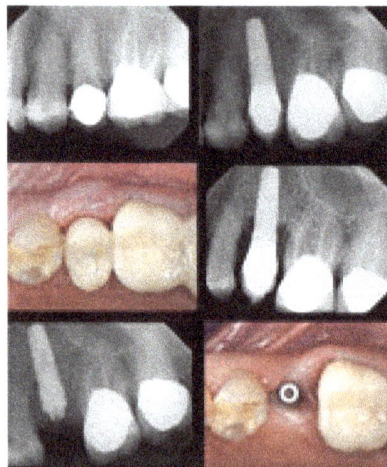

Figure 60. Top: Deep decay was under the margin of the crown on the second premolar, so the tooth was replaced with an immediately loaded provisional restoration. Center: Six weeks later, she returned with pain and gross inflammation of the marginal gingiva. A radiograph showed rapid breakdown around the collar of the implant. It was removed, and the region debrided. A fresh implant was placed with a bottleneck gingivaformer and closed after further augmentation. Bottom: Four weeks later, the inflammation in the soft tissue complex is resolving well and further healing can be expected.

9.5. Apico-implantitis

This is a problem where infection breaks down the apical bone surrounding an implant. Generally there can be two sources of the infection. The first is a residual apical infection left from a tooth in the region that was extracted previously. The second source can be from an apical infection on an adjacent tooth. Diagnosis may be difficult and access to the region for debridement can be more complex (**Figure 61**).

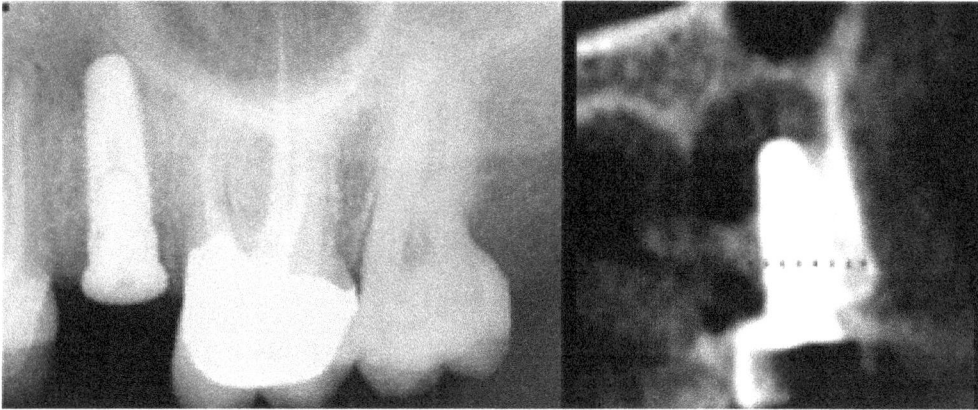

Figure 61. This implant was placed and appeared to integrate well, but a check radiograph at a later time showed apical pathology. The implant was removed, the region debrided and allowed to heal.

9.6. Sequestrum formation

Sequestra are portions of bone which lose vitality and then become a nidus of infection. Most of these occur in the mandible. Bone fragments may lose much of their surrounding support and blood supply during the extraction process or during implant placement. Most common are inter-radicular septa, followed by bone walls of adjacent teeth. Part of the issue can be that these regions may have been traumatized or even fractured during the extraction process. These can delay healing in the region, become a source of infection about an implant, and be painful. Once identified, it is best to remove the sequestrum and allow the region to heal. They can happen in any extraction socket, not just when implants are placed.

10. Summary and conclusions

Bone regeneration within four-wall sockets seems to be relatively easy to achieve. Socket regeneration is based upon using this principle. Immediate implantation is simply taking the concept one step further by stabilizing an implant in the middle of the regenerating socket. It is becoming increasingly obvious that immediate implantation procedures can be successful, that they can minimize the extent and number of surgical interventions, and return the patient to function within the shortest possible time. In addition, they help retain the supporting complex of a tooth being extracted and replaced by an implant. In comparison, traditional techniques seem increasingly outdated.

We have come to believe that it is easier to retain than regain an alveolar supporting complex. For immediate implantation procedures to be successful, it is necessary is to pay attention to some basic principles:

1. The tooth needs to be removed with minimal damage to the socket walls.

2. The socket needs to be debrided of soft tissue granulations and infected tissues.

3. Correct positioning and adequate stabilization of the implant must be established.

4. An osseous coagulum needs to surround the implant and fill the socket. Using a slow-resorbing bone graft material can help prevent ridge resorption.

5. A gingivaformer or abutment placed in the implant can provide a "tenting" effect, which assists augmentation and helps prevent early contamination of the rough surface of the implant.

6. The socket does not need to be covered with gingiva, it can be covered and protected by membranes as in socket regeneration procedures.

7. If high initial stability of the implant is achieved, then immediate provisionalization can be considered.

Author details

Peter R. Hunt* and Laura M. Ceccacci

*Address all correspondence to: peter.hunt@drpeterhunt.com

Private Practice of Implantology and Rehabilitation Dentistry, Philadelphia, USA

References

[1] Schropp L, Wenzel A, Kostopoulos L, Karring T. Bone healing and soft tissue contour changes following single-tooth extraction: a clinical and radiographic 12-month prospective study. Int J Perio Restor Dent. 2003;23(4):313-323.

[2] Hämmerle CH, Araújo MG, Simion M. Osteology Consensus Group 2011. Evidence-based knowledge on the biology and treatment of extraction sockets. Clin Oral Implants Res. 2012;23 Suppl 5:80-82.

[3] Fuentes R, Flores T, Navarro P, Salamanca C, Beltrán V, Borie E. Assessment of buccal bone thickness of aesthetic maxillary region: a cone-beam computed tomography study. J Periodontal Implant Sci. 2015;45(5):162-188. DOI: 10.5051/jpis.2015.45.5.162. Epub 2015 October 26.

[4] Meltzer AM. Immediate implant placement and restoration in infected sites. Int J Periodont Restor Dent. 2012;32(5):e169-173.

[5] Sanz-Sánchez I, Sanz-Martín I, Figuero E, Sanz M. Clinical efficacy of immediate implant loading protocols compared to conventional loading depending on the type of the restoration: a systematic review. Clin. Oral Impl. Res. 2015; 26:964–982. DOI: 10.1111/clr.12428

[6] Javed F, Romanos GE. The role of primary stability for successful immediate loading of dental implants. A literature review. J Dent. 2010;38(8):612-620.

[7] Barone A, Aldini NN, Fini M, Giardino R, Calvo Guirado JL, Covani U. Xenograft versus extraction alone for ridge preservation after tooth removal: a clinical and histomorphometric study. J Periodontol. 2008;79(8):1370-1377.

[8] Cardaropoli D, Tamagnone L, Roffredo A, Gaveglio L, Cardaropoli G. Socket preservation using bovine bone mineral and collagen membrane: a randomized controlled clinical trial with histologic analysis. Int J Periodont Restor Dent. 2012;32(4):421-430.

[9] Viña-Almunia J, Candel-Martí ME, Cervera-Ballester J, et al. Buccal bone crest dynamics after immediate implant placement and ridge preservation techniques: review of morphometric studies in animals. Impl Dent. 2013;22(2):155-160.

[10] den Hartog L, Slater JJ, Vissink A, Meijer HJ, Raghoebar GM. Treatment outcome of immediate, early and conventional single tooth implants in the aesthetic zone: a systematic review to survival, bone level, soft-tissue, aesthetics and patient satisfaction. J Clin Periodontol. 2008;35(12):1073-1086.

[11] Ferrus J, Cecchinato D, Pjetursson EB, Lang NP, Sanz M, Lindhe J. Factors influencing ridge alterations following immediate implant placement into extraction sockets. Clin Oral Impl Res. 2010;21(1):22-29. DOI: 10.1111/j.1600-0501.2009.01825.x. Epub 2009 November 13.

[12] Knoernschild KL. Early survival of single-tooth implants in the esthetic zone may be predictable despite timing of implant placement or loading. J Evid Based Dent Pract. 2010;10(1):52-55.

[13] Cosyn J, Eghbali A, De Bruyn H, Collys K, Cleymaet R, De Rouck T. Immediate single-tooth implants in the anterior maxilla: 3-year results of a case series on hard and soft tissue response and aesthetics. J Clin Periodontol. 2011;38(8):746-753. DOI: 10.1111/j. 1600-051X.2011.01748.x.

[14] Block MS, Mercante DE, Lirette D, Mohamed W, Ryser M, Castellon P. Prospective evaluation of immediate and delayed provisional single tooth restorations. J Oral Maxillofac Surg. 2009;67(11 Suppl):89-107. DOI: 10.1016/j.joms.2009.07.009.

[15] Block MS. Placement of implants into fresh molar sites: Results of 35 cases. J Oral Maxillofac Surg. 2011;69(1):170-174.

Permissions

The contributors of this book come from diverse backgrounds, making this book a truly international effort. This book will bring forth new frontiers with its revolutionizing research information and detailed analysis of the nascent developments around the world.

We would like to thank all the contributing authors for lending their expertise to make the book truly unique. They have played a crucial role in the development of this book. Without their invaluable contributions this book wouldn't have been possible. They have made vital efforts to compile up to date information on the varied aspects of this subject to make this book a valuable addition to the collection of many professionals and students.

This book was conceptualized with the vision of imparting up-to-date information and advanced data in this field. To ensure the same, a matchless editorial board was set up. Every individual on the board went through rigorous rounds of assessment to prove their worth. After which they invested a large part of their time researching and compiling the most relevant data for our readers.

The editorial board has been involved in producing this book since its inception. They have spent rigorous hours researching and exploring the diverse topics which have resulted in the successful publishing of this book. They have passed on their knowledge of decades through this book. To expedite this challenging task, the publisher supported the team at every step. A small team of assistant editors was also appointed to further simplify the editing procedure and attain best results for the readers.

Apart from the editorial board, the designing team has also invested a significant amount of their time in understanding the subject and creating the most relevant covers. They scrutinized every image to scout for the most suitable representation of the subject and create an appropriate cover for the book.

The publishing team has been an ardent support to the editorial, designing and production team. Their endless efforts to recruit the best for this project, has resulted in the accomplishment of this book. They are a veteran in the field of academics and their pool of knowledge is as vast as their experience in printing. Their expertise and guidance has proved useful at every step. Their uncompromising quality standards have made this book an exceptional effort. Their encouragement from time to time has been an inspiration for everyone.

The publisher and the editorial board hope that this book will prove to be a valuable piece of knowledge for researchers, students, practitioners and scholars across the globe.

List of Contributors

Mohammad Hosein Kalantar Motamedi
Trauma Research Center, Baqiyatallah University of Medical Sciences, Department of Oral and Maxillofacial Surgery, Azad University, Dental Branch, Tehran, Iran

Ali Hassani
Azad University, Dental Branch, and Buali Hospital, Tehran, Iran

Bahattin Alper Gultekin and Serdar Yalcin
Istanbul University, Faculty of Dentistry, Department of Oral Implantology, Istanbul, Turkey

Erol Cansiz
Istanbul University, Faculty of Dentistry, Department of Oral and Maxillofacial Surgery, Istanbul, Turkey

Fereydoun Pourdanesh, Mohammad Esmaeelinejad and Seyed Mehrshad Jafari
Department of Oral and Maxillofacial Surgery, School of Dentistry, Shahid Beheshti University of Medical Sciences, Tehran, Iran

Zahra Nematollahi
Dental Research Center, Research Institute of Dental Sciences, Shahid Beheshti University of Medical Sciences, Tehran,
Iran and Craniomaxillofacial Research Center, Azad University, Dental Branch, Tehran, Iran

Ali Hassani
Department of Oral and Maxillofacial Surgery, Implant Department, Dental Implant Research Center, Tehran Dental Branch, Islamic Azad University, Tehran, Iran

Solaleh Shahmirzadi and Sarang Saadat
Dental Implant Research Center, Tehran Dental Branch, Islamic Azad University, Tehran, Iran

Alexandra Radu
Case Western Reserve University School of Dental Medicine, Department of Oral and Maxillofacial Surgery, Cleveland, OH, USA

Michael P. Horan
The Cleveland Clinic Head and Neck Institute, Section of Oral and Maxillofacial Surgery, Cleveland, OH, USA

Esshagh Lasemi and Fina Navi
Department of Oral and Maxillofacial Surgery, Dental Branch, Islamic Azad University, Tehran, Iran

Reza Lasemi
Department of Public Health, Medical University of Vienna, Vienna, Austria

Niusha Lasemi
Department of Physical Chemistry, Vienna University, Vienna, Austria

Guhan Dergin
Dentistry Faculty, Department of Oral and Maxillofacial Surgery, Marmara University, Istanbul, Turkey

Yusuf Emes
Dentistry Faculty, Department of Oral and Maxillofacial Surgery, Istanbul University, Istanbul, Turkey

Cagrı Delilbası and Gokhan Gurler
Dentistry Faculty, Department of Oral and Maxillofacial Surgery, Medipol University, Istanbul, Turkey

Azita Tehranchi
Preventive Dentistry Research Center, Research Institute of Dental Sciences, Department of Orthodontics, School of Dentistry, Shahid Beheshti University of Medical Sciences, Tehran, Iran

Hossein Behnia
Dental Research Center, Research Institute of Dental Sciences, Department of Oral and Maxillofacial Surgery, School of Dentistry, Shahid Beheshti University of Medical Sciences, Tehran, Iran

Farnaz Younessian
Dentofacial Deformities Research Center, Research Institute of Dental Sciences, School of Dentistry, Shahid Beheshti University of Medical Sciences, Tehran, Iran

Sahar Hadadpour
Department of Orthodontics, School of Dentistry, Shahid Beheshti University of Medical Sciences, Tehran, Iran

Peter R. Hunt and Laura M. Ceccacci
Private Practice of Implantology and Rehabilitation Dentistry, Philadelphia, USA

Index

www.ingramcontent.com/pod-product-compliance
Lightning Source LLC
Chambersburg PA
CBHW050447200326
41458CB00014B/5096